MEDICINE IN CHINA
A History of Ideas

Comparative Studies of Health Systems and Medical Care

For a complete list of titles in this series, please contact the
Sales Department
University of California Press
2120 Berkeley Way
Berkeley, CA 94720

MEDICINE IN CHINA
A History of Ideas

PAUL U. UNSCHULD

UNIVERSITY OF CALIFORNIA PRESS
Berkeley   Los Angeles   London

University of California Press

Berkeley and Los Angeles, California

University of California Press, Ltd.

London, England

Copyright © 1985 by The Regents of the University of California

Library of Congress Cataloging in Publication Data

Unschuld, Paul Ulrich, 1943–
  Medicine in China.

  (Comparative studies of health systems and medical
care, Vol. 13)

  Bibliography
  Includes index.
  1. Medicine, Chinese—Philosophy. I. Title. II. Se-
ries. [DNLM: 1. Medicine, Oriental traditional—History—
China. 2. History of medicine—China.   QZ 70 JC6 U5mc]
R602.U56   1984   362.1'0951   84-2415
ISBN 0-520-06216-7 (alk. paper)

Printed in the United States of America

  5 6 7 8 9

Contents

Acknowledgments   xi

Introduction   1

1. Illness and Healing in Shang Culture   17
    1.1.   Shang Culture and Society   17
    1.2.   Responses to Illness   19
    1.3.   Harmony between the Living and the Dead   22
    1.4.   Illness as an Indication of Crisis   24
    1.5.   Illness as the Result of "Natural" Influences   25
    1.6.   Shang Healers   25
    1.7.   Concluding Remarks   26

2. The Chou Period and Demonic Medicine   29
    2.1.   Historical Background   29
    2.2.   Concepts of Demonological Therapy   34
    2.3.   The Practice of Demonological Therapy   37
    2.4.   The Concept of *Ku*   46

3. Unification of the Empire, Confucianism, and the
    Medicine of Systematic Correspondence   51
    3.1.   The Paradigm of Correspondences   52
    3.1.1.   Magic Correspondence   52
    3.1.2.   Systematic Correspondence   54
    3.1.2.1. The Yinyang Doctrine and the Issue of Syncretism   55
    3.1.2.2. The Doctrine of the Five Phases   58
    3.2.   Aspects of Confucian Political and Social Doctrine   61
    3.3.   Fundamental Principles of the Medicine of Systematic
            Correspondence   67
    3.3.1.   The Concepts of Wind and *Ch'i*   67
    3.3.2.   Structure and Function of the Organism   73
    3.3.3.   Diagnostic Principles of Systematic Correspondence   83
    3.3.4.   Classic Acupuncture: Origins and Therapeutic
            Principles   92
    3.3.5.   Concluding Remarks   99

4. Taoism and Pragmatic Drug Therapy:
   From Antifeudal Social Theory to Individualistic Practices
   of Longevity   101

   4.1.   Social Theory of Early Taoism   101
   4.2.   Early Taoism and the Question of Life and Death   104
   4.3.   The Influence of Taoism on the *Huang-ti nei-ching*   106
   4.4.   Taoist Macrobiotics and the Liberation of the
            Individual   108
   4.5.   The Origins and Early Development of Pragmatic Drug
            Therapy   111

5. Religious Healing: The Foundation of Theocratic Rule   117

   5.1.   Social Conditions during the Later Han   118
   5.2.   *T'ai-p'ing* Ideology and the Yellow Turban Revolt   120
   5.3.   Physical Existence: Tensions between Daily Life
            and the Ethos of Nature   122
   5.4.   The Five-Pecks-of-Rice Movement and the
            State of Chang Lu   127

6. Buddhism and Indian Medicine   132

   6.1.   Early Buddhism in China   132
   6.2.   Indian Medicine and the Buddhist Literature
            of China   137
   6.3.   Indian Cataract Surgery in China   144
   6.4.   The Chinese Reception of Indian Buddhist Medicine   148

7. Sung Neo-Confucianism and Medical Thought:
   Progress with an Eye to the Past   154

   7.1.   A Survey of Political and Intellectual Developments between
              the Sixth and Thirteenth Centuries   155
   7.1.1.   The Sui and T'ang Epochs   155
   7.1.2.   The Sung Epoch   161
   7.2.   Cultural and Social Trends as Reflected in Medical
              Thought   166
   7.2.1.   Reductionism and the Narrowing of Categories   168
   7.2.1.1.   Chang Chi and the Adoption of Restricted Etiology   168
   7.2.1.2.   The Cosmobiological Concepts *Wu-yün liu-ch'i*   170
   7.2.2.   Individual Contributions to Contemporary Trends   172
   7.2.2.1.   Liu Wan-su   172
   7.2.2.2.   Chang Ts'ung-cheng   174
   7.2.2.3.   Ch'en Yen   175
   7.2.2.4.   Li Kao   177
   7.2.3.   The Pharmacology of Systematic Correspondence   179
   7.2.3.1.   The Fourfold Categorization of Drug Qualities   181

7.2.3.2. The Sixfold Categorization of Drug Qualities   182
7.2.3.3. The Fivefold Categorization of Drug Qualities   185
7.2.3.4. The Determination of Primary Qualities   186

8. Medical Thought during the Ming and Ch'ing Epochs:
   The Individual in Search of Reality   189
   8.1.   Political and Intellectual Developments   189
   8.1.1.   The Ming Epoch (1368–1636)   189
   8.1.2.   The Ch'ing Epoch (1636–1912)   192
   8.2.   Medical Thought   194
   8.2.1.   The Intellectual Environment   194
   8.2.2.   The Spectrum of Conceptual Approaches   197
   8.2.2.1. Searching the Interior   197
   8.2.2.2. Searching the Exterior   204
   8.2.2.3. Searching the Past   208
   8.2.2.4. Searching Down Below   210
   8.2.2.5. Searching Far Ahead   212
   8.2.3.   Demonology, "Psychiatry," and "Psychoanalysis"   215
   8.3.   The Heterogeneity of Chinese Medicine during the
             Decline of the Empire   223

9. Medicine in Twentieth-Century China   229
   9.1.   A Survey of Intellectual Currents in the Twentieth
             Century   229
   9.2.   The Appearance and Spread of Western Medicine
             in China   231
   9.2.1.   Concepts of Modern Western Medicine   231
   9.2.2.   The Medical Missionaries: Objectives and Methods   235
   9.2.3.   Science and Scientific Medicine in Twentieth-Century
             China   242
   9.3.   Traditional Medicine in the Twentieth Century:
             Changes in Conceptual Legitimation   249
   9.3.1.   The Combination of Western and Chinese Medicine
             and the Emergence of a New Therapy   252
   9.4.   Therapeutic Plurality in Present-Day China   260

Appendix: Primary Texts in Translation   263

1. *Huang-ti nei-ching t'ai-su*   263
   1.1.   Manifestations of Winds at the Eight Seasonal Turning
             Points   263
   1.2.   The Nine Palaces and the Eight Winds   265
   1.3.   The Three Conditions of Depletion and The Three Conditions
             of Abundance   267

1.4.   The Transmission of Evil   269
1.5.   Longevity, Early Death, Firmness, and Softness   269
1.6.   Natural Phenomena That Must Be Avoided   270
1.7.   Various Statements on Winds   272
1.8.   On All Types of Winds   273
1.9.   On the Numerous Manifestations of Wind   275

2. *Huang-ti nei-ching su-wen*   276
2.1.   On the [Preservation of the] True [Influences Endowed by] Heaven in High Antiquity   277
2.2.   Comprehensive Treatise on the Regulation of the Spirit in Accord with the Four Seasons   280
2.3.   Comprehensive Treatise on the Phenomena Associated with the Categories of Yin and Yang   283
2.4.   Additional Treatise on the Five Depots   285
2.5.   Treatise on the Various Methods of Treatment That Correspond to the Four Cardinal Points   287
2.6.   Treatise on Changes in the [Assimilation of] Essence and on the Transformation of Influences   288
2.7.   Treatise on the Secrets of Mr. Yü and on the True Depots   289
2.8.   Treatise on Influences in the Depots as Patterned by [the Normal Progression of] the Seasons   290
2.9.   Blood and Influences, Body and Mind   293
2.10. On *Yao*-Illnesses   294

3. *Chu-ping yüan hou lun*   296
3.1.   Symptomatology of [the Illness] "Hit-by-Wind"   296
3.2.   Symptomatology of [the Illness Caused by] Wind-Evil   298
3.3.   Symptomatology of [the Illness Caused by] Malevolent Wind   298
3.4.   Symptomatology of Ascending Influences   299
3.5   Symptomatology of Sudden [Abdominal-Intestinal] Distress Caused by Being Hit by the Malevolent   300
3.6.   Symptomatology of [the Illness] "Hit-by-the-Malevolent"   300
3.7.   Symptomatology of a Demon Attack   301
3.8.   Symptomatology of Evil Possession   301
3.9.   Symptomatology of Nosebleeding   302
3.10. Symptomatology of Harelip   302

4. *Ch'ien-chin i-fang*   303
4.1.   Techniques of Gesticulative Magic   303

5. *Wai-t'ai pi-yao* 304

   5.1. Eight Prescriptions against an Exchange of *Yin* or *Yang* [Influences] Following a Cold-Induced Injury 304

   5.2. Forty-Two Prescriptions against Illnesses Caused by Natural [Influences], Resulting in Sweating or Similar Symptoms 307

   5.3. Four Prescriptions against Sexual Intercourse with Spirits and Demons 308

   5.4. Three Techniques to Ward Off Snakes 308

6. *Taishō Tripitaka* 309

   6.1. Sutra Containing Pronouncements of Buddha on Buddhist Medicine 309

   6.2. Sutra of the Thousand-Handed, Thousand-Eyed Avalokitesvara Bodhisattva on the Treatment of Illnesses and the Preparation of Drugs 314

7. *Ju-men shih-ch'in* 321

   7.1. Madness 321

   7.2. Fetid Breath 322

   7.3. Noises during Knee Bends 323

   7.4. Conception of a Child following Purgative Therapy 323

8. *Ku-chin i-t'ung ta-ch'üan* 324

   8.1. The Origins of Illnesses 324

   8.2. On Injuries Caused by the Evil 325

   8.3. All Injuries Caused by the Evil Originate in the Senses 325

   8.4. Integrated Treatment Using Spells and Drugs 326

9. *Chang-shih lei-ching* 328

   9.1. Exorcism of the Causes 328

10. *Shih-shih mi-lu* 333

   10.1. Direct Therapy 333

   10.2. Reverse Therapy 335

11. *Hsü Ling-t'ai i-shu ch'üan-chi* 337

   11.1. On Illnesses Caused by Demons and Spirits 337

   11.2. Illnesses Resulting from [Demon-Caused] Injuries 339

   11.3. Demon-Caused Pregnancies 339

12. *Tzu-jan pien-cheng fa* 340

   12.1. The Struggle for and against a Belief in Fate in the Medicine of Our Land 340

13. *Tsen-yang chan-sheng man-hsing chi-ping*   352
    13.1.   How to Recognize Illnesses of the Human Body   352
    13.2.   Some Insights Regarding the Use of Drugs   359

14. *Wen-hui pao*   360
    14.1.   The Evaluation of Acupuncture Anaesthesia Must Seek Truth from Facts   360

Notes   367

Bibliography: Chinese Primary Sources   391
              Chinese and Japanese Secondary Sources   394
              Western Secondary Sources   396

List of Chinese Characters   405

General Index   415

Acknowledgments

The preparation of this volume was made possible by
grant RL-0962-80 from the Translations Program of the
National Endowment for the Humanities, an independent federal
agency. I should like to thank Dr. Susan Mango, N.E.H., and
Dr. Charles Leslie, University of Delaware, for their cooperation
and support. Part of this volume was translated from a
German manuscript into English by Frank G. Lehmann and
Waltraut Lehmann, Seattle, whose assistance I gratefully acknowledge.

P. U. U.

Introduction

Ever since the seventeenth century, when early European travelers brought back from East Asia information on the peculiar technique of acupuncture and on the extensive Chinese *materia medica,* an unceasing flow of publications on health care in China has reached interested readers in the West.[1] But this information remained fragmentary and, by the end of the nineteenth century, appeared to be irrevocably consigned to the realm of the exotic at a time when Western medicine, in conjunction with the natural sciences and modern technology, seemed on the threshold of a major advance beyond all previous medical knowledge. Again today, so-called Chinese medicine has emerged as a general topic of discussion and the subject of an enormous amount of media coverage.

In recent years a steadily increasing number of both scholarly and popular publications has been devoted to this topic for a variety of reasons. Growing criticism of the nature and practices of modern medicine, in particular an awareness of the risks and deficiencies of chemical and physical therapy, has prompted some skeptics to look beyond the confines of our own traditions. News of attempts by recent Chinese administrations to structure modern and traditional therapies within one modern health care delivery system has attracted the attention of international organizations as well as of planners from countries where antagonism persists between Western and indigenous medicine. Furthermore, medical historians and medical anthropologists have begun to focus their research on China, where a wealth of written sources permits tracing a lively tradition of health care over several thousand years and where the observation of change and continuity in contemporary communities promises further insights into the nature of the human response to illness.

In this context one might ask how Chinese health care has been portrayed in Western literature. A number of basic currents can be discerned. The first current is evident in discussions that stress Chinese concepts of illness and therapy as preferable alternatives to orthodox Western medicine. Proponents of this view depict "Chinese Medicine" as an identifiable, coherent system, the contents of which they attempt to characterize. Such an approach is both ahistorical and selective. It focuses on but one of the many distinctly conceptualized systems of therapy in Chinese history, that is, the medicine of systematic correspondence, and it neglects both the changing interpretations of basic paradigms offered by Chinese authors through the ages and the synchronic plurality of differing opinions and ideas that existed for twenty centuries concerning even fundamental aspects of this therapy system such as pulse-diagnosis. Manfred Porkert might be mentioned here as a more sophisticated representative of this tendency. His publications are restricted to those facets of Chinese medicine that seem to offer— to a scientifically educated audience—superior qualities in comparison with Western medicine, whose inadequacy results, in the eyes of Porkert, mainly from its preoccupation with causative and deductive reasoning. Unfortunately, Porkert's reinterpretation of some fundamental tenets of the medicine of systematic correspondence on the basis of the Western concept of "energy" must lead to grave misconceptions on the part of those of his readers who have no access to Chinese sources themselves (see sections 3.3 through 3.3.1).

The second current in Western secondary literature on Chinese medicine has a purely historical orientation that accepts unquestioningly the "truth" of modern scientific knowledge. Proponents of this view tend to emphasize those aspects of Chinese medicine that are meaningful to current Western medical practitioners or which at least represent an obvious embryonic form of present medical thought. Authors utilizing this approach have directed their attention primarily to those historical achievements of Chinese civilization that appear to anticipate, often by centuries, corresponding discoveries or insights in the West. The search for "scientific" knowledge in surviving Chinese sources significantly influences presentations of Chinese medicine based on this view. Joseph Needham, supported by his collaborators, appears as protagonist of this current. Lu Gwei-djen's and J. Needham's history of acupuncture (*Celestial Lancets,* 1980) is the latest example of a series of studies that neglect those historical thoughts and facts in Chinese medicine that are irreconcilable with what the authors consider to be scientific, protoscientific, or at least rational. Perhaps we should recall here the demands on medical historiographers formulated by Ludwig Edelstein almost half a century ago. If we just replace the word *Greek* with *Chinese,* Edelstein's words regain their relevance immediately:

> In the historiography of Greek medicine, religious and magical healing, in general, are dealt with only occasionally and very briefly. No one will deny that, throughout antiquity, incubations played an important role, nor will it be disputed that incantations, at least in later centuries, were of great importance. But since these are factors abhorrent to modern science, they are not interesting to the modern historian either. . . . Medicine, imbued with religion and magic or freed from both of them, . . . is after all Greek medicine; Greek medical literature is, indeed, an accumulation of the most different writings. One must depict the facts as they are without prejudice and properly determine the share which each of the different forms of treatment had in reality.[2]

A third current is discernible in recent medical anthropological publications. A number of individuals have spent months or even as much as a year or two in contemporary Chinese communities outside the People's Republic of China, interviewing practitioners of traditional Chinese modes of therapy and of Western medicine and following selected patients through illness episodes, in an attempt to assess Chinese medicine in terms of both concepts and practices. These individual researchers have encountered and documented a diversity of distinctly conceptualized systems of therapy. In a number of excellent accounts, this research has shown how patients and healers act and interact and what their conceptual premises are.

Despite the wealth of data recorded, there is a pervasive element of perplexity in many of these anthropological reports with respect to the meaning of the multifaceted nature of health care in China. One possible reason for the difficulties medical anthropologists appear to have in explaining the nature of pluralistic therapy settings may be found in the lingering influence of views published by Erwin Ackerknecht in the 1940s.[3] He suggested that medical concepts should be understood as integrated aspects of culture, rather than as independent absolutes, and he initiated the "medicine as cultural system" phase of medical anthropology, a phase that has not yet been overcome.

To point out the fact that health care beliefs make sense in the context of culture represented a significant step forward from earlier notions that discriminated only between truth, science, and rapidly advancing modern medicine, on the one hand, and false, irrational, and static beliefs, stubbornly adhered to by uneducated primitives, on the other hand. The "medicine as cultural system" approach created a sensitivity toward the rationality and legitimacy of health- and illness-related beliefs in the context of an all-encompassing culture, and it greatly facilitated an understanding of the reluctance of many non-Western populations to accept modern Western medical concepts and practices enthusiastically.

Nevertheless, the limitations of the "medicine as cultural system" view are obvious when this approach is applied to complex civilizations. Ackerknecht's insights were based on an analysis of simple societies where most, if not all, members share one political, economic, and religious reality. It is in such societies that one may find the health care system representative of the culture as a whole.

The situation is different when we turn to complex societies such as China. Here one encounters, over the last two thousand years, an enormous variety of differently conceptualized systems of therapy, partly overlapping, partly antagonistic, all of which are representative of Chinese culture. This intracultural diversity cannot be explained by the "medicine as cultural system" perspective, as long as "cultural system" remains a vague concept, correlated, for instance, with "Chinese culture" or "Indian culture." Obviously, health care behavior and the ideas influencing it are part of "culture," but we need to identify variables responsible for the emergence and acceptance of differently conceptualized systems of therapy of various groups even within one so-called culture sphere.

In the present study, I wish to take a new direction, contributing not only to an understanding of the origins and long-term development of diverse health care concepts in China within the socioeconomic and socioideological context of that civilization but also to an understanding of plurality and change in health care concepts in general. This objective requires an approach that is both historical and systematic and must thus begin with the oldest available sources. In contrast to simple societies, which rarely offer any data in addition to the present, complex societies such as China, with long-established literacy, provide historical sources which enable today's researcher to trace, over many centuries, developments that form the basis of the contemporary situation. Chinese civilization offers the analyst a wealth of primary sources, reflecting concern with the experience of human illness that stretches from the fifteenth century B.C. to the immediate present. During this period of nearly 3,500 years, oracular therapy, demonic medicine, religious healing, pragmatic drug therapy, Buddhist medicine, the medicine of systematic correspondence and, ultimately, modern Western medicine either originated in China itself or were adopted from foreign cultures. The history of these seven major conceptual systems is not characterized by simple linear succession, in which practitioners exchanged each old system for a new one. Instead, the evidence reveals a diversity of concepts extending for more than two thousand years. New ideas were developed or introduced from outside and adopted by authors of medical texts, while at the same time older views continued to have their practitioners and clients.

A primary intent of this study, then, is to explore the conditions that accompanied the rise of new systems of therapy and the continued existence of old ones, and to elucidate the causes and the extent of changes that occurred over the course of time within individual conceptual systems. In this connection, I have found it useful to differentiate between two qualitatively different conceptual dimensions of the structure of medical systems, that is, between a durable paradigmatic core and a "soft coating." The paradigmatic core of any conceptualized system of health care consists of the basic paradigm accepted by the creators of a particular system of therapy. This basic paradigm supplies the fundamental causal nexus necessary to explain the occurrence of illness. In the history of medicine in China, two basic paradigms appear to have provided the entirety of all therapy systems documented with a durable core. These two paradigms, known in other cultures as well, are (1) the paradigm of cause-and-effect relations between corresponding phenomena, and (2) the paradigm of cause-and-effect relations between noncorresponding phenomena.

The former is based on a recognition that visible or abstract phenomena may be manifestations of a varying number of underlying principles. Phenomena that are manifestations of one and the same principle correspond to one another; that is to say, any change to which one particular phenomenon is subjected will also affect any corresponding phenomenon that shares the underlying principle. As will be explained in further detail in the appropriate section of this book, one may distinguish between the subparadigms of magic correspondence and of systematic correspondence. In the former, an infinite number of isolated chains of correspondence is identified in which, in general, only a small number of phenomena are linked through an underlying principle. One example would be a person and a doll resembling that person. The doll and the person are linked through the principle of their resemblance; they constitute an isolated chain of correspondence. Therefore, under certain conditions, harm done to the doll may also result in harm to the person after which the doll is modeled.

In contrast to the subparadigm of magic correspondence, the subparadigm of systematic correspondence is based on a recognition that only a limited number of underlying principles exist and that all tangible and abstract phenomena can be categorized as manifestations of one of the two (yinyang theory) or five (Five Phases of Change theory) underlying principles identified by various schools of thought. I speak of systematic correspondence here because all categories recognized by these different schools of thought are seen as constituting one intricate system of correspondences in which each and every phenomenon is systematically allotted its more or less well-defined place. The allotment of phenomena to specific principles, be it in magic or in systematic correspondence, is a result of inductive reasoning which stands in marked contrast to the methods established by modern science to arrive at sound hypotheses. The conclusion that a swallowed comb (consumed as ashes) performs the same function in the stomach as a comb that is drawn through the hair on one's head, namely the elimination of lice, is a typical example of inductive reasoning in magic correspondence. Similar, but often less obvious, logic accounts for the lengthy chains of association in systematic correspondence (see sections 3.1.2, 3.1.2.1, 3.1.2.2).

The second paradigm, that is, the paradigm of cause-and-effect relations between noncorresponding phenomena, is based on the observation that phenomena, be they tangible or not, coexist independently and that they may, under specific conditions, exert influences upon one another that may be of a harmful or beneficial nature. Thus, men and spirits share one environment; they are separate phenomena in their own rights without any intrinsic relationship. Under certain conditions the spirits may harm the humans, and vice versa. Similarly, humans may be in relationship with many other phenomena, be they wind, moisture, food, or germs. The point is that these relationships are simply temporary, recurrent, or permanent encounters between individual phenomena and that the sum of these phenomena constitutes the universe. Consequently, the paradigm of cause-and-effect relations between noncorresponding phenomena contains a stimulus to identify and, if possible, measure ever more specific relations between individual phenomena, and because of this it may support an analytical world view; efforts to explain the position of a phenomenon in an all-embracing system of correspondences may foster a more holistic, organic perspective.

It is apparent from an analysis of historical illness-concepts in China that both these paradigms played a major role in attempts to explain the occurrence of illness and also in the development of therapeutic interventions. Although the Chinese world view has been characterized by the yinyang and by the Five Phases of Change theories of systematic correspondence, it should not be overlooked that the paradigm of cause-and-effect relations between noncorresponding phenomena is equally well represented in Chinese literature. In fact, the two paradigms should be seen as complementing each other in various ways; they do not exclude each other.

Concluding this outline of the nature and contents of the durable core of Chinese therapeutic knowledge, the following list may serve as a preliminary survey of the two basic paradigms and of their respective subparadigms as they underlie the conceptualized systems of therapy discussed in this book.

1. The Paradigm of Cause-and-Effect Relations between Corresponding Phenomena
    1.1. Causation through Magic Correspondence
        1.1.1. Homeopathic Magic
        1.1.2. Contact Magic
    1.2. Causation through Systematic Correspondence
        1.2.1. Yinyang Correspondence
        1.2.2. Five Phases Correspondence
2. The Paradigm of Cause-and-Effect Relations between Noncorresponding Phenomena
    2.1. Causation through Intervention by Supranatural Phenomena
        2.1.1. Ancestors
        2.1.2. Spirits and Demons
        2.1.3. God(s)
        2.1.4. Transcendental Law
    2.2. Causation through Influence of Natural Phenomena
        2.2.1. Food, Drinks
        2.2.2. Air, Wind
        2.2.3. Snow, Moisture
        2.2.4. Heat, Cold
        2.2.5. Subtle Matter Influences
        2.2.6. Parasites, Viruses, Bacteria, and others.

The origins of the basic paradigms and of their subparadigms do not concern us here; rather I wish to examine how they were adapted to different conditions in various societies. Such adaptation supplies the durable paradigmatic core with what I call the soft coating of therapeutic knowledge, "soft" because it is flexible and subject to frequent modification. The soft coating consists, for example, of perceptions of the nature of an illness-causing agent. That is, while the paradigmatic core contains the knowledge that there exist other-than-human beings that may influence human life, the soft coating may identify these beings as permanently evil and malevolent (as in demonological medicine) or as capable of delivering both harm and cure (as in religious healing). The soft coating also includes perceptions of the functions and structure of the organism as well as the formulation of behavioral norms designed for the prevention and treatment of illness. These behavioral norms include those which, if violated, may create conditions activating any of the basic causative principles listed above.

In analyzing and comparing the conceptual contents of the different systems of therapy documented in Chinese medical texts over the past three and a half millennia and in tracing the conceptual development of single systems of ideas over extended periods of time, I have focused my attention on the soft coating of therapeutic knowledge. The question to be asked in this context is why—even within one single cultural region—different, often antagonistic systems of ideas have been developed accounting not only for a diachronic but also for a synchronic plurality of competing concepts as to the character, causation, treatment, and prevention of illness. Why is it, for instance, that some thinkers support one system of ideas, denouncing alternative systems as absurd, foolish, or—nowadays—unscientific, while the systems of thought that are denounced in these terms have their own intellectual proponents who may think about the former in similar terms? So far, attempts at comparing different systems of ideas in health care have always started from an assumption that man is confronted with a reality of illness and diseases, and that some systems of thought have arrived at a correct explanation of these phenomena while others have not. The standard approach applied is to consider the insights of one specific orthodox conceptual system as closest to a perceived truth and to investigate whether alternative explanatory systems can be reinterpreted in terms of the orthodox system. For example, African traditional treatment of psychic disorders can be reinterpreted—to a certain extent—on the basis of contemporary Western psychotherapeutic knowledge. Hence, such African traditional therapy is acknowledged as close to the truth and is integrated, occasionally, into official health care efforts by Western-medicine-oriented administrations. Another example is J. Needham's reinterpretation of a suggestion, related in older Chinese sources, for males to absorb the influences of the sun. Needham considers this as Chinese recognition of what became known in Western medicine as the beneficial effects of heliotherapy, and he concludes that the Chinese were close to the truth. It can hardly be denied that a reality of illness and disease confronts mankind—after all, a broken bone or a blind eye are convincingly real to most people— but we have, as yet, no idea as to where that reality ends and where purely constructive imagination begins. One may assume, in a general theory of cognition, that human cognitive abilities may be suitable— as a result of adaptive evolution—to interpret correctly a medium-range reality; human common sense and linguistic faculties end where we leave that medium-range reality to extend our knowledge into the depths of space or into the secrets of the smallest particles. Concepts such as "curved space" or "wave-nature of particles" can be understood by some, but to most people they make no sense on the basis of everyday experiences, and they cannot be expressed adequately with the linguistic tools that have evolved alongside these everyday experiences. Hence, some researchers in philosophy and in the theory of cognition are in a process of turning their view away from the age-old question of what is real and what is imaginary, to an analysis of mankind's cognitive abilities. I suggest that a similar turn, or revolution, should take place in the comparison of conceptual systems in medicine. Thus, at least for the time being, we should turn our back to that probable reality of illness and disease referred to above, facing, instead, those who have attempted to grasp that reality and to formulate concepts suggesting a behavior in conformity with that perceived reality. Facing into this direction we should ask ourselves what factors account for diverging, contradicting, or antagonistic systems of ideas within complex societies, within single cultural regions, and among mankind in general. Hence, in this study, I have focused my analysis on what I have called the soft coating of medical knowledge, that is, on health care-related concepts that have changed over time. I started from an assumption that variables accounting for the nature and contents of human cognition in health care might have left visible marks here.

Preliminary evidence suggested that social variables accounted significantly for the shape of the flexible elements of conceptualized systems of therapy. It therefore appeared essential, first, to identify the contents of all the different systems of therapy and, second, to determine any social significance they might have. To achieve this, I have developed a four-step methodology and applied it to the Chinese source materials. It includes a chronological, a linguistic, a structural, and a sociopolitical analysis of the systems of therapy concerned and may be outlined in detail as follows.

The chronological analysis required the tracing of concepts back to a point in time when they emerged in the literature and when they were accepted as meaningful by a group in society. Furthermore, the chronological analysis identified historical periods when specific ideas lost their appeal in society. This dating of the generation, acceptance, and fading of concepts proved to be very helpful in that the historical context provided initial clues for the identification of socioeconomic variables that changed simultaneously and may have influenced the nature and fate of the therapeutic concepts under consideration.

The linguistic analysis implied an etymological analysis of the terminology employed by the various therapy systems. In addition, it necessitated a search for parallel usage of key terms in therapeutic and other sociocultural contexts. Through this kind of analysis, important evidence was accumulated, suggesting relationships among therapeutic concepts, social facts, and sociopolitical ideologies.

These data were further corroborated by the structural analysis. It required a search for any hierarchies that might be discernible in conceptual systems of therapy. For instance, the fact that specific systems of therapy ranked the human body's internal organs and defined their respective responsibilities in a particular way suggested relationships between particular systems of therapy and particular groups.

The final methodological step, the sociopolitical analysis, required, first, an identification of the behavioral norms advocated by the individual therapy systems and, second, an investigation of the norms of conduct propagated by the sociopolitical ideologies of groups in society that sponsored or opposed a particular system of health care. Any systematized world view, be it a religion, an economic theory, or a sociopolitical ideology, including the less articulated perception of the universe in the minds of the common people, contains some specific notions concerning the reasons for crises in the society or community. In fact, the founders and propagators of Confucianism, Taoism, Christian dogma, Marxism, and even capitalism share the belief they have found the ultimate explanation of the origins of conflict and offer guidance toward social harmony. Each of these (and other) world views entails and propagates behavioral norms to be followed by all members of society in order to reach or maintain a state of peaceful coexistence. Any single individual deviating from these norms represents a threat to the social end desired by the dogmatists. The comprehensive nature of most sociopolitical ideologies is apparent not only in the efforts of their propagators to reach each and every member of society but also in their attempts to adapt all aspects of knowledge or science to their central perception of harmony and crisis. Any knowledge which, in its consequences, may contradict this central perception and the behavioral norms derived from it, will be opposed and, if possible, eliminated.

Medical knowledge constitutes a case in point. At first glance, medical knowledge may appear peripheral in relation to the goals of social ideologies. Yet, the acceptance or rejection of concepts of disease by groups in society has rarely been independent of socioeconomic and sociopolitical determinants, be they consciously considered or not. Any therapeutic system based on a distinct explanation of illness advocates a specific life-style to avoid disease and identifies specific measures to deal successfully with disease. A particular preventative life-style constitutes, together with specific therapeutic measures, the behavioral norms of any conceptualized system of health care. Important in this regard is the well-known phenomenon that different systems of therapy not only deal differently with one and the same health problem but that they, in addition, frequently recognize or emphasize quite different health problems in the first place. Each medical system organizes the abundance of initially unordered clinical pictures or possible symptoms of illness into an illustrative mosaic which in turn motivates the members of a group or society to act and interact in certain ways in specific situations. It appears to me that it is precisely this action and interaction on a personal and interpersonal basis, required by systems of therapy, that significantly accounts for the acceptance or rejection of the systems by groups in society. This required behavior may, in its consequences, contradict the behavior required by a sociopolitical ideology to maintain its specific type of social order; in fact, the maintenance or achievement of a desired type of social order may be jeopardized if such contradictions occur. The success of a sociopolitical doctrine is enhanced if such contradictions can be avoided.

To summarize, through the application to the Chinese source materials of the four-step methodology outlined above, it became apparent that two major independent variables significantly, albeit not exclusively, shape the soft coating of therapeutic knowledge and account for the acceptance—or rejection—of specific sets of ideas by groups in society. These variables include, first, specific social facts, and, second, sociopolitical notions of order and crisis. Many examples from the history of health care concepts in China, to be discussed in detail in the main sections of this book, suggest that certain images—or social facts—from our environment possess such powerful symbolic value that they, having been experienced as part of social existence, are adopted, both consciously and subconsciously, by thinkers in attempts to understand and explain individual existence. Undoubtedly, the acceptance of a particular set of therapeutic ideas by broad segments of the population is enhanced if these ideas are plausible, for the very reason that they agree with the experiences of daily life.

A similar relationship appears to exist between medical concepts concerning the causation, character, prevention, and treatment of illness, and sociopolitical ideologies that explain the causation, character, prevention, and management of social crisis. The obvious parallels in the formulation of behavioral norms by systems of therapy and by sociopolitical doctrines have, as some historical examples suggest, been created deliberately at various times by dogmatists in order to present an all-encompassing world view. Yet, such efforts seem to be the exception rather than the rule. It may well be that most thinkers who develop ideas concerning the nature of illness are unable to realize or to escape the logic of social existence. The way people live together and the way they cope with interpersonal conflicts as well as the existential guidelines they develop as a result of a desire for social order may also exert a powerful symbolic stimulus on an intellectual's conception of health and illness.

The congruity between a particular therapeutic doctrine and a particular sociopolitical ideology determines, in turn, the appeal of this therapeutic doctrine to individuals and groups. The actual therapeutic value of specific ideas, that is, their efficacy with respect to illness, seems to be of only secondary significance. The basic validity of therapeutic concepts is primarily social.

Realizing the impact of social facts and of sociopolitical ideologies on the conceptual contents of systems of therapy and on their acceptance by groups in society, we arrive at an explanation of intracultural therapeutic pluralism and of changes over time which the "medicine as cultural system" perspective cannot supply. In summary, the historical data analyzed and discussed in this book permit the following conclusions:

1. In a community where all members share the experience of one socioeconomic reality and adhere to one and the same world view, we will find only one conceptualized system of therapy that is adhered to by virtually all members of this community.

2. Plurality of concepts is inevitable in a society where different groups coexist who experience different socioeconomic realities and who differ in their perception of a desirable social system.

3. Change in dominant concepts of illness causation is inevitable in any society where basic sociopolitical change occurs; social reorganization is reflected at the level of medical thought.

4. Older conceptual systems of health care, which may have been dominant in former times, survive in social groups that continue to follow a consistent sociopolitical ideology.

5. Any group in society that, on the basis of a specific sociopolitical ideology, strives for political influence, or even dominance, will sooner or later support or create a specific set of therapeutic concepts consistent with its social norms while contradicting the ideology of political opponents.

6. In general, only intellectual dogmatists, who realize the consequences of a close relationship between one particular set of therapeutic ideas and their own ideology, as well as a minority of patients and practitioners, strive consciously for the persistence of "pure" conceptual therapy systems. In actual daily practice, eclectic and syncretic systems of therapy emerge in complex societies with therapeutic plurality.

Here, then, I wish to return to the theory-of-cognition aspects of this study. Obviously, our cognitive abilities account for many characteristics of reality as we perceive it, and, in turn, the reality we experience accounts for our cognitive abilities. While there appears to exist one general natural reality in which all humankind and its environment is embedded, within mankind in general, within single cultural regions, and within single societies, groups appear to experience different cultural realities resulting in cognitive differences in health care. These different cultural realities are formed by the different socioeconomic facts and sociopolitical ideologies referred to above. One could, therefore, speak of differing *sociorealities*. Such a term might lead, however, to reductionistic arguments, and although, in this study, the formative influence of socioeconomic facts and sociopolitical ideologies on cognition in health care is emphasized, additional variables influencing the shape of the soft coating of medical knowledge may be identified in the future. Societies constitute intricate networks of individuals and groups, interacting pragmatically as well as ideologically. It is simply inadequate, for instance, to consider society as an aggregate of various classes, each with its class-specific consciousness, as if their members lived in separate social arenas. I have, therefore, spoken only of "different realities," and it should be kept in mind that these are not necessarily separate realities. A mutual penetration of different realities within one complex society is common and can be observed, for instance, in the resort to different health care systems by a single individual. The eclectic and syncretic nature of patient and practitioner utilization of available ideas and tangible primary resources in pluralistic health care settings of complex societies is partly a result of the healers' striving for secondary resources, that is, remuneration, and of the patients' desire to maintain or regain health by all means. Eclectic and syncretic health care behavior are, thus, mainly goal oriented, not cognition based. They may, to a certain extent, be supported, however, by the fact that in complex societies many individuals witness—in daily social life—differing cultural realities. This may especially be true for changing societies where a younger generation no longer shares all the values of a parent generation— but knows of them, remembers them—or where different social groups live close enough to one another to observe the values of the others' cultural reality. The proximity of different groups in daily life may account for mutual tolerance toward, if not partial acceptance of, one another's cognitive system.

A *group* is defined here, consequently, as a cohort of persons who experience similar or identical sociocultural realities. Hence, if within one society two or more socioeconomic and sociopolitical realities exist for different people, two or more groups coexist with different cognitive abilities. This definition of *group,* which will be employed throughout this book, is not only different from the concept of "class" but is also apart from an idea of people joining together consciously for a specific purpose. Members of a group, as it is defined here, are not necessarily aware of their experience of a common reality. To put the argument to an extreme, even people living in separate geographic regions without any links, or in different historical epochs without the latter knowing of the former, may be part of one "group" if the sociocultural realities they experience are, in their essential structure, similar or identical. Consequently, one may find similar or identical concepts concerning character, causation, treatment, and prevention of illness in diachronically or synchronically separate populations without having to assume a transmission of ideas.

The methodological approach of this study has determined its organization. In each of the nine chapters of the first part of this book, I discuss, first of all, the political, economic, and intellectual aspects of the historical epochs in China that are important for an understanding of medical thought during those periods. Second, I discuss prevailing or competing systems of health care, relating them to the changing historical background in general and to social facts and sociopolitical goals of specific groups in particular. Finally, on a third level, I consider the consequences of the concepts of illness for therapy, particularly as they apply to the use of drugs. In order to allow the authors of works analyzed here ample opportunity to speak for themselves, I have augmented my presentation with numerous quotations from Chinese sources.

The second part of the book is an Appendix containing longer excerpts from primary texts, most of them translated here for the first time. All the materials in this section illustrate specific arguments in part one and are marked accordingly.

The history of medicine in China is multifaceted; no single book could describe and analyze it in its entirety. The current volume, the first of a number of independent monographs by this author on "Medicine in China" published by University of California Press as part of the series Comparative Studies of Health Systems and Medical Care, focuses on the major conceptual currents underlying Chinese health care over the past three thousand years. A second volume, *Medicine in China: A History of Pharmaceutics,* recounts the development of Chinese drug lore as documented in Chinese pharmaceutical literature since the third and second century B.C. A third volume, *Medicine in China: Nan-ching—The Classic of Difficult Issues,* offers the first philological translation of a Chinese medical classic into a Western language and traces the history of this classic through the centuries to the present time. Further volumes are in preparation.

1. Illness and Healing in the Shang Culture

1.1. SHANG CULTURE AND SOCIETY

The Shang Empire, the first Chinese dynasty to leave traces of therapeutic activities, arose approximately during the eighteenth through sixteenth century B.C. along the middle course of the Huang-ho (Yellow River), in the northeast section of modern-day Honan Province. The early history of the Shang is obscure, and the origin of their cultural achievements remains puzzling, in particular the use of horses and war chariots as well as a highly developed process of bronze casting.[1] The Shang, whose empire lasted into the eleventh century B.C., utilized a rather sophisticated early form of the script still used in China today. Some of their characters have survived to the present with a similar form and meaning. Others, however, fell into obscurity and can be identified today only with great difficulty, if at all.

The Shang period is documented by historical reports compiled during the subsequent Chou dynasty (1050–256 B.C.). But these accounts are often so strongly influenced by the political interests of later chroniclers that, if considered by themselves, they would yield a highly dubious picture of reality. A vast amount of archaeological evidence is also available, however—especially the great number of inscribed bones and tortoise shells discovered since the beginning of this century—enabling a reasonable estimation of the characteristics of Shang culture.

In order to analyze and describe the attitude of Shang society toward illness and healing, however, several methodological assumptions are necessary. Utilizing ethnological analogy, I will refer to presently existing cultures possessing a social organization similar to that of the

17

Shang; in addition, it will contribute to our understanding of this civilization to assume that a number of cultural practices, which have been documented in China only for the first millennium B.C., can be traced back to the Shang period. An analysis of the Shang system of healing must, of course, be based primarily on Shang sources. These are provided by the already mentioned bones and tortoise shells that were inscribed in approximately the thirteenth century B.C. for oracular purposes.

Shang culture was based on agriculture and livestock. Part of the population had already settled in small towns, where an upper stratum of nobility employed numerous craftsmen, but the great masses still lived as peasants in Stone Age conditions.[2] Sovereign power rested in the hands of a king.

The world view of the Shang encompassed a community composed of the living and the dead. The existence of the dead was just as much a certainty as that of the living, and it was understood that both groups were dependent upon each other. Ancestors ruled the world, but they were dependent upon the living for provisions. If the living failed to fulfill these obligations, expressions of displeasure by the departed were inevitable.

Ti was the supreme or divine ancestor. He provided the living with bountiful harvests and rendered assistance on the battlefield. Ancestors of the king were believed to have a direct influence on the actions of Ti, and it was incumbent on the king to ascertain through the oracle their will on diverse matters and, if necessary, to exert pressure by means of words or material offerings.[3] To this end, a system of communication was established, which was utilized daily to consult with ancestors regarding the weather, wars, future harvests, payment of tributes, hunting prospects, dreams, travel plans, political alliances, and, of course, lack of offspring and illnesses.[4] At first, only certain cattle bones (and later tortoise shells) were employed as a medium of communication. These were crafted in great numbers and with considerable expenditure of labor and were presented to the king. For the actual consultation of the oracle, several holes were first drilled in a bone or one of the carapaces. The king, or a diviner in his service, then made his inquiry and subjected the bone to heat, producing a series of cracks that radiated from the holes. The interpretation of these cracks by the king revealed the will of his ancestors in the matter at hand and thus provided the basis for a wide range of actions, both political and otherwise, by the ruler. It is no longer possible to determine for certain whether questions were inscribed on the bones or shells before or after the heat treatment.

1.2. RESPONSES TO ILLNESS

Turning now to the Shang behavior that we recognize today as a response to illness, it must be cautioned that available sources furnish information only about the lives of Shang kings and their immediate surroundings. At present, there is no way of determining the measures taken by the lower strata of Shang society to deal with physical distress. The surviving evidence, however, does provide a good impression of how the upper stratum of Shang society comprehended illness, and it is the history of certain concepts as they apply to specific groups that I wish to examine in the present study.

The following analysis will demonstrate that, in addition to a general awareness of illness, the Shang had already developed the notion of diseases. *Illness* is defined here as the primary experience, that is, the subjectively perceived feeling of indisposition that can lead to changes in behavior. *Disease,* by contrast, is a socially determined product, a conceptual reshaping of the primary experience of illness. Therefore, I characterize disease as a clearly defined deviation, within a specific set of ideas concerning the causation, character, and treatment of illness, from a normal state of human existence, however that normal state may be conceived. As a result, certain manifestations of illness may, in different societies, be comprehended as completely different diseases. For instance, the condition diagnosed by modern bio-chemical-biophysical medicine as a heart attack may be conceptualized in a society that practices demonic medicine as the "blow of a demon." The Shang, as I will show, were familiar with many different forms of illness, but they recognized only a very limited number of diseases, the most important by far being the "curse of an ancestor." Toothache, headache, bloated abdomen, and leg pains were only different symptoms of the same disease. To illustrate the enormous extent of the difference between Shang healing and modern medicine, it should be noted that a poor harvest and misfortune in war were also considered symptoms of this same disease—"curse of an ancestor." In the analysis that follows, it should be remembered that "disease" and "medicine" are categories that did not exist for the Shang; they arise from our own culturally determined approach. By examining an "ancestral medicine" of the Shang, I arbitrarily isolate the treatment of medical emergencies from its cultural context in the general solution of crisis situations—a differentiation not yet conceptualized by the Shang in the same manner.

Detailed indications of how the Shang perceived illness and the resulting methods of treatment and prevention can be deduced from the pictographic symbolism of certain characters as well as from the contents of the oracle texts themselves.

The character *chi* appears in oracle inscriptions as an equivalent for the modern concept of "illness." The pictograph is composed of the two elements: "man" and "bed."[5] In addition, one to four small strokes surrounding the component "man" are discernible. Various hypotheses have been advanced to explain these marks, ranging from "drops of blood"[6] and "arrowheads"[7] to "invisible pathogenic particles."[8] A comparison of additional characters in the oracle texts seems to support the meaning "drops of blood," since the small strokes were frequently used to designate blood and other fluid as well as solid bodily secretions. They are present, for example, in the pictograph for "parturition" around the character for "vagina,"[9] in a character identified as "urination,"[10] and in the symbol used for "to kill."[11] Moreover, it is possible that the drops of blood indicated in the pictograph "illness" result from injury to the sufferer. Thus, it can be argued that the entire meaning of the character would be a "person bedridden because of injury." If such a reading is accurate, this pictograph contains the original concept of illness caused by the evil intentions of a hostile third party, forcing the victim to remain in bed beyond the time necessary for rest. Such a theory of "injury caused by the evil actions of third parties" is supported, as I will demonstrate below, not only by textual usage but also by the subsequent development of the character chi. It is likely that the pictograph was given the form still valid today—a composite of "bed" and "arrow"— during the orthographic reform of the Ch'in dynasty (221–206 B.C.).

The use of the character chi in Shang oracle texts, however, indicates that the concept of illness during that period had already diverged considerably from the literal basis discussed above. One inscription, for example, reads "the king has a tooth illness."[12] It is no longer necessary that the symbol "illness" include the basic meaning of "bedridden." But, as I will show, it does retain the notion of "injury caused by evil." In addition, later oracle scribes frequently omitted the "blood" strokes around the "man" component of the pictograph.

In the oracle texts, chi was generally used in conjunction with a part of the body or bodily function. Of the approximately 200,000 oracle bones and tortoise shells discovered to date, 14 different combinations have been identified with certainty: combinations with the pictographs for head, eyes, ears, nose, mouth, tooth, neck, abdomen, foot, heel, as well as for voice, urination, and parturition.[13] Only a few such combinations have remained unclear. The combination of the characters for "illness" and "child,"[14] for example, may indicate a sick child; that of "illness" and "year, harvest" could signify either "ill year" (epidemic?) or "ill harvest."[15] Certain physical abnormalities were expressed in oracle texts without using the symbol for illness, such as "swollen abdomen"[16] and "tooth decay."[17]

Oracle inscriptions point to three causes of illness. Predominant is the concept of actions by deceased ancestors or other third parties. The following five inscription samples exemplify the overwhelming majority of oracle texts pertaining to illness:

> Question: Will there be an illness?[18]
> Question: Will there be no illness?[19]
> Tooth illness. Is there a curse? Perhaps from the deceased father-I?[20]
> The king is ill. Was he perhaps cursed by the deceased grandmother Chi? Or the grandmother Keng? Will his condition become serious?[21]
> Swelling of the abdomen. Is there a curse? Does the deceased Chin-wu desire something of the king?[22]

The influence on living persons by the hostile will of departed ancestors or others was expressed in the oracle texts by such concepts as "sent from above" or "rained down from above" whenever Ti, the deified ancestor, was himself believed to be the originator of the suffering,[23] apparently indicating the notion of a supreme "ruler on high." The pictograph *sui,* meaning "curse" or "to curse" was generally used in oracle texts pertaining to whether an illness had been caused by a direct ancestor, or perhaps by a former minister of the king.[24]

Their understanding of the causes of illness and disease led the Shang to adopt rational preventive and therapeutic procedures. If the deceased, when aroused, were able to induce illness and disease, their potential displeasure had to be forestalled with gifts. If the deceased had already carried out their curses, an attempt was made to remedy the situation, that is, to bring about the removal by means of offerings. One oracle text, for instance, reads: "Severe tooth illness. Should a dog be offered to the departed father Keng, and a sheep be ritually slaughtered?"[25]

It often appears that effort was directed solely at placating, through conjuration, the dead spirit suspected of causing the illness. Here the severity of the illness may have played a role. Three terms have been identified in the oracle literature that convey the meaning "conjuration," or "driving out by means of incantation"—*kao, yü,* and *ch'iu.*[26] In later texts, beginning in about the third century B.C., this therapeutic technique was designated *chu-yu,* "exorcism of the cause."[27]

Medicinal preparations, such as drugs made from plants, apparently found no place in the ancestor medicine of the Shang. Oracle inscriptions contain no specific drug names, and no character has been found that represents the abstract meaning "medication." Yen I-p'ing, who has studied the medical oracle texts in great detail, has pointed out several inscriptions containing the character for "wine." Based on the fact that these wines were prepared from herbs—millet, for example— Yen I-p'ing has concluded that the Shang were familiar with medicinal herbs (and recent finds in a Shang tomb have supported this conclusion).[28] However, the character "wine" appears only in conjunction with sacrificial potions for ancestors and not in what could be understood as a consciously therapeutic context.

1.3. HARMONY BETWEEN THE LIVING AND THE DEAD

The discussion of harmony between the living and the dead, the most important Shang concept pertaining to the origin, prevention, and treatment of illnesses, raises the question of why these ideas, and not others, became preeminent, at least in the ruling segment of this society. Shang culture was primarily agrarian. Ancestor worship by the upper stratum, and consequently the ancestor medicine outlined above, reflects, on a metaphysical level, a constant fear of one's fellow man, as well as a deep distrust of neighbors and even relatives. Such traits are characteristic of traditional agricultural societies of the present—Central and South America or Africa, for example; it does not appear farfetched to postulate a similar basic attitude in Shang society.

George Foster was probably the first to identify the static nature of the economic system of such cultures as an important cause of this mental climate.[29] Traditional agrarian societies are characterized by a constant level of production, year after year. In other words, we have here a situation of true zero growth, in which the resources available to the society do not expand at a steady rate. Exceptions do occur, of course, through the catastrophic effects of climate or the intervention of enemy forces, which reduce available resources, or raids into enemy territory, which produce the opposite result. A comparison of societies with a static economy and societies with a growth-oriented economy reveals that significant accumulations of wealth by individuals, families, or groups are tolerated for long periods only in the latter. The prevailing outlook in these societies—whether conscious or subconscious—is that such wealth is not gained at the expense of others, but originates from one huge, inexhaustible source, from which every person, with sufficient effort, can and may withdraw as much as he desires. The situation is perceived quite differently in those societies with little or no foreign trade and where the fields or other sources of livelihood visibly yield approximately the same amount every year. Here it is generally felt that since the total amount available to society remains constant, any enrichment of one person, family, or group inevitably occurs at the expense of all remaining persons, families, or groups. All known societies in this situation have, as a result, developed social mechanisms that in some way ensure the orderly distribution of the total product among members. As far as available sources indicate, the Shang adopted similar measures.

The ubiquitous presence of such mechanisms can be viewed as an indication of their necessity, that is, of the impossibility of maintaining a social order that assures survival and the freedom of movement without likewise adopting social conventions for the distribution of all available resources. The motivating impulse behind the establishment of such conventions seems to be the effort of individuals or entire groups to increase their share of the wealth at the expense of other individuals or groups. Mistrust is the omnipresent manifestation of a precautionary consciousness toward such efforts by others; envy is the underlying attitude of those who suspect that others have already appropriated a larger portion of available resources than they are allowed. The social conventions that arise from these attitudes aim for the continuous balance of resources in society. The egalitarian principle that opposes the accumulation of material goods by individuals or social subgroups has, in all known societies in the world possessing static economies, and even afterward in growth-oriented advanced cultures, led to the establishment of rituals whose significance appears to be the redistribution of material goods—which for various reasons have accumulated in the hands of individuals—and the compensation of the victim with an immaterial, transitory substitute, namely prestige. This is the only way to understand the fiestas in Latin America, which appear excessively costly to outside observers and which bestow the greatest glory to the most zealous spendthrift. The same is true for the *ngbaya* ceremonies in Africa,[30] the potlatch celebrations by Indians in the Pacific Northwest, and numerous similar examples. All of these rituals, no matter what additional functions they may have, help to preserve mutual goodwill among the members of a society by limiting mistrust and reducing or even completely eliminating the possibly fatal consequences of envy.

Let us now return to Shang society, where the equal distribution of resources included the dead as well as the living. The Shang buried their dead with an abundance of gifts. Carts, horses, weapons, jewelry, foodstuffs, diverse containers, and, occasionally, an entire complement of servants were to remain at the disposal of the departed.[31] Regular offerings on a smaller scale and, on occasion, more extensive presentations, such as several hundred head of livestock, were continued by the living. Since the quantities of meat left over from such occasions were subsequently consumed by the living, earthly distribution was also provided for at the same time.[32] As early as the first millennium B.C., following the decline of the Shang dynasty, similar rites of exchange survived in the winter celebrations of the peasants. Marcel Granet has fashioned his analysis of the relevant sources into a lively portrait of the "communal revelries and drinking bouts."[33] As he points out, such gatherings generally resembled fairs. Competition in gift-giving was the motivating force; in order to obligate the partners to even greater return gifts, one always had to give more than one had received. "Men competed with one another to see who was able to give his possessions away in the most ostentatious manner."[34] Those who participated in these festive occasions returned home with prestige for the coming months; the resulting hierarchy changed from year to year.[35]

1.4. ILLNESS AS AN INDICATION OF CRISIS

In the same manner that a person can suffer bodily injury in a dispute with one's fellow man, the Shang believed that the deceased, when neglected, could vent their hostilities on the living. Their weapon was the curse, and it could produce crop failure or a loss on the battlefield. But it could also result in an offending descendant being "bedridden," that is, with an illness. The first two consequences, which stand here for numerous other examples, represent a crisis in relations between the living and the dead that involves the entire community. Illness, by contrast, generally indicates a problem between a living individual and one or more ancestors, and concerns the entire population only when the king is involved. The specific measures taken to prevent or overcome such crises remained the same, regardless of whether an individual or the entire population was threatened. Thus, Shang ancestor medicine was completely integrated into the attitudes and mechanisms developed by this society to understand and solve social crises.

1.5. ILLNESS AS THE RESULT OF "NATURAL" INFLUENCES

The Shang recognized other causes for illness in addition to ancestors. In some inscriptions the deceased are asked whether "malignant wind" or "snow" produced the affliction.[36] One such inscription asks: "Question: Has the Princess Hao fallen ill because of an evil wind?"[37]

There is clear evidence on the oracle bones that the Shang believed in the existence of wind-spirits. According to the bone inscriptions, so-called *wu*-shamans could control the forces of the wind; they "either performed the rites of [the divine ancestor] Ti to cause a good wind to blow and to cause rain to the extent that it supports the growth of the crops, or they performed the rites of pacification in order to prevent or stop an evil wind."[38] It is possible that the evil wind that had to be pacified was the same entity that caused Princess Hao's illness. Evil wind, as an illness-causing spirit, may have acted in its own right, or it may have been considered to be merely a tool of Ti. Wind, if I may jump ahead here, remained, up to the present, one of the most important etiological principles in traditional Chinese medicine (see below pp. 67–72).

The oracle inscriptions mention yet another "natural" phenomenon as a source of illness: "snow." We do not know, though, whether "snow" was considered to be a spiritual entity as well or whether it was accepted as just an occasional phenomenon of the natural environment.

Finally, it should be noted that Shang oracle texts occasionally contain a character used since the Han period as a term for black magic, that is, the intentional illness-causing action of living persons that is visible only in the end result.[39] Since there is no evidence indicating exactly how Shang scribes used the pictograph known as *ku*, I will discuss it in connection with the more substantial sources of later periods (see section 2.4).

1.6. SHANG HEALERS

One aspect of Shang therapy has so far only been touched upon—the nature of its "physicians." We have encountered the wu-shamans in their function of pacifiers of (illness-causing ?) evil wind; I will have to return to this group of practitioners in the course of my discussion on demonic medicine, of which they became the central personnel.

The dominant conceptualization of illness by the Shang, which differs so greatly from modern understanding and which is most evident in the creation of practically only one disease, whose symptoms range from headache to crop failure, necessitated a type of healer totally different from what we are familiar with. Ancestor therapy neither knew nor required a physician who directed his attention to the patient and carried out medical therapy. As a consequence of their understanding of the nature and origin of illness, the Shang required only social therapy, in the sense of an adjustment of the disturbed relationship between the two large groups of society, the living and the deceased. The obligation to consult ancestors and interpret the oracle appears to have been reserved for the king alone, or for diviners in his service; he was therefore the sole practitioner of ancestor therapy. His clientele was restricted to himself and possibly the upper nobility. As already indicated, the extent to which the rest of the population was involved in ancestor therapy is unknown. Only occasionally, during epidemics and other catastrophes that transcended the concern of individuals, did the king function as the "physician" of the entire population. In every case, he was responsible for both diagnosis and therapy.

David Keightley has stressed the "powerful psychological and ideological support that ancestor worship provided for the political dominance of the Shang kings."[40] The sociopolitical significance of the "diagnoses" of oracle medicine has been demonstrated for present-day societies in which such a system has survived.[41] Although no direct evidence exists, it seems likely that the Shang king and "physician" also combined the "medical" prescripts given to the members of the upper stratum and perhaps the entire population, based on the consultation of the oracle, with his own political intentions. "If, for example, the king discovered (by means of the oracle) that his senior uncle, father Keng, was causing his toothache, he may have blamed father Keng's descendants at the court for inducing his distress."[42] Because of the kind of evidence that has survived, it is impossible to determine to what extent the sanctions resulting from such accusations and the underlying "diagnosis" may have been motivated a priori by political considerations.

1.7. CONCLUDING REMARKS

Any account of Shang therapeutic ideas, practices, and institutions must remain, because of the nature of the documents available, limited and preliminary. As the following chapter will show, the Chou dynasty, succeeding the Shang, saw the development of new concepts and techniques concerning the origin, treatment, and prevention of illness. Ancestral healing, although becoming gradually discontinued in the way it was practiced by the Shang, has persisted as an important facet of the broad range of health care strategies employed by the people of China to this day. The continued existence of beliefs in the possibility of ancestral intervention to cure or prevent illness is most notable in Chinese communities on Taiwan or in Hong Kong. The basic principle underlying the relationship between the deceased and the living is the idea of reciprocity; this notion has remained the same since the remote times of antiquity. Ancestors wish, for instance, to have their bones passed, in their grave, by good "wind and water" (*feng-shui*) influences, and are expected, in return, to guarantee prosperity and health of those descendants who arrange a suitable burial site and who cleanse and rearrange the bones in proper fashion once the corpse has decayed. Just as the human body, beginning with the third or second century B.C., was conceived as an organism whose life depended on the flow of proper influences through specific transportation channels (see below pp. 74–77), a concept of the earth as a living body containing hidden channels filled by a flow of beneficial contents was developed at about the same time. It became the task of special diviners to discover, for the establishment of tombs or other structures, favorable sites where such channels convened, and to avoid others where evil influences might be present. Hence, the belief in the potential of the ancestors for health care remained directly linked to a divination method, but the ancient technique of questioning the deceased through cattle bone and tortoise shell oracles was replaced, in accordance to views dominant in the early Han era, by a literally more down-to-earth technique of investigating the perceived properties of the world inhabited by man.

As important as the selection of suitable burial sites is the continued integration of the ancestors in the daily processes of decision making and resource exchanges among the surviving members of a lineage. Ancestral tablets, neatly arranged according to past generations in special halls or on a family altar in one's own house, are not only the focus of specified worship ceremonies signaling continuing filial piety on the side of the living; these tablets are also treated as witnesses of, and participants in, all decisions deemed important to the lineage. A lineage elder acts as link between the living and the dead; he is responsible for pleasing the ancestors by ensuring the continued adherence of later generations to the moral norms transmitted by former generations. In addition, regular offerings of, for instance, roast pig, provide further evidence of a persistent appreciation of the deceased by the living family members. The latter can expect that the former will fulfill their duties with equal attention; if the material well-being or health status of the living fails to meet a desired level, despite a sincere observation of all ritual norms, this shows that a particular ancestor has lost the power to protect later generations, for instance against evil spirits. Such a "person" will, naturally, be excluded from worship and offerings.[43]

2. The Chou Period and Demonic Medicine

2.1. HISTORICAL BACKGROUND

The organization of the Shang Empire rested on a central authority concentrated in the capital. Although it appears that the Shang king had granted fiefs to his vassals, he nevertheless maintained control by periodic expeditions through surrounding territories, reinforcing his claims to sovereignty. At the conclusion of such campaigns, the army would either leave behind a few scattered garrisons or the entire force would return to the capital. It is possible that this lack of well-organized, permanent supervision of the outlying regions of political influence was so advantageous to hostile forces that they were ultimately able to invade and destroy the Shang kingdom and establish a new dynasty. Thus the Chou, who inherited the power along the Yellow River, had first appeared in the area of present-day Kansu in northwest China. They then moved to the lower course of the Wei River, finally settling to the west of the Shang in what is today Shensi. Following their arrival, the still seminomadic Chou appear to have developed considerable agricultural skills. Of particular importance in this connection is a communally managed irrigation system. The resulting productive advantage achieved over the Shang provided the material basis for arming the Chou peasantry. With the aid of dissident Shang nobles, the even more fertile Shang territories were eventually subdued. The uncertain date of ca. 1100 B.C. is generally regarded as the beginning of the Chou dynasty.[1]

The Chou and their political system are associated with an era in Chinese history that exhibits certain parallels to the European system of feudalism. The first rulers of the new dynasty subdivided their sphere of influence into more than a thousand districts. The new capital was established not in the old Shang metropolis, but in Shensi, whence the Chou conquest had originated. The royal family proceeded to claim crown lands stretching from Shensi along the Yellow River to what is today Honan. Members of the royal family, as well as close allies, were granted fiefs in a semicircle to the east and south of this territory. Still farther to the east, separated from royal lands by this buffer zone of loyal supporters, the Chou assigned property to surviving members of the Shang ruling clan. Such favorable treatment illustrates how deeply the Chou themselves were rooted in ancestor worship; it was a matter of course that the vanquished ruling family be given the means to make the necessary sacrifices to their ancestors in a just and fitting manner. This required landholdings. The encirclement of the Shang, who perhaps considered regaining their former power, was completed with the granting of additional fiefs in the east to members of the Chou royal clan, thereby establishing a feudal system that fulfilled the expectations of its founders until the eighth century B.C. The numerous feudal lords journeyed periodically to the capital to reaffirm their loyalty to the king. They provided troops for the defense of the empire and workers for the cultivation of the royal domains; otherwise, their activities were restricted to their own holdings. A number of foreign invasions were successfully repelled during this period.[2]

The year 771 B.C. marked a turning point in the history of the Chou Empire.[3] During the bloody unrest that surrounded the succession to the throne, a decisive role was played by a foreign power whose support had been sought by one of the involved parties. After the legitimate prince had been declared successor—the king having been killed during the unrest—these allies refused to return the Chou crown lands they had occupied; for the most part, these territories remained in foreign hands. A new capital was established farther east in Lo-i, but the Chou kings now lacked the extensive landholdings required to maintain control over the entire kingdom and a preeminent role in defense against invaders. At their new residence, they gradually became dependent upon the goodwill of their vassals; during subsequent centuries their position deteriorated to such an extent that they were permitted to carry out ancestral sacrifices to the supreme celestial ruler solely for ceremonial reasons.[4]

The establishment of the new capital marks the beginning of a period that Chinese historians have designated the "Eastern Chou." The loss of power experienced by the royal family was already evident in the same century, when the Prince of Ch'u bestowed the title of "king" on his sons. Other feudal lords soon followed this example.

From this point until the unification of the empire in 221 B.C., China was plagued by an almost uninterrupted series of wars and hostilities among individual states already present in the eighth century B.C., newly formed political entities in outlying areas, and foreign peoples who staged occasional invasions. The already chaotic situation was exacerbated by countless cases of patricide, uxoricide, and fratricide within the many ruling families; this moral decay marks the decline of the Chou Empire as one of the bloodiest periods in Chinese history. The initial fragmentation of Chou territory into hundreds of small and minute units was gradually reversed by subsequent annexations and alliances. Ultimately, only a few larger states struggled for supremacy, attempting to achieve the status accorded the former Chou kings. It was only toward the beginning of the third century B.C. that the idea of a centrally unified empire arose.

As a result of a number of factors—including the introduction or invention of new technologies, the production of iron and salt, the creation of a monetary economy, and an increasingly mobile population—first one state, then another, gained prominence and power. At one point, a group of states in central China forged an alliance to oppose a common threat from the north and south. But this alliance soon disintegrated, with each member either continuing the struggle alone or seeking other allies. The center of power shifted from the central states, which between the eighth and sixth centuries had successfully resisted the almost incessant invasions from the north, to three states that had attained importance in the south. But since these aspiring powers, located on the periphery of Chinese culture, were engaged in continual wars among themselves, a balance of power emerged, which none of the states was able to upset until the third century B.C. It was only at this point that the Ch'in state was able to subdue all rivals, thereby initiating the first unification of China under a strong central authority having both administrative and military control over individual regions.[5] The final centuries preceding this event (481–221 B.C.) have been designated the period of the "Warring States" by subsequent Chinese historians, since the intensity of hostilities reached its zenith during this last epoch of the Chou dynasty.

The nature of the struggle for preeminence and, ultimately, sole control changed rapidly from a ritual and bloodless rivalry among the princes, which may have developed from the distribution of worldly prestige among the peasantry, into a murderous enmity that spared no human life when victory or defeat was at stake. The old conventions became meaningless; the opponent was no longer granted another chance to prove himself in some bloodless contest at a future date. Each side sought total triumph.[6] The ultimate objective was the complete destruction of the enemy, a goal that in earlier times would have been impossible, if only because of the common reverence for ancestors and the resulting acknowledged necessity for the continued existence of the family. Ransom was no longer demanded for the exchange of prisoners—their execution now secured the desired prestige. "The battlefield is no longer a tournament that brings honor to the participants. All that matters is success, which appears to be the result of magical skills, and not the solemn sacrifice of religious merit. The ethics of power gradually displace the old morality of honor and moderation."[7]

This transformation was brought about primarily by the unscrupulous policies of the ultimately victorious Ch'in state. Its ruler, King Cheng, heeded advisers who categorically and brutally rejected the old values of feudalism. All efforts by the legalists in Ch'in (as this school is called) were directed toward achieving economic wealth and military power for the state. To accomplish this objective, the time-honored, unwritten rites that were concerned with the social status of the individual were replaced by a codified system of laws, before which everyone, at least theoretically, was equally accountable. A system of penalties, whose severity was previously unknown, accompanied the reform of social norms. In a similar manner, the massacre of prisoners, massive threats, and misleading gifts and promises now characterized Ch'in's relationships with other states. Ch'in finally defeated the last of its opponents in 221 B.C.; King Cheng had himself proclaimed the first emperor (Shih Huang-ti) of a unified China.[8] This epochal event, however, did not end the unrest.

Although unification of the empire literally meant the destruction of all previous states, the advisers to the first emperor were fully cognizant of the fact that an aggressive program of reforms was necessary to eliminate all vestiges of the particularism that had marked the preceding feudal period. The large fiefs of numerous landowners were expropriated, and their positions were assumed by high officials. In other cases, nobles were forced to live in the capital, thereby separating them from the sources of possible reactionary movements. The entire empire was reorganized into new administrative districts, headed by military governors and civilian officials who could be replaced at any time by the imperial central government. A cultural standardization was pursued by means of a reform of the regionally diverse script; the standardization of weights, measures, and even the track width of vehicles using public roads contributed to an economic integration of the individual regions. One final measure earned the first emperor 2,000 years of contempt by Confucians, replaced only in recent times by the esteem of the Communist leadership under Mao Tse-tung. In 213 B.C., Shih Huang-ti ordered the collection and subsequent burning of all writings, except those dealing with medical care, drugs, oracles, as well as agriculture and forestry. This action was aimed primarily at historical writings that might have nurtured traditions opposing the new political direction. This was also the intention behind the simultaneous prohibition of any criticism of the present that made reference to the past.[9]

The new system was not allowed sufficient time, however, to prove itself; Shih Huang-ti died only eleven years after the founding of the first Chinese imperial dynasty. His two immediate successors had neither the power nor the skill to carry on his work and were unable to suppress opposition from feudalistic circles and revolts by conscripted laborers and state slaves. Two groups established themselves during the lengthy period of renewed strife that ensued. The first consisted of nobles seeking to reestablish their old privileges; the second was a mixed group composed of bandits, those uprooted by natural disasters in eastern China, and other insurgents, who, despite their diverse motives, were undoubtedly united by a common resistance to the harsh obligations of the peasants to state service. Liu Pang, a former village gendarme, was finally able to defeat the noble faction in 202 B.C.; history knows him as Emperor Kao-tsu, founder of the Han dynasty. Although all Ch'in laws were swiftly repealed under his rule, a return to the old social institutions did not occur. The granting of fiefs to some former allies was unavoidable, but an inheritance law and other measures ensured eventual division of the holdings.[10]

Pragmatism characterized the first decades of Han rule, as the early rulers were not guided by a specific political or social principle. The death of Emperor Kao-tsu in 195 B.C. led to renewed unrest, as the regency of the widowed empress was marked by a bloody and unscrupulous attempt to gain power and influence for her own family, while eliminating the clan of her late husband. After fifteen years of strife, the Liu family was able to regain control, and the following reigns of Wen (180–157 B.C.), Ching (157–141 B.C.), and Wu (141–87 B.C.) brought to China, for the first time in many centuries, a period of internal peace and stability. The political system that was to be characteristic of China during the following 2,000 years evolved during the reign of Emperor Wu.

Nearly 700 years of bitter strife had fundamentally changed almost every social and cultural institution of Chinese civilization. Although at the beginning of the Chou period we frequently encountered groups— ethnically, linguistically, and culturally independent, or at least only distantly related—fighting among themselves, the end of this traumatic epoch, despite the continued existence of regional differences, saw the outlines of a future homogeneous Chinese culture.

The struggles during these centuries were not fought solely on the battlefield between individual states and at court among members of the ruling family or those aspiring to rule; the emergence of Chinese culture was accompanied by diverse, frequently antithetical, philosophies which to the present day have retained a significant cultural influence, even extending beyond China to large segments of East Asia. China never again experienced a similar period of such intellectual richness; even the far-reaching upheavals of the twentieth century, with the twofold revolution from empire to republic and then to people's republic, were, in the final analysis, not really characterized by the creation of a specifically Chinese system of ideas for shaping the future, but rather by the borrowing of Western ideologies and their adaptation to Chinese conditions. The history of the rise, preeminence, and decline of certain medical conceptions in China faithfully reflects these developments in the political sphere.

A consideration of the conceptualization of illness during the Chou period therefore cannot ignore the following dichotomy. As early as the period of the Warring States, the medical ideas that gained acceptance among broad segments of the population were those that can be viewed as an immediate consequence of contemporary political conditions and social structures. These are the concepts of demonic medicine, to be discussed below. In addition, however, certain systems of ideas were developed during the Chou period that apparently exerted significant influence only after the ultimate breakdown of Chou feudalism, following the unification of the empire. These include the concepts of yinyang dualism and the theory of the Five Phases, to be discussed below, as well as the philosophies of Taoism and Confucianism and their impact on healing.

2.2. CONCEPTS OF DEMONOLOGICAL THERAPY

Following the Chou victory over the Shang, the new ruler consulted the tortoise-carapace oracle of his vanquished predecessor to determine the best location for the capital of the new empire. The use of

tortoise carapaces is also widely documented for the late Chou period.[11] Nevertheless, an obvious change in the attitude toward the
nonliving members of the earthly community resulted in a diminished
significance of ancestors and a concomitant perception of demons as
partially or even completely responsible for everyday misfortune, including illness.

The Chou adopted the so-called *wu* from the Shang, a group of
shamanlike practitioners who, according to Eichhorn, were regarded
during the Shang period "as leaders or chiefs of their clan, believed
to possess magical powers." Those responsible for sacrifices to Ti, the
supreme deified ancestor, as well as to other ancestral deities, were
undoubtedly members of the royal family. The political significance
of these and other functions, especially those concerning claims of
legitimacy by the rulers, was much too great to allow just anyone to
pursue this occupation.[12] The pictographic core of the character wu
indicates a dancer, and it was the most important responsibility of
these practitioners to ensure—by means of prolonged and ecstatic
dances and cries—the rain so vital in northern China. In addition, the
wu were required to reduce violent storms and excessive rain, as well
as to purge palace rooms of evil influences, snakes, and other poisonous creatures.[13]

The transformation of the political system that began with the Chou
period was inevitably accompanied by a change in the religious system.
Shang-ti was gradually displaced as the highest religious authority by
T'ien, the celestial deity increasingly perceived in spatial terms. The
wu lost their powerful social position and reestablished their occupation among lower segments of the population; their high status was
in part assumed by the *chu* practitioners, the "priests" or "supplicants," who during the period of the Warring States had apparently
been accorded a certain primacy in the maintenance of relations between the living and the supranatural.[14]

The prevailing view at this time appears to have been that the once
well-ordered relationships and system of communication existing between living beings and the world of deities and spirits had at first
fallen into a state of great confusion and, finally, had broken down
completely.[15] During the period of the Warring States, these attitudes
fostered, in turn, the creation of myths that recognized demons (*kuei*)
as exerting an increasingly harmful influence upon man. Wu practitioners thus found it necessary to utilize their contacts with high-
ranking, influential deities to restrain minor spirits and demons harmful to man; exorcism became their chief responsibility.[16] Three times
a year the wu played a decisive role in expelling illness-causing demons

from human settlements. In addition, they gathered around themselves clients who required individual treatment. Such practices were paralleled by the creation of myths such as the three sons of the legendary Emperor Chuan-hsü, who, after death, transformed themselves into evil, harmful demons.[17] As a result, the medical ideas we term *demonic medicine* gradually found acceptance and social preeminence.

Like ancestor therapy, the system of demonic medicine is based on a belief in the existence of beings, both visible and invisible, that inhabit the universe along with man. Unlike the Shang, however, who believed that every ancestor was associated with a specific living individual, there is no longer any direct connection between individual demons and individual persons. As I have shown, demonic medicine is based on the belief that illness is caused by the actions of evil spirits. Typical views of demonic medicine, present in literature of the first millennium A.D., are expressed in the following conditions defined as illness: "struck by evil" (*chung-o*), "assaulted by demons" (*kuei-chi*), "possessed by the hostile influence of demonic guests" (*kuei-k'o wu-chi*), and "possessed by the hostile" (*chu-wu*). A possible source for such ideas is the belief—verified for the Chou period, and perhaps even older—that each person has two souls.[18] The so-called corporeal soul (*p'o*) is present in the body from birth and perishes along with the body following death. The ethereal soul (*hun*) enters the body only much later after birth; during periods of sleep or unconsciousness it can temporarily leave the body, and after death it wanders alone through space and time. Demonic medicine perceives these unattached souls, spirits, or demons as inherently evil and thus as constantly striving to harm man. Such a view is by no means a necessary consequence of belief in demons; a concept of well-meaning or indifferent spirits is quite possible. The assumption of a permanently malicious character in these beings is fostered by a social climate that prevails in China only after 771 B.C.

At this point, it is necessary to consider another important conceptual difference between ancestor therapy and demonic medicine. According to demonic medicine, adherence to certain social conventions no longer protects an individual from future adversity (*hsieh*) or enables him to resist misfortune already present. Only when the guardian spirits associated with each individual are powerful enough, or when one is able to secure the assistance of such beings, whose position in the metaphysical hierarchy is higher than that of the attacking force, is one protected from these threats or, in the case of illness or conflict, sufficiently armed for a counterattack. The social principle reflected in this system of therapy which stands in clear contrast both to the fundamental ideas of ancestor therapy and also, as will be demonstrated below, to the Confucian-backed system of healing, can be summarized simply as "all against all." In politics as well, only the skilled employment of troops and the establishment of alliances with other states, aimed at resisting attack from third parties, ensures survival and eventual "good health." Demonic medicine thus reflects certain central aspects of the political process during the decline of Chou feudalism, including general uncertainty and the existential *angst* that seems to have marked the relationship among states as well as among individuals.

2.3. THE PRACTICE OF DEMONOLOGICAL THERAPY

The belief that demons could cause illness is widely documented in literature of the later Chou period, as well as during the subsequent Ch'in and Han dynasties. Han Fei (died 233 B.C.) expressed the prevailing attitudes of his age when he concluded: "When a person falls ill, it means he has been injured by a demon."[19] Available evidence from the Chou era, however, provides little information concerning measures taken by the sufferer himself or by medical exorcists to rid the body or surrounding environment of these evil spirits. Initially, the procedures and therapeutic techniques may have been passed down orally, or recorded on fragile materials. A remark in the *Li-chi,* the "Book of Rites" dating from the period of the Warring States, indicates that practitioners attempted to keep their skills secret.[20] During these final centuries of the Chou Empire, attempts were apparently made to combat demons with the same measures that had already proven effective in human conflicts. Several times a year, and also during certain special occasions, such as the funeral of a prince, hordes of exorcists would race shrieking through the city streets, enter the courtyards and homes, thrusting their spears into the air, in an attempt to expel the evil creatures. Prisoners were dismembered outside all gates to the city, to serve both as a deterrent to the demons and as an indication of their fate should they be captured.[21] It may well be that the ancient writing of the Chinese character *i* used for "healer" and "healing" was formed at that time. Its lower half consists of the character wu ("shaman"); the upper half combines a quiver with an arrow on the left and a spear or lance on the right. The entire character thus depicts exactly the type of practitioner active in the rituals described.

By the late Chou or early Han period (206 B.C.–A.D. 8), more subtle methods to ward off demons or to enlist the help of spirits to cure an ailment appear in medical sources still extant today; they may, of course, have been developed much earlier. Donald Harper's recent brilliant analysis of the *Wu-shih-erh ping fang*, a fragmentary manual recommending a broad spectrum of (as the title states) "prescriptions against fifty-two ailments," and of other texts unearthed from the Mawang-tui graves of 168 B.C. near Ch'ang-sha, Hunan, in 1973, has brought to light a hitherto unknown sophistication of demonological (in conjunction with magical) concepts and practices that must have been a result of intellectual efforts by the best minds of the educated strata of Chinese society. Twenty-seven prescriptions (almost 10 percent of the total number of prescriptions) listed in the *Wu-shih-erh ping fang* are based on spells. For instance, to treat an affliction that may be identified as "lumping," the unknown compiler of the script suggested the following:

> Wait for lightning in Heaven and then rub both hands together, face the lightning, and chant an incantation to it saying, "Sovereign of the Eastern Quarter, [Sovereign of] the Western Quarter, [. . .] preside over the darkness and darken this person's stars." Do it twice seven times and [   ].[22]

As Harper pointed out, "it was a general belief in Han times that alimentation under a starry sky caused the growth of small lumps in the flesh. The hard essence of the stars transferred under the skin is yet another process of cosmic replication, similar to the effect of the moon on the growth of the pearl inside an oyster. . . . Because of the astral etiology of the ailment, the magical act employed to cure it exploits a flash of lightning and the incantation calls upon the Sovereigns of the Eastern and Western Quarters to 'darken the person's stars'; i.e., to remove the skin lumps which the stars have caused to appear."[23]

The incantations and maledictions listed in the *Wu-shih-erh ping fang* echo various categories of magic applied to demonology. "Several spells are simple summons for divine assistance, others invoke the assistance of spiritual agents and then threaten the spiritual perpetrator of the ailment with extermination."[24] Breath magic, including spitting and spouting, accompanies verbal spells because it was believed that "spitting saliva or spouting substances out of the mouth is like blowing out a stream of fire," a stream of fire which communicates chanted incantations to the spiritual world just as the burning of talismans transfers the written word to a metaphysical destination.[25]

A number of prescriptions in the *Wu-shih-erh ping fang* list non-verbal exorcistic techniques, such as the "steps of Yü," which I will discuss below with the first texts providing detailed information on their practice. All these nonverbal techniques combine demonological with magical concepts; they include, in addition to the "steps of Yü," "examples of magical transfer in which the ailment is transferred into an intermediate object, and the object is then safely discarded." "Beating the patient with exorcistic instruments is used in treating inguinal swellings. The list of magical weapons includes the following: thuja pestle, iron hammer, hemp cloth, and rammer."[26] Further examples are exorcistic archery and magical entrapment, as well as the demon-deterring employment of animal feces applied as therapeutic ointment or bath.[27] Finally, concepts of magic correspondence accounted for the specification of certain days, or times of day, as being most suitable for performing various exorcistic rituals.[28]

The use of talismans is documented in the *Wu-shih-erh ping fang* too; by the early Han period the entire population, from emperor to simple citizen, wore—in part as a fixed component of official dress—flat, rectangular pieces of wood, jade, or gold, secured to the waist, the forearm, or on a hat. Such pieces carried an inscription on both sides announcing that a deified ruler of antiquity had admonished his ministers to transform the object into a spear that could prevent all epidemics and serious illnesses. A word list compiled between 48 and 33 B.C. designated such amulets "projectiles against demons resembling a child" (*she-ch'i*) and "banishers of evil" (*pi-hsieh*), that "eliminate all kinds of misfortune."[29] Some 150 years later, the author of the etymological lexicon *Shuo-wen* (ca. A.D. 100) wrote the following in connection with the term *hai-szu*, which was also used for amulets: "they are used to drive out [evil] influences and demons."[30] The first written work devoted to amulet medicine may have been compiled at about the same time. This work, which has not survived in its original form, was, according to legend, authored by Chang Tao-ling (34–156), the somewhat shadowy founder and first "pope" of organized Taoism. Around A.D. 200, sources indicate a further development in efforts to combat and destroy demons in the human body; at the time, exorcistic inscriptions on paper or silk were usually burned to ashes and administered in a potion.[31] Amulets, also termed *seals* (yin) or *talismans* in Chinese, were now composed like official documents, bringing the world of demons into the administrative hierarchy of imperial bureaucracy. Talismans were already in use during the feudal period. It was customary for a prince who had assigned a task to one of his subjects, to break in two a piece of wood or jade inscribed with an appropriate text, and retain one of the pieces for himself. The remaining half was then presented to the person delegated with the task, to serve as proof of the official nature of his mission. The contractual and official character of charms is also evident in demonic medicine.

Exorcists prepared talismans resembling official documents, in which a command was given by a high official within the demon hierarchy to lowly evil spirits responsible for illness in humans. The inscriptions on these charms were generally in the form of intertwined, vertically arranged signs and symbols. The heading was generally a character signifying "assignment" or "command." Since the prestige of the "issuer" of the command was decisive for its therapeutic or preventive efficacy, the talismans contain the likeness or name of influential deities believed able to repel evil spirits. Such illustrations frequently included the god of thunder with his lightning bolts, the sun, moon, various stars, and commanders of celestial armies, or renowned magicians. Since demonic medicine was adopted by several groups during the first century A.D., especially by various Taoist sects and by Buddhism (verified in China since A.D. 65), the founders and other personalities associated with these two religions are also named as "issuers." In addition, the talismans contain characters that indicate the nature of the command, such as the admonition "to depart," "to sink," "to come here," and "to kill" another demon. These are followed by a designation of the "curse," "evil," or "misfortune" to be eliminated and, finally, by a phrase generally found in official documents, such as "obey the law" or "respect this command." Taoist charms frequently conclude with the words "quickly, quickly, this is an order" or "as swift as fire!" An additional procedure was also intended to simulate the power structure of human society. Imperial decrees were prepared with vermillion ink on yellow paper, and a seal was then affixed. In place of the imperial seal, Taoist exorcists affixed the seal of Lao-tzu or Chang Tao-ling on similar yellow paper. The talisman achieved its greatest efficacy, however, only when the characters had been written with a genuine cinnabar brush that had been removed from the desk of a secular administrative official.[32]

The use of medicinal drugs to expel or destroy demons in the body appears to be as old as demonological therapy itself. Here, too, magic concepts appear to have guided the application of such substances in a demonological context. The *Wu-shih-erh ping fang* offers numerous instances of attempts to cure demon-caused illnesses by means of natural or man-made drugs. They include aromatics, prepared animals or parts of animals, herbs, a woman's menstrual cloth, and others.[33]

The *Sou-shen hou-chi* of the third or fourth century A.D. contains the following depiction of a "hitherto unused" method in the struggle against evil spirits; the story related reminds us of a similar event recorded in the *Tso-chuan* for the sixth century B.C.[34] and may well refer to a time when the use of drugs against demons was a novelty:

Li Tsze-yü, though still young, was an able medical expert, whose perspicacity and spirit his contemporaries extolled. Hü Yung was governor of Yü-cheu, and resided at Lih-yang when his younger brother fell ill; his heart and his belly ached severely for more than ten years, and he was almost dead, when one evening he overheard a specter from behind the screen accosting the demon within his belly. "Why do you not kill him immediately?" it said; "if you do not, Li Tsze-yü when passing along here will strike you with something hitherto unused, and this will cost you your life." On which the specter in the belly said: "I do not fear him." Next morning Hü Yung sent somebody for Tsze-yü; he came, and no sooner did he pass through the gate than the patient heard within himself a plaintive voice. The doctor entered, saw the sufferer, and said: "this is a demoniacal disease." Taking a red ball, compounded of eight poisonous substances, out of his linen box, he gave it the sick man to swallow, and through his belly immediately rolled a thundering noise; several times he had a copious discharge of diarrhea, and then he was quite well.[35]

The use of medicinal substances for the treatment of demon-related illnesses was continually refined in subsequent centuries. In approximately A.D. 600, Chen Ch'üan compiled the *Ku-chin lu-yen fang,* a collection of prescriptions containing the following recommendations for possession:

Pills for the five kinds of possession

Additional names: spirit and mountain recluse pills; pills worth a thousand times their weight in gold; pills that bring about a turning point in suffering caused by possession; pills that control fate; pills that kill demons.

They cure ten thousand illnesses, [drive out] and [eliminate] illnesses caused by possession, as well as abdominal pain and belching. In addition, the prescription is effective against the harmful effects of cold, seasonal illnesses, and epidemics

Cinnabar—pulverize
Arsenopyrite—burned for a half-day in earth
Realgar—pulverize
Croton seed—discard the skins, roast
Hellebone—roast
Aconite root—subject to dry heat

use 2 *fen* of each of the above ingredients

Centipede—broil, remove the feet

Press these seven ingredients through a sieve and combine with honey
to form pills the size of small beans. The correct dose is one pill daily.
This will result in a cure. If the suffering is not relieved, an additional
pill should be taken at midnight. This will certainly end all complaints.
One pill should be carried on one's person at all times to ward off future
misfortune. Pork, cold water, fresh-bloody things, and fox meat are to
be avoided [during the treatment].[36]

Empirical evidence supported the assumption that certain drugs
were effective against spirits. This was especially true for poisons,
which could harm man, or whose destructive effects had at least been
observed in insects. They were worn as charms or burned as a fu-
migant. One of the earliest prescriptions pertaining to the fumigation
of demons was recorded by Sun Ssu-miao (581–682?) in his treatise
on alchemy, *Tan-ching yao-chüeh*.[37] It contains, in addition to such
toxic ingredients as realgar (As_2S_2) and arsenic trisulfide (As_2S_3), substances that, when burned, produced acrid fumes, such as sulfur, and
those that already possessed a penetrating odor, such as musk. Another
group of the nineteen ingredients in the prescription is composed of
drugs that on the basis of their external appearance or medicinal effect
were compared with weapons in the war against demons and given
appropriate names. Sun Ssu-miao refers to the "demon arrow" (*kuei-
chien*), which is also known as "divine arrow" (*shen-chien*) and "protective spear" (*wei-mao*). The myrtle flag plant was used in demonic
medicine possibly because its ideogram was composed of two sun
symbols, and it was therefore assumed the substance contained the
concentrated power of the sun. Because of their fragrance, orchids
found use in exorcistic rites, as did numerous tree resins, which were
seen as the coagulated blood of the plant. When such resins were taken
medicinally, the vital spirit of the tree, which was also coagulated in
this blood, destroyed the demons in the body of the patient.[38]

The *Ch'ien-chin i-fang*, a compendium prepared late in life by Sun
Ssu-miao, contains thirty-two drugs effective against demons.[39] In his

various medical and alchemistic treatises, Sun Ssu-miao not only re-corded instructions for the medicinal treatment of demon-caused ail-ments but the twenty-ninth and thirtieth chapters of the *Ch'ien-chin i-fang* also comprise the oldest collection of demonic medicine spells continuously handed down through the centuries until our present time, under the title "Classic of Interdictions" (*Chin-ching*). Sun Ssu-miao had had a comprehensive education that included both the nat-ural sciences and medicine, and he was influenced by both Taoist and Buddhist traditions. In the preface to the "Classic of Interdictions" he wrote:

> It is said that, when the clear had not yet been separated from the turbid, when night and day were still one, and the division [of the universe] into heaven and earth had just taken place, it was possible to distinguish warm and cool, the four seasons were separated, cold and heat were sent down to earth and created, the three sources of light shone forth; light and shadow alternately grew and died out. The five characteristics were given to man, and the surface of the body was given the ability to absorb and obstruct. Thus Lao-tzu spoke: "I must suffer greatly because of the fact that I have a body. If I did not have a body, how could there possibly be any cause for suffering?" From this it can be seen that form and matter are conducive to illness. If one contem-plates this in peace, it can be seen that only formlessness can avoid suffering. If not even the holy men on this earth are able to free them-selves from suffering, how can it be done by the candle in the wind?[40]

With these words, Sun Ssu-miao touched upon a central thesis of demonic medicine that is not without sociopolitical significance. He has expressed here the conviction that illness and suffering are natural and unavoidable. Such a view ran counter to the already existing medicine of systematic correspondence, which was based on the belief that illness could be avoided by means of an appropriate way of life. But the conduct advocated by the medicine of systematic correspon-dences for the preservation of good health conformed, as I will dem-onstrate in chapter 3, to a large degree with the norms of Confucian political philosophy for the maintenance of harmony and order in society. By emphasizing the inevitability of illness and the need for a healing system devoted to the treatment of existing suffering, Sun Ssu-miao implicitly questioned the necessity of following certain moral dictums recommended for the preservation of good health by Con-fucian doctrine, as well as by certain Taoist sects.

The spells in the "Classic of Interdictions" resemble the structure of the talismans. The exorcist, or the sufferer himself, seeks an alliance with supranatural authorities, whose assistance, it is hoped, will expel or destroy the demons. In an opening chapter, Sun Ssu-miao explains in great detail various methods that are first needed to acquire the skill of reciting effective spells. These include ritual fasting and cleansing that served to purify the body and mind, as well as breathing techniques needed to absorb the vigorous influences of the sun, moon, and stars. The "Step of Yü" played an important role in the magical conveyance of internal and external forces. In order to avert a drought, Yü, a legendary ruler of antiquity, had offered himself as a sacrifice to God. But the god had accepted only half of his body, leaving Yü paralyzed on one side. To achieve his real objective—the founding of the Chinese Empire and the prevention of an imminent world flood— Yü had to perform a magical-ritual dance, which alone radiated sufficient power for the successful realization of such a momentous ambition. Because of his paralysis, Yü could only dance on one leg and had to drag the other behind him.[41] His success is documented in the literature of the first millennium B.C., where the "Step of Yü" appears as an essential component of rites designed to secure the assistance of a suprahuman power (see appendix 4.1).

Only someone who had successfully performed all these preparatory ceremonies, which were also associated with particularly favorable times of the day and year, was able to heal diverse afflictions by means of spells. A selection of the diseases and illness-causing agents listed in the "Classic of Interdictions," for which Sun Ssu-miao was able to offer useful spells, illustrates the spectrum of indications:

Hostile influences of demons; seasonal epidemics caused by heat; alternating attacks of heat and cold [yao afflictions]; boils and swellings; numbness of the larynx; toothache, eyeache; danger of suffocating by choking; difficult childbirth; hemostasis; possession; harassment by evil animals, tigers, wolves; snake venom; scorpions and wasps; robbers and thieves.

Two representative incantations are presented here in their entirety:

Interdiction of the hostile influence of demonic guests.
I am responsible for the wine sacrifice of the celestial master [i.e., Chang Tao-ling]; Heaven and earth have sent me. On my body I transport [the authority over] the celestial soldiers: 100 times 1,000 times 10,000 times 100,000 [of them] stand before and behind me, are lined up to my left and right. Which spirit would dare to alight here! Which demon would dare be present! Only a legitimate spirit should appear here! Evil demons—depart quickly! Quickly, quickly, this is an order![42]

Interdiction of intermittent fevers [i.e., the *yao* illness].

I ascend a high mountain. I look down into the water of the sea. A dragon with three heads and nine tails lives in the water. He subsists on nothing but *yao* demons. In the morning he devours 3,000 of them; at night 800. If his hunger is not yet stilled, he dispatches emissaries to drag in more demons. Amulets and drugs penetrate the five granaries of the body; the *yao* demons should retreat. Those who do not submit will be put in chains and delivered to the lord of the river. Quickly, quickly, this is an order![43]

One additional weapon in the arsenal utilized by Chinese physicians against demons cannot be ignored—acupuncture. In his *Ch'ien-chin i-fang,* Sun Ssu-miao cited the physician Pien Ch'io, purportedly active in the fifth century B.C., and indicated the exact location of thirteen puncture points for the needle treatment of demon-related illnesses that Pien allegedly had recommended.[44] The thirteen puncture points bear such revealing names as "demon camp," "demon hearts," "demon path," "demon bed," or also "demon hall." The needles used to penetrate a "demon heart" in the treatment of an individual were analogous to the spears used by exorcists at the time of Confucius (551–479 B.C.), when they ran through the streets gesturing in the air, in order to free the inhabitants from the threat of evil spirits. Surviving sources do not indicate with certainty whether demonic medicine actually utilized acupuncture during the late Chou or Ch'in periods, as Sun Ssu-miao's reference to Pien Ch'io would imply; in fact, no reference to therapeutic needling at all has been found in any Chinese text prior to 90 B.C. But the possibility that acupuncture originally had purely demonic medicine functions should not be excluded. I will return to this issue in a discussion of the possible sources of needle therapy (see below pp. 92–99).

We have now seen the wide range of therapeutic measures developed in the fight against illness-causing demons. All of these methods for the prevention and treatment of illnesses subsequently became a permanent part of medical care in China and continue to be practiced today, both outside of the People's Republic and, as recent mainland press reports indicate, in the People's Republic (although it is impossible to determine the extent of such practices). The longevity of these concepts should not be sought so much in their roots in popular Taoism and Buddhism, but rather in the general prevailing social atmosphere of existential uncertainty which made such concepts attractive to the great rural population until the present century.

2.4. THE CONCEPT OF *KU*

During its 2,500-year history, demonic medicine was developed and differentiated in a multitude of ways. Universal belief in the existence of evil forces that occupied transcendental sphere was transformed by numerous regional and supraregional attitudes and adapted to the specific empirical experiences of individual groups.[45] An informative example is provided by the concept *ku,* which is described throughout the medical literature of the first and second millennia as one of the many causes of illness, and which also found both preventive and therapeutic consideration. The ku, a worm spirit, deserves special attention because it is a possible example of how the universal encounter of a region or epoch with actual parasite infestation, transformed by demonological concepts and the influence of social experiences, developed into an explanatory model that was able to convince both the educated and uneducated for many centuries.

Ku appears in several variations in Chinese literature, but the basic concept is as follows. A human "host" fills a container with various poisonous insects, worms, or snakes, which after a period of time, generally 100 days, destroy or devour one another until only one animal remains. It is assumed that the survivor contains the concentrated poison of all the original beasts. The human host then places this last animal, along with another, into a vessel containing water, where the two mate. The seed of the male floats on the surface and constitutes the so-called ku poison. The host picks up the seed with the eye of a needle and must now locate, on the same day, a person to whom he can administer the ku seed in food or drink. As soon as the recipient has swallowed the ku seeds, they develop into worms that resemble their parents. The worms gnaw on the viscera of the victim, producing pain, a swollen abdomen, progressive emaciation, and, ultimately, death. The proof of ku poisoning is visible following the demise of the victim, when worms crawl out from orifices in the corpse. As a reward for providing the ku parents, which are merely manifestations of a spirit that can only reproduce in this manner, with a secondary host, in which the seeds can mature, the ku spirit presents the primary host with all possessions of the deceased victim. If the primary host is unable to find a secondary host the same day, or he permits some sort of harm to befall the ku worm, he is killed by the ku spirit. For this reason the primary host may even find himself forced to select a relative from his own household as the victim, if no stranger appears on the day the ku seed was produced. There is only one way for a primary host to rid himself of the obligation to the ku spirit. He must gather together in a basket a large amount of valuable objects, such as silk, silver, and gold, and the ku worm, leaving it in a field or at an intersection. The person who finds this treasure and is unable to resist taking it home, is considered the new primary host by the ku spirit. If someone notices too late what an unfortunate burden he has acquired, he can free himself from the resulting obligation only by returning the basket with its original contents, plus about 30 percent interest, to the place it was found, or to a similar location.[46]

Medical literature considered the ku spirit, which could also appear in the form of a dog, frog, or other animals, to be the cause of various illnesses. As a result, there are numerous preventive, diagnostic, and therapeutic measures designed to protect against this danger.

A simple method of prevention, when eating outside of the home, was to have the host first sample the proffered meals. Another technique was to stir the food with bronze chopsticks. If the meal had been poisoned, the chopsticks turned black. Innkeepers had daily contact with numerous strangers and were continually suspected of being in league with a ku specter. To ensure that entering an inn did not entail any risk, it was advisable first to clean the soles of the shoes on an inner wall of the establishment or to spit on the floor. If the dirt produced in this manner disappeared immediately, or if the place seemed suspiciously clean, one could be certain that a ku spirit was at work, and it was a good idea to look for different lodging.

To diagnose whether someone was suffering from ku poisoning, the patient was asked to spit into water; if the spittle sank, the result was positive. Another method was for the victim to place a pea into his mouth. If it became soft and lost its skin, ku poison was present.

Prescription literature was filled with antidotes. All known Chinese conceptual systems of healing dealt with the ku phenomenon and developed therapeutic strategies that were in accord with their basic principles. The Buddhists recommended prayers and conjurations, thus utilizing the same methods as practitioners of demonic medicine. In pharmaceutical literature, drugs of a plant, animal, or mineral origin were described as effective against ku poisoning. Adherents of homeopathic magic recommended the taking of centipedes, since it was known that centipedes consume worms.

The familiar character for ku, a vessel with two (three since the Ch'in period) snakes or worms, appears, as I indicated in the previous chapter, as early as the Shang period on oracle bones and tortoise carapaces inscribed in the fourteenth century B.C. From the second century until the last imperial dynasty, laws prohibited, under severe penalties, the production and use of ku poison.

It appears that the attitudes toward ku outlined above are rooted in the observation of certain symptoms of human illness—swollen abdomen, emaciation, and the presence of worms in the body orifices of the dead or living. Such symptoms allow a great number of possible explanations and interpretations; in my view, very specific social conditions are necessary for the rise and general acceptance of the ideas encompassed by the concept ku. Particularly striking is the constant fear of one's fellow man, an omnipresent suspicion that is reflected in the view that some people are constantly striving to take over the possessions of others. This is, of course, the social atmosphere of envy that one can still see today in societies whose organization and economic structure can be equated in principle with the corresponding structures of the Shang. But the concept of ku is unknown outside of China. Instead, one finds what may be its conceptual equivalent, the "evil eye," present in all "envy societies." From the Shang texts themselves, one learns little more about contemporary views on ku than that it was a cause of illness. Sources from the Chou period are only slightly more informative. The *Tso-chuan* contains two different examples of illness resulting from the effects of ku, and it is significant that in both cases, the victims had been guilty of "excesses."[47] A text from the fourth century A.D. is the first to describe the preparation of ku as a means to obtain the wealth of others; the oldest surviving description of the production process itself dates from the sixth century.[48] The lack of early evidence tells us little about the actual age of attitudes toward ku, but it does seem certain, as Feng and Shryock recognized, that

> the practice of *ku* extended at one time over the whole area included in China proper . . . even in the medieval period [third to seventh centuries], Chinese observers remarked on the prevalence of the practice in southern China, and from the T'ang period on, the practice appears to have been more and more confined to aboriginal tribes of the south.[49]

The nature of ku poisoning thus changed over the course of centuries from an internal threat to a conflict between the Chinese and their less civilized neighbors, a relationship under constant strain. In the south, non-Chinese peoples suffered continually under the incessant expansion of the Chinese Empire. The cultural gulf between the southern tribes and the approaching Chinese was obvious. The conquered territories were administered by Chinese officials, and the original inhabitants either exterminated or driven out, or tolerated in enclaves under Chinese suzerainty. Whether consciously or subconsciously, there were sufficient grounds for the Chinese to expect some kind of resentment and retaliation from their disadvantaged neighbors, and it is not surprising that these fears eventually took the form of etiological concepts.

Chinese children were the preferred victims for ku poisoning by members of non-Chinese tribes, as the following remarks from the nineteenth century indicate:

> During the fall, the Miao women carry pears in cloth bags, selling the pears to children. Many children are poisoned by ku in this way.[50]

Reports about the purported poisoning of Chinese administrative officials by local inhabitants may also reflect the subliminal expectations of retaliation:

> The chiefs of Yüan-chiang have handed down the method of producing ku. This medicine is not beneficent, but is poisonous. An astonishing fact is that when a new magistrate arrives, the people must prepare a feast to welcome him, and they poison him then. The poison does not become effective during his term of office, but the pupils of his eyes turn from black to blue, and his face becomes pale and swollen. Then some months after he leaves office, his whole family dies.[51]

Reports of ku poisoning in China often contain the implied desire of the disadvantaged to live under the same conditions as those who are better off. However, the ku concept contains suspicion of clean and wealthy households. In this manner, a stigma was gradually attached to those who were wealthy and clean, since they had possibly achieved their position only with the aid of criminal methods, such as the use of ku. These kinds of attitudes lead to precautionary methods similar to those found in societies where the "evil eye" is prevalent, such as the concealment of possessions and a preference for neglected external appearance.

As the legal measures of individual dynasties demonstrate, administrative officials viewed ku as a reality, as late as the nineteenth century. The primary host was considered a criminal; a person guilty of the despicable act of preparing and administrating ku poison was executed, occasionally with his entire family, in a gruesome manner. In addition to the obvious desire to punish severely criminal practices that could result in the death of the victim, it is possible that Confucian distaste for the accumulation of material goods, and above all for the resulting social mobility, contributed to this attitude. Indeed, the penalties for the use of ku poison appear to have been more severe than those for other forms of murder.

In contrast to the obvious attitude of the authorities toward the primary host, some reports depict the criminal as a victim much like the secondary host. The desire for wealth, symbolized by the picking up of the filled basket from the road, and the envy of others that induces someone actually to produce a ku worm, are viewed here as the real "disease." The healing of this suffering is only possible through the dissolution of the voluntary or involuntary pact with the ku spirit— a costly undertaking since one has to give away more than was received in the first place. Thus, envy and greed, which are supposed to result in gain, are ultimately punished by death or, in the case of a successful treatment, by the loss of possessions.

3. Unification of the Empire, Confucianism, and the Medicine of Systematic Correspondence

The concepts of demonic medicine mirror human experiences during the period of the Warring States; the increasing amorality and continuing uncertainty of personal and collective existence were reflected in the way the age perceived the nature of illness and its prevention and treatment. The conceptual characteristics of the medicine of systematic correspondence also evolved in part during the declining Chou dynasty. The major difference, however, is that the medicine of systematic correspondence reflects ideas and sociopolitical structures resulting from efforts to overcome the chaos of the Warring States and from the subsequent conditions accompanying the first unification of China.

On the one hand, the theoretical foundations on which the medicine of systematic correspondence was based can only be understood in light of this sociopolitical background. On the other hand, this system of healing integrated several paradigmatic world views which, today, are associated with traditional Chinese science in general. Altogether, the conceptual framework of the medicine of systematic correspondence was composed of the following elements: (1) magical beliefs in the unity of nature, (2) the yinyang and the Five Phases theories, (3) concepts of demonic medicine, (4) concepts of finest matter influences as the basis of life, and (5) certain structural characteristics of the united empire. I will deal with these five points in detail, as well as touch upon certain aspects of Confucianism in order to reveal some conceptual parallels between this political and social doctrine and the medicine of systematic correspondence.

3.1. THE PARADIGM OF CORRESPONDENCES

The paradigm of correspondences combines two sets of concepts whose close conceptual relation justifies the common designation. These are the concepts of magic correspondence and the concepts of systematic correspondence. Both are based on the same principle, namely that the phenomena of the visible and invisible world stand in mutual dependence through their association with certain lines of correspondence. The paradigm of correspondences concludes that manipulations of one element in a specific line of correspondence can influence other elements of the same line. The lines of magic correspondence are usually separated from one another and cannot exert systematic mutual influence. In the science of systematic correspondences, however, magical concepts have been refined and combined with elements from the yinyang doctrine and the theories of the Five Phases, and all lines of correspondence have been integrated into one detailed system of mutual correspondence.

3.1.1. Magic Correspondence

Just as the concepts of demonology, of which demonic medicine may be considered an integral part, have been present in all known civilizations of the past and present, including East Asia, China also shares with numerous other cultures a belief in magic and, consequently, in concepts of a magical system of healing. Since Frazer's studies at the beginning of this century, two fundamental concepts of magic have been distinguished—contact magic and homeopathic magic.[1] Contact magic is based on the view that a contact or former union between two elements creates a relationship in which a manipulation of one of the elements, which are now spatially separated, produces a visible effect upon the other. In societies where contact magic is practiced, the possession of part of a fingernail, hair, or even a placenta, for example, brings with it the power to influence the fate of the person from which the object came.

Homeopathic magic, in contrast, rests on the principle that like corresponds to like. It is believed that harm inflicted upon the image of a person results in harm to that person himself, despite the fact that the two might be separated by great distances. It is also believed that eating a walnut, for example, can be beneficial to the brain, since the two objects have similar appearances. The *Liu-t'ao*, a work by Lü

Wang containing material from the late Chou and Han periods, provides the following example:

> After King Wu had replaced [the rule of the] Yin [with the rule of the Chou], Marquis Ting stayed away from court. The grandfather [of King Wu] then drew a picture of Ting on a bamboo tablet and shot three arrows into it. Ting fell ill and a soothsayer spoke: "This is the result of a curse that emanates from the Chou. The situation is serious!" [Marquis Ting] then surrendered himself and his entire territory. The grandfather sent an emissary who removed an arrow from Marquis Ting's head on the first day, an arrow from his mouth on the second, and an arrow from his abdomen on the third. The Marquis' illness was gradually healed.[2]

The *Shan-hai ching* (Classic of the Mountains and the Seas), compiled between the eighth and first centuries B.C., includes certain remarks in the description of foreign lands that may represent early examples of the transfer of concepts of homeopathic magic to physiological processes:

> There is an herb there . . . that produces no fruit. It is called *ku-jung*. Those who consume it will have no children.[3]
>
> There is an animal there whose appearance resembles that of the wild cat. . . . It combines both the male and female sex. Whoever consumes it will not become jealous.[4]

Medical literature of the last two thousand years, especially the works devoted to drugs, often recorded therapeutic measures derived from homeopathic magic. Two examples may suffice here. In the *Shen-nung pen-ts'ao ching chi-chu,* an herbal compiled from older sources, T'ao Hung-ching (452–536) recommended that women in labor be given a potion consisting of wine and the ashes from charred crossbow strings, and that these strings be wrapped around the abdomen to hasten delivery and to enable the placenta to exit the body.[5] Li Shih-chen (1518–1593), the second great author of Chinese *materia medica* literature, described the internal use of charred wooden combs as a remedy for abdominal swelling resulting from the consumption of lice.[6]

The practical application of homeopathic magic in the daily life of the Chou was not restricted to the problems of individual suffering; belief in the macrocosmic interrelatedness of all things also permitted measures designed to preserve and influence collective existence. An example of this was the rain ceremony performed during periods of drought. Shamans had to carry out an exhausting dance within a ring of fire until, sweating profusely, the falling drops of perspiration produced the desired rain.[7]

3.1.2. Systematic Correspondence

During the last centuries of the Chou period, homeopathic magic already experienced a significant conceptual development in China. It was recognized that not just one, two, or a limited number of elements form a line of correspondence, but that most, if not all, natural occurrences and abstract concepts can be incorporated into a single system of correspondence. The basis for this step was provided by the doctrines of yinyang and the Five Phases, both of which can be considered logical and systematic extensions of homeopathic magic.

The emergence, and rise to conceptual dominance in Chinese natural philosophy, of the ideology of systematic correspondence marks one of the most decisive periods of Chinese intellectual history. Although the paradigm of cause-and-effect relationships between noncorresponding phenomena was well represented in China too as a basis for an explanation of the onset of events, or of change, the holistic and inductive type of thinking associated with the notion of systematic correspondence of all phenomena certainly played the major role as far as Chinese medicotheoretical literature is concerned.

The origins of this innovative development, beginning with the late Chou, are not sufficiently documented in ancient Chinese sources to allow for any definitive identification. The possibility of a foreign stimulus cannot be excluded. It is commonly accepted that the rise of philosophy in the Ionian sphere, that is, the step from *mythos* to *logos,* dates back to influences originating from some other cultural center, farther to the east. Ionian Greek philosophers took up what they learned from outside, developed it further, and gave to it its characteristic Greek appearance. They were not ashamed of having assimilated outside thoughts; on the contrary, they were proud to have refined what was brought to them in a rudimentary state.[8] About two centuries later, a similar development occurred in China, and the doctrines conceptualized by Chinese philosophers were as innovative in Chinese intellectual history as the ideas of Anaximander, Empedocles, and Democritos had been in Greece. A philosophical impulse may have spread from one unknown source somewhere between Greece and China, carried by its revolutionary strength, never, though, to fill a previously existing void in its original form but always to be modeled and to be adapted to local conditions, corresponding to the specific intellectual milieus it met. Thus, it would be too simplistic to search for a Chinese Empedocles or for a Chinese Democritos. The travel of ideas is different from the travel of merchandise. The latter can be handed on, from one region to the next, by different means of transportation, without itself undergoing any change. Ideas must be transmitted by the head, and, of necessity, will undergo change. Where could a foreign idea be accepted, assimilated, or transmitted without being influenced by the particular situation it meets, by the changing languages that serve as its means of transportation, and by the preconditioned patterns of thought cherished by the final receiver?

The distinct feature of emerging Greek and Chinese philosophy in the second half of the last millennium B.C. is the attempt to explain the phenomena of the perceptible world as natural occurrences, without referring to mysterious forces such as gods or ancestors. The world is now understood by some intellectuals in its own right, and together with a probing into its structure, the central problem of coming-into-being and passing-away is approached conceptually.

3.1.2.1. The Yinyang Doctrine and the Issue of Syncretism

In approximately the fourth century B.C., one Chinese philosophical school appears to have based its understanding of the relationships between all phenomena on the empirical evidence that indicated that much in the surrounding world is dualistic or complementary in nature. The result was a dualistic line of association which encompassed numerous natural phenomena and abstract constellations, viewed as manifestations of two opposed yet complementary categories that spanned all existence. The cyclical patterns evident in the movement of the tides, and in the alternation of day and night, may have led these thinkers to a world view marked by a characteristic dynamic underlying apparent stability and continuity. Natural events were explained by a model of the ceaseless rise and fall of opposite yet complementary forces.

These opposing forces were designated by the symbols yin and yang, which had originally meant only "shady side of a hill" (yin) and "sunny side of a hill" (yang). The *Shih-ching*, a collection of ancient folk songs from the first millennium B.C., contains what are possibly the first beginnings of the yinyang lines of association. Yin is associated here

with "cold," "cloudy," "rain," "femininity," "inside," and "darkness," while yang symbolizes a line of correspondence associated with
"sunshine," "heat," "spring," "summer," and "masculinity."[9] In the
yinyang doctrine, the terms *yin* and *yang* no longer retain any specific
meaning themselves; they function merely as categorizing symbols
used to characterize the two lines of correspondence.

One indication of the close relationship of the yinyang doctrine to
homeopathic magic is the concept, common to both, of the correspondences among phenomena encompassed by the lines of correspondence. Just as the drops of sweat from the shaman compelled a
corresponding drop of rain from the heavens, so too the condition or
change of condition of one element in the yin (or yang) line of correspondence had to affect other members of the same line. Since these
lines also had macrocosmic implications, the association of natural
laws and moral-normative concepts was inevitable (and possibly intended). In the words of Marcel Granet:

> The most important concern of the state, upon which hinges the pres-
> ervation of natural and social order, is the marriage of the prince. If
> the union of the king and queen is not complete, the order of the universe
> is disrupted. If one partner oversteps his rights, eclipses of the sun and
> moon occur. "The son of the heavens controls the movement of the
> masculine principle [yang], his wife controls the movement of the fem-
> inine principle [yin]."[10]

The quotation cited here is taken from the *Li-chi,* the Confucian
"Book of Rites" dating from the Chou period. Rarely is the continuity
and, simultaneously, the transition of the old magical notions to the
expanded yinyang doctrine and even to the moral conceptions of the
Confucians, which we will later encounter in the form of *te* (power
of virtue), so clearly delineated as in this brief passage.

Probably the oldest textual document of a comprehensive application of the yinyang doctrine to medicine is the *Huang-ti nei-ching.*
This is a heterogeneous collection of eighty-one treatises (some are no
longer extant) whose earliest portions pertaining to the concepts of
systematic correspondence may date from the second century B.C.
Their contents provide clear evidence that various subschools had
emerged already by that time, arguing on the basis of differing interpretations of the yinyang paradigm. We recognize one school which
offered a fourfold subcategorization by subdividing the two categories
yin and yang into yin and yang subcategories, allowing for a more
subtle differentiation between concrete or abstract phenomena. Thus,

the yin category was regarded as containing a yin-in-yin (i.e., mature yin) phase and a yang-in-yin phase, while the yang category contained a yang-in-yang (i.e., mature yang) phase and a yin-in-yang phase. This fourfold subcategorization was applied, for instance, to the course of the annual seasons. Summer represents the pure yang phase; in autumn the yin phase of winter begins to emerge within the remaining yang phase of summer, and so on. Of course, many other applications for this theory were conceptualized, and I will discuss one of them, a pharmacological application, in more detail later on (see section 7.2.3.1).

A second school appears to have favored a sixfold subcategorization of the yinyang paradigm, propagating three subcategories for yin and yang each. These include a great-yang (*t'ai-yang*) phase, a minor-yang (*shao-yang*) phase, and a yang-brilliance (*yang-ming*) phase as subcategories of yang, and a great-yin (*t'ai-yin*) phase, a minor-yin (*shao-yin*) phase, as well as a ceasing-yin (*ch'üeh-yin*) phase as subcategories of yin. A few instances of the application of this sixfold subcategorization to therapeutic and physiological issues will be provided below (see section 7.2.3.2).

While contradicting each other, both of these schools appear to have agreed in their rejection of a second major paradigm of systematic correspondence, that is, the Five Phases doctrine which shall be outlined in the following paragraph. However, I may point out here already one of the characteristic traits of the history of ideas in Chinese medicine. Whenever antagonistic subparadigms emerged within one of the major paradigms, the resulting contradictions appear to have been solved only rarely, if ever, in a manner familiar to the historian of medicine and science in the West. Although we may witness, in the literature, sufficient traces of heated argumentations between the schools propagating opposing views, after a while the issue was resolved neither in a dialectical sense in that a more advanced synthesis was created out of thesis and antithesis nor in a (Kuhnian) revolutionary sense in that a more recent paradigm achieved prevalence and dominated a subsequent era of "normal science" until it was replaced by the next revolutionary paradigm. The unique feature of the Chinese situation—and this should receive more attention from historians and philosophers of science—is the continuous tendency toward a syncretism of all ideas that exist (within accepted limits). Somehow a way was always found in China to reconcile opposing views and to build bridges—fragile as they may appear to the outside observer—permitting thinkers and practitioners to employ liberally all the concepts available, as long as they were not regarded as destructive to society. The oldest and at the same time most intriguing example of this attitude—repeated again and again in subsequent centuries up to the present time—is the history of the yinyang and Five Phases schools as it is documented in the *Huang-ti nei-ching*. The *Huang-ti nei-ching* should not be approached as a classic from which one may distill a homogeneous system of ideas based on stringent concepts and terminology. Rather it should be understood as a collection of the teachings of numerous schools of various times, ranging from eras predating systematic correspondence (see the discussion of wind etiology below) to various interpretations of the yinyang and Five Phases doctrines and, finally, to attempts to link all these within one all-encompassing conceptual structure. This all-encompassing structure is a fascinating edifice in that it demonstrates the desire and ability to link structural elements that would not seem to fit at first glance. The problem of how to overcome the incongruity between the even numbers of the various yinyang categorizations and the odd number of the Five Phases doctrine, for example, was resolved either in that one of the Five Phases was recognized as being central or neutral, allowing for a yinyang categorization of the remaining four, or in that a sixth phase was conceptualized, allowing for three yin and three yang phases. It must be emphasized, however, that pure yinyang and Five Phases doctrines continued to exist side by side and that such syncretistic constructs, and various others, were applied only when necessary for a specific argument; they remained possible but not stringent facets of a complex and heterogeneous theoretical system. One of the basic difficulties in interpreting traditional Chinese medical terms and concepts today in a Western language results directly from this syncretistic trait of Chinese medical history. Identical terms were often employed to denote very different concepts, and at no time was a standardization attempted which might have led to a dominating or stringent interpretation of even the core concepts by a majority of dogmatists and practitioners.

3.1.2.2. The Doctrine of the Five Phases

Tsou Yen (ca. 350–270) is generally considered by Chinese historians as the creator of the second natural philosophy that influenced the system of correspondences and, consequently, the medicine of systematic correspondence. Tsou Yen, or whoever was the real initiator of this doctrine, had selected, for reasons unknown, the number five as the basis of his theory of association; his school arranged concrete natural phenomena and abstract concepts not into two, but into five lines of correspondence. Tsou did not use abstract terms as central symbols, but rather chose five tangible natural phenomena: metal, wood, water, fire, and soil. They constitute an easily understandable foundation for the five lines of correspondence, conveying at the same time a number of mutual relationships among various lines. The best known of the total of sixteen are the relationships of mutual destruction and of mutual generation. They can be expressed symbolically in the following manner:

> Water overcomes fire; fire melts metal; metal—in the form of a knife, for instance—overcomes wood; wood—as in a spade—overcomes soil; soil—as in a dike—subdues water.
>
> Water/watering produces plants and trees, that is, wood; wood brings forth fire; fire produces ashes, that is, soil; soil brings forth metal; when heated, metals produce steam, that is, water.[11]

The categorization of numerous natural phenomena and abstract concepts in five separate lines of correspondence was designated with the term *wu-hsing,* translated here as "Five Phases" to reflect the dynamic notion inherent in the Chinese term *hsing* (literally "to proceed"). Although the translation of wu-hsing as "Five Elements" ought to be avoided in general, it should be pointed out that ancient Chinese sources do indeed refer to water, fire, metal, wood, and soil as substantial necessities of the human environment, adding grain as a sixth "element." Thus, the *Tso-chuan* stated:

> Heaven created the Five Materials (*wu-ts'ai*); the people use them all. To eliminate but one would not be possible.[12]

And elsewhere:

> The Six Treasuries and the Three Businesses, they are called the Nine Achievements. Water, fire, metal, wood, soil, and grain are called the Six Treasuries (*liu-fu*); rectification of the people's virtue, the conveniences of life, and the securing of abundant means of sustentation, these are called the three businesses.[13]

The *Shu-ching* stated:

> Virtue is seen in the goodness of the government, and the government is tested by its nourishing of the people. There are water, fire, metal,

wood, soil, and grain: these must be duly regulated; there are the rectification of the people's virtue, the conveniences of life, and the securing of abundant means of sustentation, these must be harmoniously attended to.[14]

Later, in the *Shih-chi,* compiled about 100 B.C., the term *wu-te* is also used in connection with the activities of Tsou Yen.[15] This implies a relationship between the doctrine of the Five Phases and homeopathic magic, since *te* signifies the magical force exerted, for example, by a properly performed ritual on the appearance of a desired natural event or, in Confucian terms, by morally faultless behavior on the harmony of society and of the universe.

Various schools shared a belief that the number five underlies natural phenomena, and it was inevitable that differences of opinion would arise concerning the assignment of occurrences to specific categories. Like the yinyang duality, the Five Phases encompassed certain elements whose association with one of the five possible categories was beyond all doubt. For the rest, this system was based on purely subjective perceptions, and the lack of objective criteria led to significant discrepancies in the classification of phenomena to individual lines of correspondence adopted by different schools. Thus it is not surprising that already during the Han period, a few thinkers seized upon the contradictions and inconsistencies of these theories, as well as on the arbitrariness of arrangements, to reject, in a sometimes sarcastic tone, the entire system. The well-known critique by the empiricist Wang Ch'ung (first century A.D.) provides a good example:

The sign *yin* corresponds to wood, and its proper animal is the tiger. *Hsü* corresponds to soil, and its animal is the dog. *Ch'ou* and *wei* likewise correspond to soil, *ch'ou* having as animal the ox, and *wei* having the sheep. Now wood conquers soil, therefore the tiger overcomes the dog, ox and sheep. Again, *hai* goes with water, its animal being the boar. *Ssu* goes with fire, having the serpent as its animal. *Tzu* also signifies water, its animal being the rat. *Wu,* conversely, goes with fire, and its animal manifestation is the horse. Now water conquers fire, therefore the boar devours the serpent, and horses, if they eat rats [are injured by] a swelling of their bellies. [So run the usual arguments.]

However, when we go into the matter more thoroughly, we find that in fact it very often happens that animals do not overpower one another as they ought to do on these theories. The horse is connected with *wu* (fire), the rat with *tzu* (water). If water really conquers fire, [it would be much more convincing if] rats normally attacked horses and drove them away. Then the cock is connected with *ya* (metal), and the hare with *mao* (wood). If metal really conquers wood, why do cocks not devour hares? Or again, *hai* stands for the boar [and water], *wei* for the sheep [and soil], and *ch'ou* for the ox [also earth]. If soil really conquers water, why do oxen and sheep not run after boars and kill them? Furthermore, *ssu* corresponds with the serpent and fire, *shen* with the monkey and metal. If fire really conquers metal, why do serpents not eat monkeys? [On the other hand] monkeys are certainly afraid of rats, and are liable to be bitten by dogs, [yet this is equivalent to] water and soil conquering metal [—which is not in accordance with theory].[16]

But the voices raised in protest remained ignored. By the time of Wang Ch'ung, the theories of the Five Phases had already become a part of Confucian philosophy, which in the meantime had been elevated to political and social orthodoxy. Official recognition of such a critique was impossible as long as Confucianism retained its powerful cultural authority.

Let us now turn to a brief overview of Confucianism itself, the social doctrine whose dominant influence for most of two thousand years made the medicine of systematic correspondence the official and orthodox system of healing, a situation that continued into the twentieth century.

3.2. ASPECTS OF CONFUCIAN POLITICAL AND SOCIAL DOCTRINE

The life of Confucius (551–479 B.C.) coincided with the formation of numerous philosophical schools, which, confronted with the prevailing social chaos, advanced widely diverging social theories. Attempts were made to convince the rulers of competing states that the application of these ideas to practical politics would reunify the empire, leading to peaceful coexistence among men. The best-known of these schools were the Legalists, whose views, as I have shown, were influential in the Ch'in state and who considered the force of law and threat of punishment to be the guiding principle of government; the Moists, who had developed a concept of universal love; the Taoists, who saw the violation of the natural course of events as the principal cause of the disintegration of society and considered the ideal rule to involve as little governmental intervention as possible; finally, the Confucians, whose ideas will be discussed in greater detail below.

Based on his own experience, Confucius concluded that the real cause underlying the obvious social unrest was the discrepancy between the expectations associated with social roles and the actual conduct of members of society, including the ruler, whose behavior was expected to be exemplary. The objective of the harmonious society envisioned by Confucius was therefore to bind individuals and groups to precisely defined social roles and to regulate permanently the relationships between these roles by means of a hierarchical, tightly-knit nexus of mutual obligations. *Cheng-ming* ("rectification of names") was the maxim used by Confucius to express the view that designations of status should in reality correspond to the conduct of those on which they were bestowed; a king must conduct himself in a manner befitting a king; otherwise he does not deserve the title and forfeits his mandate. Confucian notions of a firmly established hierarchy by no means excluded the social mobility of individuals commensurate with abilities; the roles of ruler, minister, scholar, entrepreneur, and farmer were fixed. The individual was allowed the possibility of exchanging one role for another.

In Confucian social doctrine, the social relationships among those fulfilling these roles were bound by customs and rites. As Franke and Trauzettel have emphasized, "the great achievement of Confucius [was] the transformation of traditional rites, which contained no individual elements, but which were practiced in a strictly collective manner as a communal cult, into an individualized, personalized ethic."[17] According to Confucius, the force *te,* which earlier ages had ascribed to magical influences, now emanated from morally impeccable conduct, based upon justice, human virtue, filial piety, and righteousness of the superior man. The superior man, however, was no longer determined automatically from birth, but by the acquisition of certain qualities. Confucius believed in the innate ability of man to learn and demanded that the prince, for example, should be the person who best embodied virtue.[18] Custom and ceremonial regulated the five fundamental individual relationships between ruler and subject, father and son, husband and wife, elder brother and younger brother, and between friends; but a more general code of conduct also aimed to preserve a harmonious society. A central concern of these more general principles was expressed in the dictate "follow the mean." Confucius taught that excesses in any area disrupt social order and are therefore to be avoided.

The call for a primacy of ability over birth in filling positions of leadership and other roles, a completely revolutionary concept for the period of hereditary feudalism by the nobility, in conjunction with the highly idealistic foundation of this doctrine, may have contributed to the almost universal rejection Confucius experienced from ruling parties in his native state and during his travels to various courts. Only the expansion of Confucian concepts by the philosopher Hsün-tzu in the first half of the third century B.C. produced a political and social theory whose suitability for the stabilization and preservation of a united China was acknowledged, particularly by the advisers of the Han emperor Wu (156–87 B.C.). None of the other competing political philosophies appeared prepared to create the bureaucratic apparatus required to govern the united empire, whose officials were largely independent of familial, regional, and feudal ties and solely responsible to a central authority.

The work of Hsün-tzu (fl. 238 B.C.) deserves special attention at this point, since it reveals perhaps most clearly the intellectual interconnections between the particular strain of Confucianism that later achieved state orthodoxy, on the one hand, and the concepts of the medicine of systematic correspondence, on the other. A symbolic indication of this close relationship is provided by a passage from Hsün-tzu that reappears almost verbatim in the oldest surviving work on the medicine of systematic correspondence, the *Huang-ti nei-ching*, (The Yellow Emperor's Classic of Internal Medicine), the nucleus of which may have been compiled shortly thereafter.[19] Hsün-tzu remarks:

> The true ruler begins to put [his state] in order while [a condition of] order [still prevails]; he does not wait [until] insurrections [have already erupted]. (*Chün-tzu chih chih fei chih luan yeh*)[20]

The corresponding passage in the *Huang-ti nei-ching* reads:

> The sages do not treat those who have already fallen ill, but rather those who are not yet ill. They do not put [their state] in order only when revolt [is underway], but before an insurrection occurs. (*Sheng-jen pu chih i-ping chih wei-ping pu chih i-luan chih wei-luan*)[21]

It is uncertain whether Hsün-tzu experienced the unification of the empire under Ch'in Shih Huang-ti. He lived near the end of the period of the Warring States and advocated a political philosophy based heavily on the moral tenets of Confucius, but that was also influenced by the quietism of earlier Taoists and the realism advocated by the Legalists. The eclectic nature of his remarks may help explain why two of his pupils, the already-cited philosopher Han Fei-tzu (see section 2.3) and the statesman Li Ssu, the most important adviser of Ch'in Shih Huang-ti, became known as Legalists. Hsün-tzu differed from

Mencius, his great predecessor in the elucidation and refinement of Confucianism, primarily through his belief in the innately evil nature of man. But Hsün-tzu taught that in spite of this, every man can raise himself to moral greatness by studying the classics and taking ritual guidelines seriously.[22] Like an all-encompassing connective link, adherence to ceremonial customs promised health and prosperity to the individual and the state alike:

> If a person utilizes his body and his nature, his insight, understanding, and mature consideration in the manner prescribed by custom, order and success will ensue; otherwise, the result is unpredictability and upheaval, idleness and unruliness. If the consumption of food and drink, clothing, lodging at home and outside of the home, as well as movement and rest are carried out in the manner prescribed by custom, one will achieve harmony and order; otherwise one is subject to attack and betrayal, and illnesses will occur. If a person arranges his appearance and demeanor, his coming and going, as well as his manner of movement in accordance with custom, he will achieve elegance; otherwise barbaric crudity, depravity, vulgarity, and savagery ensue. This means that man cannot live without ceremony, the concerns of daily life cannot be successfully concluded without ritual; without rites, the state cannot exist in peace.[23]

Closely allied with this emphasis on the ceremonial was Hsün-tzu's conviction that man had the ability to shape his own destiny, largely independent of external circumstances. The individual and society may be threatened by certain natural processes, but they can protect themselves by carrying out appropriate measures:

> A permanent regularity underlies the changes of the heavens. Change does not take place because the [benevolent ruler] Yao once lived, and it was not destined to end when the [evil tyrant] Ch'ieh appeared. He who approaches [the laws] of heaven in an orderly fashion shall be blessed with good fortune; he who approaches the [laws] of heaven with disorder, shall suffer misfortune. He who supports the fundamental principles [of the state] and exercises restraint in all outlays, shall not be impoverished by heaven. Heaven shall not allow those to fall ill who ensure that the vital necessities of life are present in sufficient quantities, and that the appropriate efforts are made at the correct time. He who in his life follows the *tao* without prejudice and without doubts, cannot suffer harm from heaven. Floods and droughts will bring him neither hunger nor thirst; cold and heat will not cause him to fall ill. Strange beings can send him no misfortune. But if the fundamental principles

[of the state] are neglected and outlays are marked by wastefulness, heaven will prevent prosperity. If the replenishment of provisions is insufficient for the needs, and appropriate efforts are made only rarely, heaven cannot bring forth abundance. Heaven shall not bless those who turn their backs on the *tao* and cultivate an improper life. He shall hunger before floods and droughts come; he shall fall ill before cold and heat oppress him. He shall suffer misfortune before strange beings have seized him! He shall experience the seasons [with the same regularity] as a well-ordered life, but unlike a well-ordered life, he shall be plagued by misfortune. This person should not be angry with heaven for his fate; the path he himself has chosen is the cause![24]

Although Hsün-tzu alluded in the quotation just cited to "strange beings," demons and spirits were just as foreign to such a world view, which taught individual responsibility for personal existence within the context of impersonal natural laws, as were those who believed that such beings had the ability to influence human destiny or the course of nature. Even Confucius had been extremely reticent in comments concerning the afterlife. Hsün-tzu was much more straightforward in his agreement with those contemporary philosophers who maintained doubts about the existence of any gods, spirits, or demons; his rejection of such notions and related rituals was unambiguous:

One prays for rain and it rains. What is the connection between the two events? I say: none at all! If the sun or moon are consumed [i.e., during an eclipse], [someone beats the drums to] rescue them; if a drought comes, one prays for rain; if an important decision is to be made, the soothsayers and shamans are consulted first. But no one has ever achieved any success through such activities! Everything is purely ornamental. The true ruler recognizes it as decoration; the folk believe in the involvement of spirits.[25]

Confucianism was thus oriented completely around the organization of earthly social life. In place of divine or other transcendental laws, Confucian political doctrine incorporated the theories of yin-yang, and especially the Five Phases, to explain social and political changes. Orthodox historical thought accounted for the rise and decline of individual dynasties by means of the flow and ebb of individual phases, which were in part determined by human conduct, in the pentacycle.

A fragmentary work by Tsou Yen, the purported founder of the doctrine of the Five Phases, contains what is probably the oldest link between these natural-law views and the historical succession of various ruling houses:

> When some new dynasty is going to arise, Heaven exhibits auspicious signs to the people. During the rise of Huang Ti (the Yellow Emperor) large earth-worms and large ants appeared. He said, "This indicates that the element Soil is in the ascendant, so our color must be yellow, and our affairs must be placed under the sign of Soil." During the rise of Yü the Great, Heaven produced plants and trees which did not wither in autumn and winter. He said, "This indicates that the element Wood is in the ascendant, so our color must be green, and our affairs must be placed under the sign of Wood." During the rise of Thang the Victorious a metal sword appeared out of the water. He said, "This indicates that the element Metal is in the ascendant, so our color must be white, and our affairs must be placed under the sign of Metal." During the rise of King Wen of the Chou, Heaven exhibited fire, and many red birds holding documents written in red flocked to the altar of the dynasty. He said, "This indicates that the element Fire is in the ascendant, so our color must be red, and our affairs must be placed under the sign of Fire. Following Fire, there will come Water. Heaven will show when the time comes for the influences of Water to dominate. Then the color will have to be black, and affairs will have to be placed under the sign of Water. And that dispensation will in turn come to an end, and at the appointed time, all will return once again to Soil. But when that time will be we do not know."[26]

Because of the magical tradition underlying their ethical outlook, the adoption of such a theory of history by the Confucians by no means signaled the adoption of a fatalistic world view. The force arising from the moral conduct of the ruler could bring about an earlier or later termination of the heavenly mandate, and thus an earlier or later transition to the next phase in the dynastic succession. This aspect of the theories of the Five Phases achieved its characteristic, lasting form in the first century A.D. Each action, it was understood, that diverged from a moral norm led to aberrations in the cosmic order. The conduct of the emperor, for instance, could stimulate the growth of trees, the formation of storms, and irregularities in the course of planets. The same was true for the conduct of lower officials and citizens. Each of the official dynastic histories of Confucian China includes extensive chapters enumerating exceptional events and unusual occurrences of the past and analyzing their significance for the growth and decay of the dynasty in question.

The sociopolitical linking of the natural philosophy of the Five Phases with the ethical norms of Confucianism is obvious; the medicine of systematic correspondence paralleled this development.

3.3. FUNDAMENTAL PRINCIPLES OF THE MEDICINE OF SYSTEMATIC CORRESPONDENCE

3.3.1. The Concepts of Wind and Ch'i

During the course of the last three centuries B.C., unknown authors began to develop a system of healing whose theoretical principles corresponded closely to the social-political order advocated during the same period by Confucian political ideology. As a consequence, this system of healing—in its rise to medical orthodoxy, in its tradition down to the present, and, ultimately, in its displacement by Western medicine in the past decades—was continuously dependent on the interests and fate of Confucianism itself. With the elevation of Confucianism to orthodox political doctrine by the Emperor Wu, the Han period theoretical foundations of this ideology remained fixed for a long span of time.

The system of healing whose theoretical principles transferred the sociopolitical conceptions of Confucianism to the medical sphere rested on a syncretic doctrine that was influenced, as already indicated, by concepts of demonic medicine, the theories of yinyang and the Five Phases, homeopathic magic, concepts of finest matter influences as the basis of life, as well as by structural elements associated with the unification of the empire.

Demonic medicine and the political reality of the feudal period reappear in both terminology and concepts of the medicine of systematic correspondence. The body may be "hit" (*chung*) by outside agencies; it therefore possesses "guards" (*wei*) and "army camps" (*ying*)[27] to deal with intruders. But attacks from external enemies are not the only source of crisis; the internal components of the body may fight one another as well. Thus, although the individual functional units of the organism are seen as mutually depending upon one another, as soon as one of them displays signs of weakness, those who are in a position to do so will "subdue" (*k'e*) their neighbors or "seize" (*ch'eng*) their territory. The forces disposed of by the individual units are regarded as "proper" (*cheng*) as long as they do not overstep their boundaries; they are termed "evil" (*hsieh*) as soon as they invade territories other than their own.

A casual reading of the texts of the medicine of systematic correspondence reveals that here, too, diseases occasionally are caused by the "malevolent" (*o*) but it is, in particular, the term *hsieh* ("evil," "harmful") that is used for all pathogenic agents. However, the meaning of the old terms has been transformed. Evil itself is no longer embodied by demons, but rather by abstract as well as empirically visible influences and emanations. The new designation representing these influences and emanations in the medicine of systematic correspondences is *ch'i*. Consequently, in the medicine of systematic correspondences, the agents of illness are not represented by the character combination *hsieh-kuei* ("evil demons"), but rather by the combination *hsieh-ch'i* ("evil influences," "evil emanation"). If demonic medicine was based on the view that man is constantly subject to the action of demons, the medicine of systematic correspondences assumes that man must live in harmony with the influences and emanations of all conceivable natural phenomena. The conceptual transformation of the belief in the illness-causing activities of demons parallels the skepticism with which Confucians viewed the existence of such beings.

It appears, however, that the concept of ch'i did not replace the concept of demons directly, but only after some mediating idea had paved the way. I suggest that changes in the old Chinese belief in the illness-causing potential of wind (see above p. 25) mark a transition, during the final two or three centuries B.C., from demonological concepts to an idea of influences and emanations originating from the natural environment of substances. It appears worthwhile to follow these changes in detail.

By the close of the third century B.C., techniques of divination were developed in China that did not—as had been the case during the Shang and later during the Chou dynasty as well—revolve around the interpretation of an abstract milfoil oracle or the consultation of ancestors (utilizing tortoise carapaces or cattle bones). Rather, they were based upon the observation of natural phenomena, primarily wind and rain.[28] Evidence from the second century B.C. indicates that wind was perceived as a demon,[29] but it appears that, possibly at the end of the third or beginning of the second century B.C., an alternative concept arose. In this view, wind was exclusively a natural phenomenon but was nonetheless perceived as a portent of future events that was activated as a response of the heavens to the travels of T'ai-i, the head of the demon-spirit hierarchy. T'ai-i is mentioned in the essay "Chiu-kung pa-feng" of the *Huang-ti nei-ching t'ai-su* (called *T'ai-su* hereafter; see appendix 1.2); the earliest historical source for T'ai-i as the "supreme celestial spirit" is the biography of Emperor Wu-ti (reigned 140–86 B.C.) in the *Shih-chi,* compiled around 100 B.C.

As the basis for their forecasts, the T'ai-i soothsayers utilized a belief in the eight palaces in the eight principal directions of the compass, which T'ai-i would occupy in a certain order on the so-called *pa-cheng* dates, namely, the first day of spring, summer, autumn, and winter, the autumn and spring equinoxes, as well as the winter and summer solstices. If the wind on these days came from the direction in which T'ai-i happened to be residing, it was the so-called wind of repletion and was considered an auspicious omen. If the wind blew from the opposite direction, however, it was regarded as an unfavorable sign. Textual evidence suggests that the development of these concepts was undoubtedly influenced by agricultural experience with wind during seasons that were critical for the future harvest. Such experiences find their expression in predictions about higher or lower grain prices during the coming year in another essay of the *T'ai-su,* that is, the "Pa-cheng feng-hou" (see appendix 1.1). They may be related to a recognition that winds from specific directions during certain times of the year are responsible for a subsequent abundant or insufficient harvest, and that wind is thus responsible for situations of repletion or depletion, of sufficient food or hunger, and of well-being or illness. The texts reveal that such concrete experiences served as the basis for more abstract conclusions. The wind-soothsayers were able not only to forecast the future of individual social strata and the outcome of military ventures but also to predict which emotions would dominate during subsequent seasons.

Of the writings in Book 28 of the *T'ai-su,* the treatise "Pa-cheng feng-hou" is apparently the oldest, reflecting the origins of the medical application of the T'ai-i wind-oracle. On the basis of, at first, only the winter solstice and the first day of spring, the significance of the wind direction for the future welfare of the populace is indicated. In addition, the treatise mentions the wind-oracle on the first day of the year as well as on a specific day of each month. Of significance is the notion of the inevitability, of the external determination of illness, as soon as someone is struck by a depletion-wind. The apparent inability of man to escape the assaults of depletion-wind is reminiscent of the fundamental concepts of demonology, even going beyond the latter with this feeling of being completely at the wind's mercy. Against demons it was at least possible to do battle, but how is it possible to escape wind?

Chinese thinkers of the time appear to have concerned themselves with this question, and they were obviously aware of the fact that there are serious as well as minor illnesses, that some people remain healthy although many others have to suffer, and that some people fall ill apparently without coming into contact with the wind. The corresponding discussions and discoveries are indicated in a further *T'ai-su* essay, that is, the "San-hsü san-shih" (see appendix 1.3). Conceptual innovations included here suggest, first, that it was possible to avoid the wind—although how this can be done was not elucidated in detail—and, second, that the severity of illness depended on various combinations of repletion and depletion both in man's environment and in his organism itself. Thus, the treatise "San-hsü san-shih" contains the first hints that it is the physiological condition of the organism that creates the predisposition for possible injury by wind. Accordingly, the susceptibility of the organism to injury is dependent upon three different factors. These are, first, the so-called decline of years. Yang Shang-shan (seventh century) explained this statement in his commentary to the *T'ai-su*. In this view, human life, following the seventh year of life, passes through additional phases of nine years each. The transitional points from phase to phase, namely the sixteenth, twenty-fifth, thirty-fourth, forty-third, and so on, years, are considered critical years in which one is particularly susceptible to illness. These years were apparently viewed as "low points,"[30] hence the designation "decline of years." Whether Yang Shang-shan's commentary conveys the intended meaning of the authors of the *T'ai-su* treatise cannot be determined conclusively. The supposition that it invokes some kind of concept of critical years of life may, however, correspond to the substance of the passage.

The second factor that brings about repletion or depletion in the organism is the dependence of the physiological rhythm on the rhythm of the changing phases of the moon. The full moon produces a repletion with strength within the body, while a new or waning moon signifies a period of weakness, of susceptibility to injury.

The third factor, finally, is the first and only one that appears to concede to the individual some influence over the condition of his health. "When a person loses harmony with the season" (see appendix 1.3), this produces a depletion. The text says nothing more on this subject, and it can only be surmised that what is meant is perhaps the adaptation to the demands of the climate of individual seasons or a certain life-style during the critical years of life.

If all three factors are negative, that is, if a person in the "decline of years" loses "harmony with the seasons" during the new moon, the result is a threefold depletion and the greatest vulnerability to the depletion-wind. Between the critical years, during the full moon, and at a period of harmony with the season, man is afforded his greatest protection against the wind.

The etiology of wind, on the basis of the discussion so far, had no connection to the theoretical foundation of systematic correspondence; neither the concept of yinyang nor the doctrine of the Five

Phases was adopted into the discussion up to this point. The first half of the essay "Shou yu kang jou" (Long Life, Early Death, Firmness, and Softness) of the *Huang-ti nei-ching ling-shu* (see appendix 1.4 and 1.5) changed this. In this treatise the organism and its illnesses have already been completely integrated into the yinyang categories. For the first time the wind appears as an illness restricted to the yang-region of the body and a new term for a corresponding injury to the yin-region was introduced, namely, *pi*. If yin- and yang-regions are both affected by symptoms that can be traced to the influence of wind, cold, and dampness, the result is a *feng-pi* illness.

Wind etiology was subsequently liberated from all vestiges of its demonological underpinnings and integrated into the purely nature-based system of correspondences. In the *T'ai-su* essay "T'ien-chi" (Natural Phenomena That Must Be Avoided; see appendix 1.6), the dependence of the physiological rhythm on the phases of the moon is demonstrated even more clearly than before, and the essay "Chu-feng tsa-lun" (see appendix 1.7) attempts to eliminate doubts that wind in fact represents the primary source of illness and rejects the view that demons might be a factor in one or another mysterious case.

The essays "Chu-feng shu-lei" and "Chu-feng chuang-lun," also of the *T'ai-su,* document the continuing integration of wind concepts into systematic correspondence; the former points to the yinyang doctrine, the latter alludes to the Five Phases (see appendix 1.8 and 1.9). In addition, the term "wind" now appears with increasing frequency as a designation of various illnesses themselves that are caused by wind. Depending on how the injury had occurred or how it manifested itself, it was possible—to cite only a few examples—to distinguish among stomach-wind, brain-wind, or liver-wind, as well as discharge-wind.

As a spirit or demon, the wind resided, according to various indications in Han and pre-Han literature, in caves, tunnels, or valleys. Chapter 6 of the *Huai-nan tzu* contains an explicit reference to *feng-hsüeh* ("wind caves"). The term *hsüeh* ("caves," "holes") is used in acupuncture literature to designate those holes in the skin through which the so-called *ch'i* is able to penetrate into the body (as well as flow out) and at which it was deemed necessary to apply needles in order to influence the inner ch'i. This represents yet another significant step that marked the entire subsequent history of medical therapy of systematic correspondence.

Here, too, one is restricted to conjecture, but the most likely interpretation from the perspective of available sources permits the conclusion that, in addition to the concept of wind as a pathogenic agent, a more general and comprehensive concept was introduced, namely, of environmental influences that affect the organism from outside but are present within the organism as well. These environmental influences were designated with the term *ch'i,* the etymology of which is of some interest. The character ch'i consists of two distinct segments; a pictogram indicating "rising vapor" is placed above the pictogram of "rice" or "millet." Hence, the entire character should be read as "vapors rising from rice (or millet; i.e., from food)." The more general reading of "vapors rising from food" is supported by an alternative version of the character, cited by the etymological dictionary *Shuo-wen* of around A.D. 100, which combines the two segments mentioned above with a third indicating "food" (i.e., radical 184). In this context it should not be overlooked that during the fourth century B.C., Greek Hippocratic medicine developed (or accepted from elsewhere) the concept of φῦσαι ἔκ τῶν περιττωμάτῶν as its central pathogenic idea. Surprisingly enough, this phrase has exactly the same meaning as the ch'i pictogram, that is, "vapors rising from food."[31] This simultaneous appearance of an identical concept in both China and Greece is probably coincidental but, nevertheless, noteworthy. At any rate, in China the pictogram ch'i, possibly created to correspond to an etiological concept, was used in the literature of the third and second centuries, in a broader context; its meaning included related ideas and phenomena such as "that which fills the body," "that which means life," "breath," and "vapors" in general, such as clouds in the sky, or even "wind." As early as the late Chou or beginning Han period, substance or tangible matter was believed by at least one author to consist of dispersible finest vapors, designated with the term *ch'i.* Ch'i was considered to float through the air and, together with blood, through the organism. Hence, I translate it with "finest matter influence" or simply "influence," with a substance or matter connotation in mind. This may not yet be an ideal rendering, but the choice of this term and the argumentation on which it is based should demonstrate that the customary translation of ch'i by some Western (and Asian) authors as "energy" represents a basic misconception that is not supported by Chinese ancient sources.

With the development of the idea that environmental influences in general had an illness-causing potential, the central significance of wind in the origin of disease was relativized. From then on, the wind represented only one of many environmental influences, although for many authors and for many centuries to come, it was the most important. As a consequence, the concept of depletion and repletion also required a new definition. When questioned by Huang-ti about this subject, Ch'i Po replied: "When evil influences are present in great number, this is repletion. When the [proper] influences [of the organism] are lost, this is depletion."

This statement can be regarded as the conclusion of a development in which notions of wind can be assigned the role of a transitional or intermediate concept. To be sure, wind etiology was unable to eliminate demon etiology, and influence etiology was unable to eliminate wind etiology; all three interpretive models continued to exist concurrently.

In conclusion, I return to the question of whether it is possible for the individual to avoid illness. The notion of external pathogenic agents, which characterizes demonology, appears at first to be the distinguishing attribute of wind etiology as well. The recognition that an accommodation to the demands of the season reduces the probability of illness signaled a change to an at least partial acceptance of the self-responsibility for illness. Finally, the medicine of influences, which made the well-being of the organism dependent upon the proper balance of the body's own influences and those absorbed from outside of the body, arrived at the view that the individual was solely responsible for his well-being. The commensurate conduct of one's life that brought about the harmony of all influences, guaranteed health. Since not only foods, drinks, the effects of climate, or similar concrete phenomena but also music, emotions, and morals affected the balance of influences, it became imperative to avoid extravagance in every sphere of life. Unlike the proponents of demonic medicine, the followers of a medicine of influences grounded in systematic correspondence were convinced that it was worthwhile to subject oneself to rules of conduct in order to remain in good health. This was the basis for the reintroduction of morality into the understanding of well-being and illness. Climatic influences emanating from the points of the compass, from the stars, from food and drink, from heaven and earth, from rain and wind, from heat and cold, and from numerous other phenomena were no longer inherently evil. Survival in this field of influences was possible if man adapted himself—by means of a lifestyle based on well-defined norms—to the system of influences and emanations and did not contravene it.

3.3.2. Structure and Function of the Organism

In the early 1970s, the excavation of three ancient graves near Ch'ang-sha, the capital of the province of Hunan, yielded a wide range of artifacts, obviously arranged as a rather complete set of household items that should accompany the buried persons in their afterlife. Among these finds were fourteen manuscript texts with medical contents; they provide us, as the oldest immediate sources of ancient Chinese medicine extant today, with valuable data on the knowledge that had developed in China at the close of the third century B.C.[32]

The texts discovered at the so-called Ma-wang-tui site reflect not only the magical and demonological concepts and practices dominating Chinese health care during Chou times (and, as far as the lower social strata were concerned, for a long time to come), but also a variety of concepts and practices related to the nascent medicine of influences. These include the beginnings of the medicine of systematic correspondence as well as early evidence for the cultivation of breath, grain avoidance techniques, and physical exercises to support the flow of the influences through the organism. The latter three facets came to be associated later with Taoism and will be discussed there. The idea of a vital importance of external (and internal) influences to human life appears to have developed alongside a new understanding of the structure and functions of the organism where these influences displayed their effects. In this context, two of the Ma-wang-tui texts deserve our special interest; these are the *Tsu pi shih-i mo-chiu ching* and *Yin yang shih-i mo-chiu ching*. As the titles (formulated by a research team organized to analyze the Ma-wang-tui manuscripts) suggest, both these texts refer to a total of eleven vessels[33] permeating the body.[34] These vessels are depicted as separate entities; some of them are categorized as yang, others as yin. They occupy specific locations in the body, although the two manuscripts are somewhat at variance here. Both texts, though, name six vessels originating from the feet and extending upward, in some instances to the head, and five vessels originating from the hands and extending into the chest or to the head. Nothing is said in these two Ma-wang-tui texts on the nature of the contents of these vessels, and it is only on the basis of other Ma-wang-tui scripts—notably the *Mo-fa*[35]—that one may conclude that these vessels were filled with the kind of vapor called ch'i. Each of the eleven vessels is associated with a list of specific symptoms or illnesses, and it is, again, only the *Mo-fa* ("Vessel [treatment] techniques") which suggests that these symptoms or illnesses represent a deficiency or surplus of the contents of these vessels.

This information may be compared with corresponding data offered by the *Huang-ti nei-ching* texts, that is, the earliest medicotheoretical texts handed down to our own times through the centuries. The ideas of the *Huang-ti nei-ching* texts concerning structure and function of the organism are markedly different from those of the Ma-wang-tui scripts. If we assume that a historical development led from the latter to the former, and if we take into regard the information on the ideas of the physician Shun-yü I of the second century B.C. as recorded by the historian Ssu-ma Ch'ien in the *Shih-chi* (compiled around 100 B.C.), it appears as if the ideas concerning structure and function of the vessels in the organism as laid down in the *Huang-ti nei-ching* texts were conceived during the late second or early first century B.C. In contrast to the Ma-wang-tui texts which, to repeat, suggest but the possibility of depletion or repletion in eleven isolated vessels, Ssu-ma Ch'ien quotes the physician Shun-yü I as believing in a movement that may occur within each single vessel, a movement that may cause deficiency or surplus of contents in perhaps the upper or lower section of any given vessel. It is only the *Huang-ti nei-ching* that informs us of a third stage in this succession of ideas in that it consistently refers to twelve vessels—now called "conduits" (*ching*) or "conduit vessels" (*ching-mo*)—which are linked to each other and which are passed by a continuous circulatory flow of specific substances. The *locus classicus* has the following wording:

> The Emperor asked: "I should like to hear which influence (*ch'i*) causes man's depots [i.e., organs, see below] to suffer from sudden pain." Ch'i Po replied: "The flow in the conduit vessels never stops; [it moves] in an annular circuit without a break. When influences of cold enter the conduits, [this flow] is retarded. [The contents of the conduits] congeal and do not move. If [the influences of cold] settle outside of the vessels, there will be only a little blood [moving; if they] settle within the vessels, the *ch'i*-influences cannot proceed. As a result there is sudden pain."[36]

Obviously this is a straightforward concept of circulation in the organism. This concept, however, differs from contemporary Western ideas in various respects. It is not clear exactly what kinds of substances were thought to circulate and where exactly they were thought to flow. It may be, as Epler has pointed out, that an earlier concept of blood-filled vessels was supplemented by a concept of vessels filled with ch'i-influences—at some time between the late third and early first century B.C.[37] Perhaps two different schools developed, one advocating the circulation of subtle influences in the vessels, while the other one preferred a belief in the flow of blood. A third, syncretistic school may have suggested the simultaneous circulation of both ch'i and blood in identical vessels, while yet another school may have believed in two simultaneous systems of circulation, in separate vessels. The *Huang-*

ti nei-ching texts contain passages that may be interpreted as traces of all four of these differing perspectives. As is characteristic of the history of ideas in Chinese medicine, the resulting contradictions appear never to have been discussed to a point where one homogeneous system of ideas and terminology concerning circulation might have emerged. Rather, as in so many other instances, the *Nei-ching* presented different concepts and terms, partly overlapping, partly antagonistic, which came to be transmitted as such through the centuries down to our own times. We may say, though, that according to one belief, so-called constructive influences (*ying-ch'i*) circulated through the vessels while so-called protective influences (*wei-ch'i*) circulated outside of the vessels. Some authors appear to have assumed that the "constructive influences"—generated by stomach and spleen—served the functions of generating the blood and of nourishing the entire body, while others expressed the view that the "constructive influences" are identical with the blood. Similarly, the "protective influences" were equated by some authors with the influences controlled by the lung, and these would be the same influences that circulate in the twelve conduit vessels. Acupuncture, the dominant therapeutic technique introduced by the *Huang-ti nei-ching* texts, is always directed at the conduit vessels where the needles are supposed to affect the movement of the ch'i-influences, not the blood. The opening of superficial or deep-lying vessels for bloodletting appears in the *Nei-ching* too; it seems to predate the manipulation of the ch'i-influences (see below), and was recommended in later centuries of the first and second millennium A.D. by only a few authors, for instance in the treatment of leprosy.[38] In pulse diagnosis, the throbbing movement that can be felt at the wrist is caused, in the view of Western medicine, by the pulsating flow of blood. Some passages in the *Nei-ching* correspond to this view. The traditional Chinese diagnostician, though, should perceive here, first of all, the flow of the ch'i-influences.

No force or "motor" responsible for the ongoing circulatory movement in the body was mentioned in the *Huang-ti nei-ching* texts. There is, however, a conceptual link between the heart and the vessels in general, in repeated phrases such as "the heart masters the vessels," or "the blood belongs to the heart."[39] Similarly straightforward passages refer to links between the ch'i-influences and the lung, with inhalation and exhalation being considered as the entering and leaving of the body of ch'i. The *Huang-ti nei-ching* texts contain absolutely no indication as to a conceptualization of either the heart or the lung as fulfilling any kind of a pumplike or bellowlike function.[40]

The question to be asked here is how a conception of a circulation of ch'i and blood could emerge in ancient China, and why such a conception appears to have developed at some time during the second or early first century B.C.

Obviously, the so-called conduit vessels occupied a central position in early Chinese notions of physiology and pathology. The twelve conduit vessels introduced, for instance, in the treatise "Ching-mo" of the *Huang-ti nei-ching ling-shu* include three so-called hand-yin conduits extending from the chest into the hands, three hand-yang conduits extending from the hands to the head, three foot-yin conduits extending from the feet to the chest, and three foot-yang conduits extending from the head to the feet. While in the Ma-wang-tui texts only four of the eleven vessels were linked explicitly to an organ, each of the twelve conduit vessels named in the *Huang-ti nei-ching* was associated systematically with one of altogether twelve organs. In the *Huang-ti nei-ching* texts, and in the medicine of systematic correspondence in general, these organs are divided into two groups with different functions. These are, first, the *tsang* (kidneys, liver, heart, spleen, lung, and heart-enclosing network, all of them defined as situated in the interior parts of the body, and hence classified as yin entities), and, second, the *fu* (stomach, small intestine, large intestine, bladder, gall, and Triple Burner, all of them defined as situated in the exterior sections of the body, and hence categorized as yang entities). The Triple Burner is the only organ lacking a verifiable anatomical counterpart. It appears to be a late addition to the list. It is not mentioned in texts prior to the Han era and may have replaced the throat, which was mentioned as the sixth fu in a text of the second century B.C.[41]

All the tsang and fu are interrelated through the system of the twelve main conduits as well as through a network of secondary and tertiary ducts. In a sick organism the flow of the ch'i-influences and of the blood through all these conduits and ducts may at least locally be interrupted for a while without necessarily entailing death for the patient. Life depends, first, on primordial influences (*yüan-ch'i*) which are innate in the organism and which may be depleted before time, leading to death, if wasted through excessive consumption, and, second, on influences assimilated from outside. In addition, the organism produces specific ch'i itself, such as the "constructive influences" (*ying-ch'i*) and "protective influences" (*wei-ch'i*). Health of the body can be maintained as long as external influences enter the organism in sufficient quantities and in balanced proportions, are conveyed to the tsang and fu and, finally, are eliminated—as far as superfluous remaining portions are concerned—from the body.

This, then, is the nucleus of a very complex and highly sophisticated system of physiology and pathology. I should not go into further details here (some will be provided in the subsequent paragraphs in passing, and also by the translations in the appendix)[42] because this would immediately require a discussion of different schools offering different interpretations of many of the basic concepts. The medicine of systematic correspondence was subject to conceptual changes and diversifications through the ages and has at no time represented a homogeneous system of ideas. Already its classic scripture, the *Huang-ti nei-ching,* is a compilation of heterogeneous, partly antagonistic texts. It does not provide the reader with a coherent set of ideas concerning the causation, character, treatment, and prevention of illness as seen from a perspective of systematic correspondence, but rather with a section of an ongoing process of a multilinear formation of thoughts. Possibly because these thoughts originated from inductive logic, throughout the centuries we rarely find agreement between different authors on more but the most fundamental concepts. I shall return to this issue in the discussion of developments during the second millennium A.D. (see chapters 7 and 8).

Although what I have called *organs* so far, and a network of transportation channels, occupy the central position in the physiology and pathology of systematic correspondence, an exact understanding of body structure was never developed by this system of healing—I may even say, was never systematically aspired to (at least until one or two centuries ago). Certain indications of an anatomical familiarity with the organism are already evident in the earliest texts of the medicine of systematic correspondence. The twelfth treatise of the *Huang-ti nei-ching ling-shu,* "Ching-shui," possibly compiled during the first century B.C. or A.D., contains the statement that the conditions and dimensions of the organs and blood vessels can be determined by a postmortem examination. This remark is apparently based on actual experience, since, in treatise 31 ("Ch'ang-wei"), the unknown authors of this work presented their readers with detailed information concerning the length, diameter, circumference, and capacity of several internal organs. Specific results from a dissection were also given in section 42 of the *Nan-ching,* the "Scripture of Difficult Issues," possibly compiled only shortly later. In addition to morphological findings, this passage includes detailed measurements of the weight of the liver, heart, spleen, lung, kidneys, gall, stomach, large and small intestines, and urinary bladder.

After the Han dynasty, medical authors, especially of the second millennium A.D., continued to discuss the nature and location of internal organs. However, an anatomical approach was never again pursued seriously.[43] It was only in the eighteenth century that Wang Ch'ing-jen dedicated his entire adult life to an attempt to convince Chinese physicians that a conception of function is meaningless without an understanding of actual structure (see section 8.2.2.5). Seen from the Han dynasty, though, Wang Ch'ing-jen's voice lay almost two thousand years in the future, and for the time being Chinese medical philosophy of systematic correspondence preferred to base its understanding of health and illness on a perception of physiological processes that appears to have been derived from analogical conclusions rather than anatomical evidence. In other words, with a rudimentary knowledge of tangible internal organs and various other anatomical entities, such as blood vessels, muscles, uterus, and brain, as a substratum, the medicine of systematic correspondence focused its interest on a definition of various functional entities in the organism, on an assessment of the linkages between these functional entities, and, finally, on an analysis of their relation to the macrocosmic whole of which they were considered an integral part.

If the physiology and the pathology of the medicine of systematic correspondence do not rest on an attempt to analyze a tangible organic substratum, but represent a system of relations and functions derived from conclusions by analogy, the factors stimulating and guiding these analogies cannot have originated from within the human body. Instead, they should be searched for in the environment of the philosophers who created these ideas.[44]

The impulse behind this completely novel—one might even say, revolutionary—understanding of structure and function of the organism is easily discerned in the unique circumstances surrounding the unification of the empire, which, during the third and second centuries B.C., produced social and economic institutions that had usually been present earlier only in an embryonic form, if at all. The decreasing number of competing states struggling for sole control of China and the inception of the Ch'in and Han dynasties were marked by fundamental changes in the economic system. During the feudal period, human settlements had been small and largely self-sufficient. Cities whose outer walls achieved a length of one mile were accused of extravagance. Shih Huang-ti, the founder of the Ch'in dynasty, quickly moved 120,000 families into the capital of the united empire![45] The emergence of such densely populated centers was only possible with the concomitant development of a monetary economy, an increase in trade, and a calculated expansion of transportation. The standardization of weights, measures, coins, and script, including even the track-width of carts, on a national scale, as well as the forced construction of roads and canals, contributed to this development. To a significantly greater degree than before, the construction of granaries was necessary to assure continuous supplies to urban populations separated from agricultural production centers. During the Han period the government would purchase grain inexpensively when supplies were plentiful, store it in granaries, and sell it when prices began to rise, a system that attempted to free the urban population from a predictable dependency on the vagaries of grain delivery.[46] During the feudal period, it was believed that grain should not be allowed to cross regional borders;[47] the Ch'in government, however, consciously pursued a policy that stimulated trade in foodstuffs on a national scale. Centers of population that had been largely isolated during the Chou period were increasingly brought into contact with one another by the cultivation of intervening territories. The result was a previously unknown mobility of goods and people.[48] The general aspirations of both state and men were based on the rapid development of new technologies, which, through mines, smelters, and saltworks, enabled the large-scale exploitation of ore and salt resources. The construction of the Grand Canal by Shih Huang-ti has been hailed as "one of the greatest hydraulic engineering achievements of the world."[49]

One may well conclude that all these structural changes that accompanied the unification of China were sufficiently innovative to supply intellectuals of that time with the concept of an integrated complex system, the individual parts of which can function only as long as their relations with the remaining parts are not disturbed. The well-being of the system as a whole depended on the exchange of resources among its individual parts.

The symbolic value of the newly structured social and economic environment may have been significant enough to have been transferred, consciously or subconsciously, by thinkers concerned with health and illness to an understanding of structure and function of the human organism; hence the physiological and pathological basis of the medicine of systematic correspondence accurately reflected these structural innovations.

A consideration of the terms used to designate the major structural elements of the organism reveals a significant etymology. A literal translation indicates that the organism was composed of "storage facilities" or "depots" (tsang) and "grain collection centers" or "palaces" (fu). These "depots" and "palaces," as I shall translate them henceforth, were linked by a system of conduits or transportation channels which were designated with terms such as *ching* and *lo,* among others of less significance. These terms do not yet appear in the medical texts unearthed from the Ma-wang-tui graves of 168 B.C.; they seem to have been the result of conceptual developments that took place between the writing of the Ma-wang-tui manuscripts and the compilation of the *Huang-ti nei-ching* texts, where they were employed in a medical context for the first time. The term *ching* designates, in this context, the main transportation channels which form an ongoing link between all six depots and six palaces, thus creating a one-way circuit. The term *lo* is used to designate conduits linking the major transportation channels with each other, thus creating a complex network. In addition, *sun*-vessels are mentioned occasionally as sub-branches of the lo-ducts. A small number of further transportation channels cut across this system of ching-, lo-, and sun-conduits, with the *ch'ung-mo* ("through-way vessel"), the most important of them, feeding all the other vessels and running through the entire organism like a Grand Canal.

All important elements of the transformed state economy—granaries (i.e., "depots") and centers of consumption (i.e., "palaces"), as well as the transportation network necessary for the exchange of resources among these entities—were represented in the organism. In this regard even the existence of the anatomically indeterminable "Triple Burner" becomes comprehensible. The triple burner was considered an organ (the debate about how it really did "look" was never solved satisfactorily) that, simultaneously at three locations in the body, contributed to the transformation of raw materials, by means of heat, into useful products. The logic of the economic allegory virtually compelled an organic parallel to the smelters and saltworks so vital to the state, even when the existence of such a structure could not be definitely proven. Similarly, the concept of the transportation channels, or conduits, reflects a transfer of an understanding of the vital importance of waterways to the state to a conception of the vital importance of the flow of specific substances through the organism to the human individual. It is needless to emphasize the role irrigation engineering played in China throughout its documented history. The

Li-chi (first century B.C.), the *Kuan-tzu* (second century B.C.?), the *Lü-shih ch'un-ch'iu* (third century B.C.), and also Wang Ch'ung (first century A.D.), to name but a few early examples, stressed the importance of hydraulic works. To open clogged waterways, to drain floodings, to irrigate the soil were among the most important responsibilities of the government to ensure richness of the land and abundance of its products.

In the context of irrigation and water control, we find many of the terms used by the *Huang-ti nei-ching* to designate the system of transportation channels within the organism, including "gutter" (*hsü*), "ditch" (*tu*), "to pour" (*kuan*), "to irrigate" (*kai*), and "underground passage" (*sui*). The term *ching,* designating the twelve major transportation channels, directly refers to the large rivers (*ching-shui*) running from the mountains through the country into the ocean,[50] while the term *lo,* designating the network ducts in between the major channels reflects the gutters (*lo-chü*) designed to drain a city's waters into the large rivers passing nearby.[51]

The central symbolism seen by Chinese philosophers in all these and other environmental facts was summarized by the Confucian author of the *Lü-shih ch'un-ch'iu* when he wrote, in the third century B.C.:

> Flowing water and the pivot of a door do not rot because of their constant movement. The relationship between form and influences (*ch'i*) is the same. If the form does not move, the essence (*ching*) does not flow; if the essence does not flow, the influences will stagnate.[52]

Consequently, the conception of the significance of ceaseless flow was transferred to the organism. A prior knowledge of liquid blood moving in surface and deeper-lying vessels may, as a result, have been extended—under the compelling evidence offered by the transformed social and economic environment—to a conception of liquids and goods, that is, blood and finest-matter influences (ch'i), circulating through the transportation channels of the organism.

Since we have no clues indicating that the passage quoted earlier from the *Huang-ti nei-ching,* referring to a circulation of ch'i-influences and blood through the organism, was legitimated by any anatomical proof, we may hypothesize that the "recognition" of this circulation in China at some time during the second or first century B.C. was stimulated by environmental symbolism. We might even go so far to claim that, given the means to observe anatomical structures available at that time, this "discovery" might have been prevented by other, less accurate insights if systematic dissections had been performed.

3.3.3. Diagnostic Principles of Systematic Correspondence

The symbolism reflected by the physiology of the influence-medicine reappears in the pathology of this conceptual system. In the state, disruptions occurred—especially as the result of a failure in the transportation system or an obstruction of canals, whether due to human sabotage or natural catastrophes—which interrupted the harmonious flow of goods from outside and within the country. Disturbances of this kind could lead to deficiencies of supplies in a population center and to surpluses in production centers or storage facilities. The opposite situation, the all-too-rapid depletion of the latter and an excess of supplies in the former, likewise meant a disturbance of the harmonious circulation of goods. Similarly, depletion (hsü) and repletion (shih) in the body's depots (tsang) and palaces (fu), as well as obstructions in the transportation channels (ching) are the three central diseases in the medicine of systematic correspondence. They are primarily a result of the inability—or willful negligence—of man to adapt his behavior to the influences of his environment. At rest and at work, in eating and drinking, in their senses and desires, so criticizes a passage in the *Huang-ti nei-ching,* men violate the "correct" (cheng) course of things, thus providing an open invitation to the influences of "evil" (hsieh).

A method existed, however, that enabled man to protect himself against all of the influences that the body did not require—and which were thus "evil" if they managed to enter the organism—or, if an irregularity had already appeared in the equilibrium of influences, to regain his health. This knowledge was based on an understanding of the correspondences between the structure and functions of the organism, on the one hand, and the phenomena of the macrocosmic environment, on the other hand. The link was provided by the lines of association of yinyang dualism and the Five Phases which encompassed the depots, the palaces, and the conduits, inside and outside, front and back, upper and lower sections of the body, the spirit and the blood, the two souls hun and p'o, all emotions, and, of course, the multiplicity of influences (ch'i) that enter the body from outside or which are present in the body itself. Since, furthermore, every cardinal direction, the sun, the moon, and the stars, the time of the day, the seasons, food, color, sound, and odor, and so forth were all incorporated into the system of correspondences, it was possible to assess a code of behavior on the basis of both natural and moral-normative principles that represented the harmonious assimilation of all vital influences and provided protection against all evil influences. Conversely, in cases of illness, the color of specific regions in one's face, the condition of the skin of the lower arms, the pitch of one's voice, and the odor of one's breath, the longing for food with specific taste, and the condition of body orifices and sensory organs, one's emotional state, and last but not least, the condition of the movement in the conduit vessels indicated which of the depots, palaces, and transportation channels had been affected by an irregularity of influences and, hence, which influences had to be increased or drained, or where an obstruction had to be cleared.

It is important to mention the special contribution made by the *Nan-ching* (Classic of Difficult Issues) to the examination of the movement in the conduit vessels for diagnostic purposes in particular and to the systematization of the rather heterogeneous body of knowledge accumulated in the *Huang-ti nei-ching* texts in general. The *Huang-ti nei-ching* texts contain—for instance, in the discussion of wind as a cause of illness—numerous passages with concepts predating systematic correspondence, and they contain, furthermore, numerous treatises marked by early formative stages of the development of systematic correspondence where, for instance, the antagonism between schools advocating the yinyang paradigms and those advocating the Five Phases paradigm is still recognizable. In contrast, the *Nan-ching* should be considered *the* mature classic of systematic correspondence. In the history of this particular conceptual system it occupies a prominent place since it appears to be the only ancient work we know of that combines a high degree of innovative thinking with a consistent— in the Chinese sense—body of thought. The application of the paradigms of systematic correspondence was not limited, in this work, to the introduction of a new set of diagnostic patterns; the *Nan-ching* offered new ideas in physiology, pathology, and treatment as well.

The eighty-one chapters of the *Nan-ching,* called *nan* ("difficult issue," or "question"), are structured as dialogues, each consisting of one or more sets of questions and answers. The questions often quote terms or passages that appear in the *Huang-ti nei-ching* too, asking for their interpretation. However, the answers, in general, fill these terms or passages with entirely different meanings and concepts. The terminologies employed in the *Huang-ti nei-ching* and in the *Nan-ching* appear similar, if not identical, on first glance, but in fact the two convey different ideas. The *Nan-ching* is the Chinese medical classic that provoked the largest number of commentaries in subsequent centuries. It is safe to say that in terms of intellectual importance and influence, the *Huang-ti nei-ching* texts, with their unsystematic, heterogeneous, and partly pre-systematic correspondence contents, were pushed almost into oblivion during the first millennium A.D. by the *Nan-ching*. Commentators and authors of separate works acknowledged, accepted, and further developed concepts introduced by the *Nan-ching*. It was only after the Sung era that conservative commentators arose who considered the *Huang-ti nei-ching*—the older text—as the one and only source of truth, and who lacked any understanding for the innovative character of the *Nan-ching*, which had been compiled to transcend the *Nei-ching*. Hence these authors, among them, for instance, the famous Hsü Ta-ch'un of the eighteenth century, interpreted the *Nan-ching* on the basis of the *Nei-ching* and could not help but criticize the former whenever it seemed to misrepresent the ideas of the latter. Ever since, the *Nan-ching* has been termed a "commentary" compiled to elucidate more difficult issues of the *Huang-ti nei-ching* text, an erroneous and quite misleading characterization that has been accepted by Western secondary literature as well.[53]

One of the major contributions of the *Nan-ching* may be seen in its solving the contradiction between the "discovery" of ch'i-circulation in the organism, on the one side, and certain diagnostic (and therapeutic) principles outlined in the *Huang-ti nei-ching* texts, on the other side. In the Ma-wang-tui scripts, as I have pointed out repeatedly, the eleven vessels named were considered separate entities, each being associated with a distinct set of symptoms indicating an illness of that particular vessel. We may assume that the eleven vessels had to be examined individually in order to determine the nature of their respective illnesses, that is, whether they suffered from depletion or repletion. In contrast, in the *Huang-ti nei-ching* texts, the twelve conduits were known to be connected to each other, forming an extensive circuit passed by ch'i. Still, the individual movement in any of the twelve conduit vessels—which were now, in fact, simply sections of the entire circuit—was regarded as an important parameter for determining the presence, the nature, and the location of an illness in the organism. Hence, the *Huang-ti nei-ching* refers to numerous points on all the twelve sections of the conduit circuit, spread all over the body, where the movement in (or of) the conduits can be felt, and where specific diagnostic data can be obtained. Of special importance are the *jen-ying* holes on both sides of the larynx, and the *ch'i-k'ou* holes near the wrist of both hands. It is the merit of the unknown author (or authors) of the *Nan-ching* to have conceived and published, possibly during the first century A.D., the theoretical consequences of the "discovery" of the circulation of ch'i for diagnosis. If the contents of the conduit circuit do indeed circulate through the entire organism, there is no point in checking the condition of this movement at various locations and for each conduit separately; it should suffice to conduct this examination at one location only. The location chosen was the "influence-opening" (ch'i-k'ou) at the wrists, an idea introduced in the first of the eighty-one chapters comprising the *Nan-ching*. However, when it was understood previously that the condition of the influences in each depot or palace, and in each of the twelve conduits associated with the depots and palaces, could be assessed by feeling the movement in each of the conduits individually, a method had to be discovered now to obtain similarly detailed information on each functional unit in the organism from the one location at the wrists. The first twenty-two chapters of the *Nan-ching* offer the solution to this problem.

In a manner characteristic of ancient Chinese scientific thinking, the *Nan-ching* developed numerous diagnostic patterns, all based consistently on the doctrines of systematic correspondences; however, these patterns were not necessarily compatible with one another. While the resulting intricate diagnostic system cannot be outlined here in all its details and ramifications, a survey of some of its central features may suffice to illustrate the reasoning of the *Nan-ching* author. The following diagram (fig. 1) uses the example of an illness in the heart to show the basic pathophysiological assumptions supposedly guiding a Chinese physician when prescribing an appropriate treatment for a patient on the basis of the concepts outlined by the *Nan-ching*.[54]

The heart is depicted here as one of the Five Phases. The Five Phases are related to, and may influence, one another in various ways, with the so-called sequences of mutual generation and of mutual destruction (or mutual control) being considered as the major parameters offering an understanding of the mutual interaction of the five depots in the organism (the sixth depot, i.e., the heart-enclosing network was disregarded in the context of the Five Phases paradigm). Five external evil influences were known to be capable of harming the organism, and each of them was believed to be able to enter the body through but one specific depot.

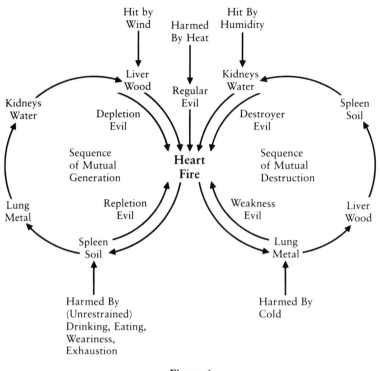

Figure 1

Heat corresponds to fire and so does the heart. Hence evil influences of heat can enter the organism only through the heart. Similarly, both wind and the liver correspond to the phase of wood; hence wind will always harm the liver first. Humidity and the kidneys are associated with the phase of water; hence humidity will always harm the kidneys first. Cold and the lung are associated with the phase of metal; hence cold will always harm the lung first. And, finally, the evil influences associated with unrestrained eating and drinking, weariness, and exhaustion, as well as the depot spleen correspond to the phase of soil. Hence such influences will always harm the spleen first. However, the individual depots that have been affected by wind, heat, humidity, and so forth may transmit these evil influences to other depots in the organism, and when a physician is confronted with a patient he must find out the current situation of this transmission. He has to examine whether the illness is still in the stage of primary affection.

In the case of the heart, the physician might realize that the patient was harmed by heat, and if these heat-influences were still confined to the heart, the heart would be diagnosed as being hit by its "regular evil." If, however, the heart was recognized to be subject to a secondary affection, the physician would have to determine the source of the evil influences within the organism, and label the illness accordingly. In the sequence of mutual generation of the Five Phases, wood generates fire. The liver, accordingly, is the mother depot of the heart. Evil influences transmitted from mother to child are called "depletion evil"; they need a therapeutic approach that differs from a "repletion evil" which is present when evil influences were sent from the child depot, in this case from the spleen. If the affection originated from the kidneys, it should be labeled as "destroyer evil" since water (associated with the kidneys) is capable of destroying fire (associated with the heart), according to the sequence of mutual destruction of the Five Phases. Prognosis in such a case is rather bleak. However, if the lung had been harmed by cold first, and had then transmitted these influences to the heart, this would constitute a "weakness evil." Since fire can overcome metal, but not vice versa, prognosis in this case would be rather favorable.

Consequently, the physician should treat the depot where the illness is situated at the moment of diagnosis, but he should also take care of the depot affected primarily; the latter must have some problem, otherwise it could not have been affected by evil influences from outside. Finally, the physician should be able to determine which depot might be affected next. Once he understood all this, he could prescribe the treatment needed to cope with this particular case successfully. The issue to be solved as a necessary consequence of the "discovery" of the circulation of ch'i-influences through the organism was how to gain all the data necessary to assess the status of a given patient through examining the movement in his conduit vessels at one single location only.

According to the concepts of systematic correspondence, like corresponds to like. Hence, as is illustrated by figure 2, the fact that the body has an upper half (yang) and a lower half (yin), a left side (yang) and a right side (yin), as well as the location of the lung (top), heart (next to top), spleen (center), liver (next to bottom), and kidneys (bottom), should be reflected in the movement of the influences through the conduit circuit at any given location. The location most convenient for an examination and, as one Ch'ing commentator suggested, the ones most suited in the context of Confucian prudishness,[55] were the wrists of the hands. In addition to their former designation, these locations were now called *ts'un-k'ou* ("inch-opening"); the location at the wrist of the left hand was called *jen-ying* (which contributed to some confusion, see above p. 86), whenever it was deemed necessary to distinguish between left and right.

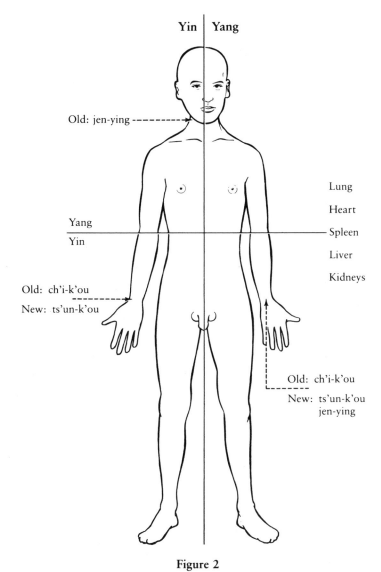

Figure 2

The various patterns offered by the *Nan-ching* to assess the condition of the individual depots through an examination of the movement in the vessels include, among others, the one diagrammed in figure 3.

The "influence-opening" of either the right or left hand could be touched slightly. This would enable one to perceive a movement in the vessels revealing the condition of lung and heart, both of which are located above the diaphragm. Pressing down to the bone and slightly lifting the finger would enable one to examine the condition

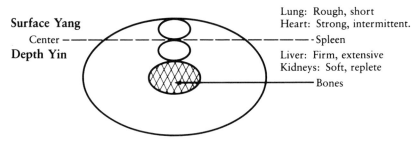

Figure 3

of liver and kidneys, both of which are located below the diaphragm. The movement in the vessels indicating the condition of the spleen could be examined in the center (see fig. 3).[56]

Another pattern offered by the *Nan-ching* (fig. 4) distinguished five different levels and recommended five different degrees of pressure to be exerted by one's fingers (degrees that had to be calculated in accordance with the weight of increasing amounts of beans) in order to reach the individual levels where movements indicative of the condition of the corresponding depot could be felt.[57]

In addition to these longitudinal patterns, cross-sectional patterns were developed. Figure 5 shows a lower arm in an upright position. The palm (above) is separated from the wrist by the so-called fish-line. The influence-opening at the wrist is divided by an imaginary line called gate; the gate corresponds to the diaphragm. The movement in the vessels that can be felt in a nine (uneven number = yang) fen section above (= yang) the gate reveals the condition of lung and heart; the movement in a one-inch (equaling ten fen, even numbers are categorized as yin) section below (= yin) the gate reveals the condition of liver and kidneys.[58]

In another, slightly more complicated pattern, longitudinal and cross-sectional patterns are combined. Here (fig. 6) the movement indicating the condition of lung and heart is to be felt in the nine-fen section near the surface (= yang), while the movement indicating the condition of liver and kidneys is to be felt in the one-inch section in the depth (= yin).[59]

While it did not matter whether one used the wrists of the left or right hand to apply the diagnostic patterns mentioned so far, by far the most intricate pattern suggested by the *Nan-ching* distinguished between information that could be obtained from the jen-ying location at the wrist of the left hand (yang) and information that could be

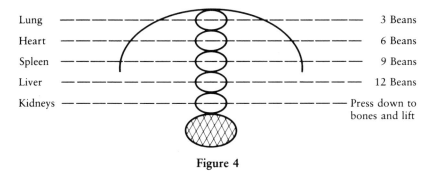

Lung   3 Beans
Heart   6 Beans
Spleen   9 Beans
Liver   12 Beans
Kidneys   Press down to bones and lift

Figure 4

obtained from the ts'un-k'ou location at the wrist of the right hand (yin). This pattern, as did some others, redefined the gate-line as a section of its own, and allowed the physician to obtain data not only on all the six depots but also on the six palaces (see fig. 7).[60]

In addition to diagnostic patterns relying exclusively on an examination of the movement in the vessels, the *Nan-ching* recommended patterns that linked the vessel movement to a wide range of further symptoms. Figure 8 depicts one of these patterns, where correspondence between complexion, vessel movement, condition of the skin of the lower arms, the five pitches, and so forth signals health, while any deviation from this schema indicates illness. The application of this pattern involves an examination of the vessel movement at the wrists, too, but the differentiation among nine-fen, one-inch, and gate-section (or line), or among longitudinal levels, are not necessarily of concern here.[61]

The physician, then, was free to choose among all these different patterns which were only indirectly compatible with one another in that all of them were based on the concepts of systematic correspondence. The individual patterns could not, in most cases, be reconciled with one another; some even appear to exclude others. But the "either/or" question that might be posed by a scientist used to deductive reasoning obviously did not concern a Chinese theoretician or practitioner who thought in terms of systematic correspondence. It cannot be stressed enough that this phenomenon is one of the basic characteristics distinguishing traditional Chinese thought from modern Western science, and it is in this context that one should regard all those attempts as questionable and misleading that try to eliminate this distinctive feature of traditional Chinese thought by artificially isolating a coherent and—in the Western sense—consistent set of ideas and patterns from ancient Chinese sources.

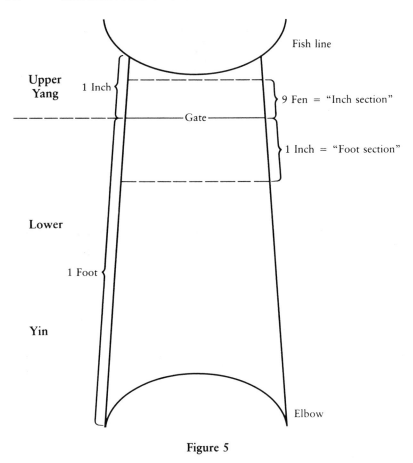

Figure 5

3.3.4. Classic Acupuncture: Origins and Therapeutic Principles

Acupuncture is a technique whereby the movement of the ch'i-influ-ences through the body's transportation channels is regulated. As such, it is described for the first time by Ssu-ma Ch'ien in his biography, in the *Shih-chi* (of 90 B.C.), of a physician named Shun-yü I. This man was accused of malpractice, and one cannot but infer that the tech-niques he used were unfamiliar to those who accused him and asked him for explanations. In the course of two trials, one allegedly in 167 B.C. and the following in 154 B.C., Shun-yü I defended his practices. As the cases quoted in his biography suggest, Shun-yü I knew about the movement of the ch'i in the organism, but a concept of circulation does not appear yet. Acupuncture needles, in the opinion of Shun-yü I, were suitable to cause influences which had moved unduly upward

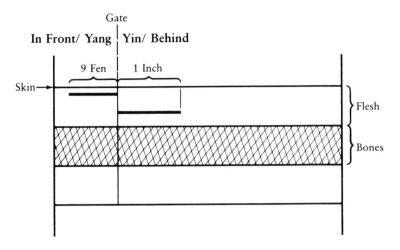

Figure 6

in the organism to descend again (and vice versa); to cause inflow and outflow of ch'i; to affect evil influences which had entered the organism, and to reverse a movement of influences contrary to their proper course. Apparently, some of the points on the skin used by Shun-yü I to insert the needles lay on recognized transportation channels, others not.[62]

With the compilation of the *Huang-ti nei-ching* texts, only slightly later than Shun-yü I's lifetime, acupuncture was considered useful—in addition to the indications mentioned by Shun-yü I—in stimulating the circulation of ch'i through the body by exerting an influence on the function of the depots and palaces as well as on obstructed transportation channels.

When, in 1973, numerous medical texts were unearthed from the Ma-wang-tui graves of 168 B.C., for the first time textual evidence became available which definitively predated the *Shih-chi* and the *Huang-ti nei-ching*. It is obvious, as various analyses have shown, that the Ma-wang-tui texts reflect early phases of traditions which reappear, in more refined stages, in both the *Huang-ti nei-ching* and the *pen-ts'ao* literature.[63] The Ma-wang-tui texts are impressive because of the broad range of concepts and techniques recorded and recommended, including moxa-cauterization, oral spells and magic rituals, gymnastics, sexual practices, drugs, massage, cupping, bathing, and fumigation, based on the paradigms of magic and systematic correspondence, on demonological concepts as well as, presumably, on straightforward experiences. The use of pointed stones is recommended several times

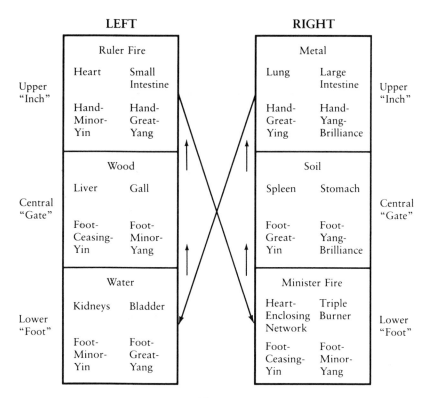

Figure 7

for opening abscesses and once for applying hot pressure to hemorrhoids. Moxabustion, that is, the burning of powderized mugwort plants on the skin, is recommended as the sole stimulus for influencing the contents of the eleven vessels. No specific points are suggested for the application of such treatments; obviously, the treatment directed at a specific tract had to be performed on that tract, wherever possible or most convenient.

The absence of acupuncture in the Ma-wang-tui texts is quite conspicuous. If virtually the entire range of available paradigms and curative means was brought together for assistance in the buried person's afterlife, why should the relatives or officials responsible for furnishing the grave have left out acupuncture? It is hard to believe that they harbored an aversion specifically against this one technique, and it is quite legitimate to assume that acupuncture was unknown to them.

The origin of acupuncture in China is not clear. No known Chinese source prior to the *Shih-chi* (90 B.C.) contains any reference to the technique.[64] Of course, one can, as several Chinese and Western au-

Five Phases		Wood	Fire	Soil	Metal	Water
Five Depots		Liver	Heart	Spleen	Lung	Kidneys
Correspondence Between	Color	Virid	Red	Yellow	White	Black
	Vessel Movement	(In the Depth) Tense Stringy	At the Surface Strong Dispersed Vast	In the Center Relaxed Intermittent	At the Surface Rough Hairy Short	In the Depth Soft Stony Smooth
Correspondence Between	Vessel Movement	Tense	Frequent	Relaxed	Rough	Smooth
	Skin	Tense	Frequent	Relaxed	Rough	Smooth
Five Pitches		Shouting	Laughing	Singing	Wailing	Groaning
Five Odors		Rank	Burnt	Aromatic	Frowzy	Foul
Five Tastes		Sour	Bitter	Sweet	Acrid	Salty

Figure 8

thors have done, cast the net rather wide and consider the existence of bamboo or bone needles in Chou China as sufficient evidence for the presence of acupuncture at the same time; and one also can accept early references to pointed instruments used for opening abscesses to drain the pus from them as references to acupuncture.[65] In contrast to such an inclusive definition, though, the *Huang-ti nei-ching*—the classic scripture of acupuncture treatment—clearly distinguishes, in a discussion of the origins of different therapeutic techniques, between the treatment of boils and ulcers with pointed stones (originating in the East) and the treatment of cramps and numbness or paralyses with needles (originating in the South) (see appendix 2.5). In fact, no available evidence supports the assumption of a sudden monolinear development of the *Huang-ti nei-ching* acupuncture—a rather sophisticated therapeutic approach—from primitive petty surgery such as the opening of abscesses.

Elements clearly recognizable in ancient Chinese literature as possible sources of a multilinear development toward acupuncture include the following: First, the practice, already mentioned, of opening abscesses. This practice in turn may have originated from demonological concepts. I have alluded in the previous chapter to public health measures based on demonological concepts practiced by Chou communities. Just as one attempted to kill invisible spirits responsible for all kinds of public problems by stabbing with swords and lances into the corners of streets, yards, and houses, the belief that demons took refuge in the organism, causing various illnesses there, may very well have suggested the pricking of afflicted body parts with lances and swords of a minor scale, that is, with needles.[66] As we have seen, only one Chinese source known, that is, the *Ch'ien-chin i-fang* of the early seventh century, directly refers to a demonological background of acupuncture; this source cannot be accepted as primary evidence, though, because its distance from the events is too great.

Second, related to the concepts and practice of opening abscesses are the concepts and practice of bleeding, or bloodletting. In the *Huang-ti nei-ching* texts, a development of the purpose of needling is clearly discernible.[67] It ranges from a strongly mechanistic and organic release of bad blood to a stimulation of the flow of ch'i-influences. Several treatises refer to needling as a means to induce bleeding, without mentioning ch'i. The practitioner is explicitly instructed to stick a needle in a given site so that blood flows out. In some other treatises, the removal of noxious elements was supplemented with the therapeutic goal of restoring a proper equilibrium of blood and ch'i; subsequently this notion was replaced by the indication of needling as a means to drain surpluses and to fill depletions—now of ch'i only—without removing anything from or adding anything to the body other than the needles. In due course, the vascular basis of needling lost its significance, while the conceptualization of a system of specific insertion points as a late addition to the *Huang-ti nei-ching* texts, formed the basic tenets of acupuncture as they are known still today. As Epler concluded:

> These concepts appear in part to be from an external theoretical structure which is suddenly imposed on a body of medical thought and practice, . . . [and] the mechanistic, recognizably organic concepts are submerged under a system of cosmological correspondences which could not have evolved from the body of data accumulated through the practical use of needling.[68]

Third, moxa-cauterization had obviously been chosen first as a technique to influence the movement of ch'i in the individual vessels, as is documented by the Ma-wang-tui texts. Perhaps the original meaning of the character ch'i, that is, "rising vapor," suggested an application of heat to stimulate its movement.

Finally, one might speculate about a foreign element which entered the stage to provide the catalyst for the fusion of all these separate elements in front of a variegated background composed of sociopolitical ideals, socioeconomic facts, and cosmological reasoning. Liu Tun-yüan, the discoverer of the Han reliefs depicting Pien Ch'io as a human-headed bird, suggested that the latter could have been influenced by the Indian *gandharva* myth which may somehow have reached the East China coast.[69] The gandharvas, human-headed birds known in India since Vedic times, were traditionally regarded as skilled physicians.[70] Maybe some healers adopted not only the bird-human disguise but also an innovative technique that came along with it!

Returning to the facts, in the second century B.C. acupuncture was adopted, supplementing moxa-cauterization, as the dominant conceptually integrated therapeutic technique of the medicine of systematic correspondence.

We have seen above that the *Huang-ti nei-ching* texts, although referring to the circulation of ch'i through the organism, had not yet perceived the far-reaching diagnostic consequences of this "discovery." The same applies to needle treatment. The *Huang-ti nei-ching* texts name a large number of holes which are located all over the body on the twelve conduit vessels. The texts claim that through an insertion of different kinds of needles into these holes, all the therapeutic effects were achievable that might be desired in case of illnesses such as "repletion evil," "depletion evil," or others conceived by the influence-medicine. Just as unknown as the origins of acupuncture in China per se is the origin of the knowledge of the more than 300 holes mentioned in the *Huang-ti nei-ching* as suitable for needling. Their sudden presence in Chinese medical literature can hardly have resulted solely from experiences with abscess opening by means of pointed stones; if this knowledge developed in China itself, the pricking of painful or swollen locations all over the body with symbolic lancets in a demonological context may have led to an awareness of numerous physiological effects to be achieved this way. The fact that the courses of the eleven vessels outlined in the Ma-wang-tui scripts differ from one another, and that the conduits described in the *Huang-ti nei-ching* differ again from the courses recorded in the Ma-wang-tui scripts, indicates historical changes (or a simultaneous existence of various schools) resulting from differing experiences with the technique of needling. Consequently we may assume that the selection of the holes recommended by the *Huang-ti nei-ching* texts was empirically rather than theoretically legitimated.

It was again the author of the *Nan-ching* who must have realized the logic contradiction between the concept of circulation on the one hand, and the practice of needling "individual" conduits—as if these constituted separate entities with distinct illnesses—on the other hand. The *Nan-ching*, therefore, disregarded the conventional circuit-needling outlined by the *Huang-ti nei-ching,* and concentrated, instead, on a system of acupuncture that was legitimized solely by the paradigms of systematic correspondence. Certain aspects of the *Nan-ching* system of needling can also be found in the *Huang-ti nei-ching* texts; the author of the *Nan-ching* may have adopted and further systematized them. One can, however, not exclude the possibility that later authors editing the *Huang-ti nei-ching* texts added some of the *Nan-ching* innovations to them.

The *Nan-ching* system of acupuncture located six short hand- and foot-conduits in the forearms and in the lower legs, respectively, each with but five holes.[71] These conduits were not considered as parts of the larger conduit circuit, although their holes do appear on the conventional conduits too. Rather, these short conduits of the forearms and lower legs were conceptualized as streams, originating from the hands or feet and submerging into the tissue near the elbows and knees, respectively. The names of the twelve short conduits of the *Nan-ching* are identical with the designations of the twelve conduits listed in the *Huang-ti nei-ching,* that is, hand-great-yin conduit of the lung, and so forth. The holes located on the short conduits, though, have generic designations in addition to their individual names. The first holes are called "well"; the remaining four holes are called "brook," "rapids," "stream," and, finally, "confluence." Each of these five holes on each conduit is associated with one of the Five Phases and with yin and yang, and hence with one of the depots and palaces. To apply the needles at these few holes in order to transform diagnostic insights gained by feeling the movement in the vessels at the wrists into therapeutic action, required not only proficiency in the theories of systematic correspondence; it required, in addition, a firm belief that these theories worked independently of traditional experience.[72] However, while the diagnostic innovations introduced by the *Nan-ching* gained wide acceptance in subsequent centuries and have remained, in theory at least, the dominant diagnostic tool of the practitioner of the medicine of systematic correspondence to this day, the *Nan-ching* system of acupuncture did not receive much attention later on. Acupuncture therapy has continued to rely on circuit-needling. The resulting im-

manent conceptual incongruity in the medicine of systematic correspondence may present today's historian of science with questions that
touch on the very validity of the theoretical foundations of this healing
system; it appears not to have constituted an epistemological problem
in China at any time.

Before I conclude this outline of basic ideas of the medicine of
systematic correspondence, a few words must be written on the status
of drugs in this therapy system. Natural substances must have been
widely used as drugs by the end of the Chou era; the *Wu-shih-erh
ping fang,* a fragmentary prescription text unearthed from the Ma-
wang-tui site, provides ample evidence of a large materia medica applied
in a context of sophisticated and complex pharmaceutical techniques.[73]
And yet, a pharmacology of systematic correspondence was not developed prior to the early second millennium A.D. This issue will have
to be discussed in detail in chapters 4 and 7, but I may at this point
already indicate one major reason that may account for the astonishing
fact that the medicine of systematic correspondence did not, during
its formative phase, integrate a rich body of knowledge concerning
the therapeutic utilization of pharmaceutical substances which existed
in the population and cannot have been without positive effects.

The belief in drugs as valuable preventive and curative means re-
leases man from a perceived necessity to follow a specific life-style as
the basis of health. In the system of correspondence, this "health" was
defined as an integrated personal and social health. The one of these
two aspects was guaranteed by the other, and both were maintained
through a behavior in conformity with a specific ethic. If personal
health could be secured by means of drugs, the link with social health
was severed and social order was no longer guaranteed because what
better stimulus could be thought of to compel an individual to follow
a strict code of moral norms than the reward of personal health! The
concept of acupuncture differed from that of drug application in that
it constantly reinforced the system of correspondences, providing stimuli only where man had not been able, owing to his own negligence
or external conditions, to balance his existence in the proper way.

3.3.5. Concluding Remarks

The preventive and therapeutic principles of the medicine of systematic
correspondence make plausible the preeminence of this system of healing in Confucian society. The structure of the human organism and
the functions assigned to its individual elements reflect a complex social

organism founded on the wide-scale movement of goods both internally and to and from the outside. They further reflect the bureaucratic apparatus of a state in which a wide variety of tasks have been delegated to a responsible ruler and his many civil servants. This is no longer the small feudal state and principality of the waning Chou period, but rather the Confucian-Legalist administration system of the united empire. Consequently we read in the *Huang-ti nei-ching:*

> The Yellow Emperor asked: "I should very much like to hear about the relative importance of the twelve depots and their mutual relationships." Ch'i Po replied: "That is truly an informed question! Let me answer it immediately. The heart is the ruler. Spirit and enlightenment have their origin here. The lung is the minister; the order of life's rhythm has its origin here. The liver is the general; planning and deliberation have their origin here. The gall is the official [whose duty it is to maintain the golden] mean and what is proper; decisions and judgments have their origin here. The heart-enclosing network is the emissary; good fortune and happiness have their origin here. The spleen and stomach are officials in charge of storing provisions; the distribution of food has its origin here. The small intestine is the official charged with collecting surpluses; the reformation of all things has its origin here. The kidneys are officials for employment and forced labor; technical skills and expertise have their origin here. The triple burner is the official in charge of transportation conduits; water channels have their origin here. The urinary bladder is the provincial magistrate and stores body fluids; once the influences [of the latter are exhausted through] transformation, they may leave [the bladder].
>
> "If the ruler is enlightened, peace reigns for his subjects. He who carries out his life on these principles is assured of longevity; he will never be in danger. He who rules the empire in accordance with these principles will bring forth a golden age. If, however, the ruler is not enlightened, the twelve officials are endangered; streets shall be closed and all traffic interrupted. Form will suffer great harm. He who carries out his life on these principles will bring down misfortune. He who rules the empire on such principles shall endanger his entire clan."[74]

4. Taoism and Pragmatic Drug Therapy: From Antifeudal Social Theory to Individualistic Practices of Longevity

4.1. SOCIAL THEORY OF EARLY TAOISM

As I have previously indicated, the teachings of Confucius and his successors were not the only ideological reaction of Chinese intellectuals to the disruptive circumstances prevailing during the period of the Warring States (481–221 B.C.). One of the numerous alternative systems of ideas offering elucidation of the causes and the promise of reversing the period of decadent decline was Taoism. Since proponents of this philosophy of nature and society also had a direct influence on the conceptualization and practice of Chinese healing, I will now discuss those aspects of Taoism that were significant for the development of Chinese medicine.

The designation *Taoism* generally groups together differing, sometimes even antithetical, intellectual currents that do not have much more in common than a conception of the *tao,* the unfathomable law of nature. Confucianism also referred to the tao, but the concept meant something like the correct manner of human coexistence in society. This points to one of the fundamental differences between the two doctrines. If the Confucians believed they could derive an understanding of man from a study of man himself, the highest of all creatures, the Taoists felt that the observation of nature also provided insight into man, a creature that in the final analysis was no better than the lowest worm. But the Taoists were not so much concerned with an understanding of man himself as with the knowledge of how man can best conform to the laws of nature. Thus, "no active intervention" (*wu-wei*) is one of the central and best-known Taoist precepts. Whereas

101

Confucians trusted implicitly in the moral power (te), resulting from adherence to a detailed system of rites, to rectify the political situation, the Taoists of the fourth, third, and subsequent centuries B.C. explicitly rejected such submissive infringements, basing their own doctrine on the potential (te) that arises from adaptation to the Way of Nature (tao). The title and contents of the Taoist classic *Tao-te ching* clearly express these conceptions. Adaptation, conformity, passivity, and weakness—not independent action, control, and intervention—were the values derived from these ideals. Three passages from the *Tao-te ching,* in the words of the author, Lao-tzu, serve to illustrate these points:

> Man is weak and pliant when he is born,
>   solid and strong when he dies.
> Herbs and trees are soft and lush when they germinate,
>   parched and hard when they die.
> For that which is solid and powerful is a part of death,
>   that which is soft and weak is a part of life.
> Therefore, if the weapons are powerful, victory is impossible;
> A strong tree attracts the notice of the woodcutters.
> Strength and power lie below; weakness and softness stand above.[1]

> In all of the world nothing is more pliant than water.
> And yet it has no equal in resiliency against that which is hard.
> It cannot be changed by anything.
> That which is weak conquers that which is strong; that which is soft
>   conquers that which is hard,
> The entire world knows this,
>   but no one can act accordingly.[2]

> In guiding mankind, in service to Heaven,
> There is nothing better than limitation.
> For only limitation leads to early submission.
> Through early submission, great stores of potential can be accumulated,
> By acquiring great stores of potential, man is equal to every situation.
> If man is equal to every situation, he knows no bounds.
> If no one knows our limits, we can take possession of the empire.
> He who controls the productive forces of the empire can endure.
> This is the deep root and solid foundation,
>   the natural law of eternal existence and infinite contemplation.[3]

These passages illustrate, better than any description I could give, the transition from the Taoist doctrine of the contemplation of nature and the understanding of general underlying principles, to a political application of these ideas. As I have already shown, Confucius and his followers based their efforts to restore social order on the view that individual members of society no longer conducted their lives in accordance with the positions assigned to them by the feudal hierarchy. But it was the establishment of this hierarchy and the assignment of positions itself that Taoists considered the cause of all misfortune and decadence. Confucian virtues such as "benevolence" (*jen*) and "righteousness" (*i*) were explicitly condemned as inadmissible instruments of bureaucratic intervention in the natural harmony of human relations. One of the most vivid and expressive documents of this opposition to Confucian doctrine is an ironic passage in the *Chuang-tzu,* a work by the early Taoist philosopher Chuang Chou (369–286 B.C.), who blames the ancient "bringers of culture," so revered by Confucians, for the current deplorable state of society:

> Huang-ti began to confuse the mind of man with "benevolence" and "righteousness." In their great exertions to satisfy the physical needs of man, Yao and Shun scraped away the hair from their legs. They attempted to achieve benevolence and righteousness within themselves; they expended their spirits, in order to mark out law and measure, and still they did not accomplish their objectives. . . . When the age of the historical dynasties dawned, the world was in for a real shock . . . the uniform share that all men had in the great potential was destroyed, and the natural order of things burned and sank. . . . The world loved [Confucian] wisdom and became insatiable in its desires. The executioner's ax and saw carried out their task. Death was dealt out according to guidelines. Men proceeded with hammer and chisel and the world was torn asunder and driven into extreme disorder. All this came to pass because the mind of man had been confounded. For this reason the sages today crawl into the caves of the sacred mountains and the princes in their palaces tremble with fear. The corpses of the executed lie about in great numbers; the chained and bound crowd [the streets], and when someone is sentenced to flogging, he must first watch and wait his turn. And the Confucians and Moists stand on their toes and wave their arms among the hordes in chains and bonds. Oh, what an enormous affront to mankind! Oh, why have they not recognized that all this sacredness and wisdom caused these chains and that all the benevolence and righteousness created these bonds![4]

The political attitudes underlying these comments brought the Taoists into a glaring contrast not only with the Confucians but also with representatives of the prevailing feudal system. One can often read that the mere existence of such a social form rests only on pillage and exploitation. One example, in the words of Chuang Chou, argues: "If someone steals a hair clasp, he is executed. If someone steals an empire, he becomes prince!"[5]

These views resulted in the suggestion for a solution to the social crisis of these centuries offered by the early Taoists of the waning

Chou period. They advocated the return to a primitive, collective community, without private property or social stratification.[6] They rejected the form of human coexistence that we designate with the modern term *society*, that is, a form of organization which—unlike the primitive cultural categories of hunter and forager, as well as of farmer and livestock breeder—is characterized by regular contact with strangers. The long-term, regulated inclusion of strangers into a community, and thus the formation of a society, is only possible if neutral and authoritarian powers are created at the same time, which all participants view with equal confidence.[7] This cultural advance, in turn, is unthinkable without the simultaneous codification of norms that regulate the contact among strangers; formal institutions supplement and gradually replace the informal organization of members of the community who both know one another and are mutually dependent, based on the bonds that have developed over time. The writings of the early Taoists seem to indicate that they felt this "society" could be reversed and that the feudalistic society of a large empire could return to numerous small communities, which maintained neither hostile, nor peaceful and commercial relations among themselves. It was only in this manner that the element of the stranger, with its accompanying consequences for social organization, could be eliminated. Lao-tzu wrote:

> Let there be a small land with few inhabitants: even if there were inventions that would reduce the amount of labor tenfold or one-hundredfold, the people would not use them; the people would die twice before they would depart from this place. Perhaps there would be boats and wagons, but no one would travel in them; perhaps there would be weapons, but no one would practice with them. There would be no writing, except for knots in a rope; the people would be satisfied with their food, content with their clothing, happy with their shelter, and would take delight in their [simple] customs. The closest settlement might be so near that one could hear the roosters crow and the dogs bark, but the people would grow old and die without having gone there.[8]

4.2. EARLY TAOISM AND THE QUESTION OF LIFE AND DEATH

Lao-tzu and Chuang Chou, who recorded such thoughts at approximately the same time, assumed that the form of human life they portrayed had at one time actually existed in the past. Not only did they recognize the implications that a communal organization had for the regulation of political conditions, but they also expressed their understanding of the consequences of simple life for the existence and well-being of the individual. Chuang Chou introduced the term *chen-jen*, the "true man," to designate the sages who in antiquity had been able to live under these conditions in complete harmony with the tao. Important for this discussion is the attitude attributed to the true man toward the question of illness and death. Chuang Chou considered one of the fundamental attributes of the true man to be the recognition that the human form was no more and no less than a temporary manifestation of an existence undergoing continual transformation. The physical form of this existence emerged from a noncorporeal period and eventually returned to this form until the unfathomable creator bestowed upon it a new, and not necessarily human, form. The true man, who had comprehended this situation, therefore stood above the fears surrounding life and death that motivated decadent men.

To recognize the ways of nature, and to understand how they must relate to the actions of man: that is the goal. Understanding the ways of nature is brought about by nature itself, and the understanding of the [natural] action of man is attained by recognizing that which is knowable, and thankfully enjoying that which is inaccessible to man. To complete the years of life and not suffer an early death half-way along: these are the fruits of knowledge. . . .

What is meant by "the true man"? . . . The true men of antiquity did not dream while sleeping and experienced no fear upon awakening. Their meals were simple, their breathing deep . . . The true men of the [ancient] past knew no strong desire for life and no aversion to dying. Their appearance [in the physical world] brought them no joy, their return [to the world of formless existence] was accompanied by no resistance. They departed in serenity, they arrived with tranquility. They neither forgot their origins, nor pursued their end; they accepted their fate and were pleased with it; and unmindful [of death], they returned [to the world beyond]. . . .

Life and death are destiny; that they are as eternal as day and night is due to the nature of things; that there are limits that man cannot exceed, is due to the general conditions that determine the existence of all creatures . . .[9]

Four men spoke to one another: "He who is able to transform non-action into a head, life into a body, and death into a tail, and has understood that death and life form a single body, shall be our friend." The four looked at each other, laughed, and were friends from that day on. After a while, one of them—Tzu-yü—fell ill, and another—Tzu-ssu—came to visit him. "Truly, the Creator is great," said the sick man, "see what he has done to me. My back is so crooked that my bowels lie all the way up, my cheeks are at the same level as my navel, my shoulders are higher than my neck, and my hair grows away from Heaven. The natural course of all my bodily functions has been disrupted. And yet I still possess my mental equilibrium." He then dragged himself to a well in which he could view his reflection and called out: "Oh, that the Creator has injured me in this way!" "Are you afraid?" asked Tzu-ssu. "No," replied Tzu-yü, "what is there to fear? I shall soon be released. My left shoulder shall become a cock that will announce the dawn, my right shoulder a crossbow with which I can hunt ducks. My behind will serve as a pair of wheels, and with my soul as a horse before me, I shall travel in my own wagon. Why should I need other vehicles? I received life because it was my time, and I now depart from it in accordance with the same law. Content with the natural course of these events, I am affected by neither joy nor grief. I am simply suspended, as it was said in antiquity, in mid-air, unable to free myself, bound by the web of all things. But all things have been subject to heaven [for all eternity]—why should I fear [a return to the Creator]?"

After a while, another of the four—Tzu-lai—fell ill, and lay, fighting for breath, while his family stood crying around him. Tzu-li, the fourth friend, came to visit him. "Leave, begone!" he cried to wife and children. "You are hindering his release!" Then he said, casually leaning against the door, to his friend: "Truly, the Creator is great! I should like to know what he intends to do with you, where he will send you. Do you think he will make of you a rat liver or a snake shoulder?" "A good son must go where his parents send him," replied Tzu-lai. "And Yin and Yang are the parents of man. If they make known to me that it is time for me to die, and I resist, it means only that I am impious—how could I reproach them for that? . . . When it is time, I shall fall asleep, and when the time comes, I shall awaken again."[10]

4.3. THE INFLUENCE OF TAOISM ON THE *HUANG-TI NEI-CHING*

Chuang Chou found efforts to prolong the physical form of existence beyond the time allotted by the Creator just as ridiculous as the grief surrounding the departure from one form of existence into another. He compared the breathing techniques practiced by some of his contemporaries to other arrogant measures of false "sages."[11] But the reference in the first of the two passages cited above, in which the true man, based on his understanding of the course of all things, is accorded the possibility of "completing the full measure of his life, and not dying prematurely half-way" cannot be ignored. This notion of a firmly allotted lifetime, which the ancient sages were able to utilize fully (while men of the present are summoned halfway to the goal) and references to a simple, communal form of organization in antiquity based upon the natural course of things, are recorded in a therapeutic context in several chapters of what is probably the most renowned work of traditional Chinese medicine, the *Huang-ti nei-ching* (The Yellow Emperor's Inner Classic). The literal quotation from the writing of Chuang Chou, as well as inclusion of the concept of the true man (chen-jen), indicates the close intellectual connection of these chapters with early philosophical/political Taoism. A further manifestation of this relationship is the form that the entire work takes—a dialogue between the legendary Yellow Emperor Huang-ti, a personality probably included for the first time in the mythical succession of prehistorical rulers by the early Taoists,[12] and several of his advisers and ministers.

The first chapter of the surviving version of the *Su-wen* (Pure Questions) section of the *Huang-ti nei-ching* refers to the one hundred years that men in antiquity were able to live with full possession of physical and mental faculties, while fifty years was the norm for old age in the present (see appendix 2.1). In addition, we read of the seven times seven years allotted to the female life cycle and the eight times eight years allotted to the male life cycle. Nevertheless, this significant work cannot be viewed in its entirety simply as a Taoistic text. The *Huang-ti nei-ching* is also, in fact, the literary expression of the medicine of systematic correspondence that we discussed in conjunction with Confucianism. If we look more closely at the numerous chapters of this work, keeping in mind the conceptual symbolism of the medical notions of the cause, nature, treatment, and prevention of illness, we discover once again that the *Huang-ti nei-ching* constitutes a rather heterogeneous compendium of diverse systems of ideas. The above-mentioned comments in the first chapter of the *Su-wen* ("Shang-ku t'ien-chen lun"), which reflect early Taoist conceptions, represent a striking contrast to thoughts recorded, for instance, in the section "Ling-lan mi-tien lun," which provide an allegorical description of detailed administrative structures (ruler, minister, general, official) and organizational forms of state economy (storage facilities, centers of consumption, smelters, transportation canals, construction, and defense). In addition to these ideologically rather transparent deliberations, oriented on either early Taoist ideals and attitudes or Ch'in and early Han structures, numerous sections are devoted solely to a discussion of systematic correspondences. But these, too, are not totally value-free. Let us recall Lao-tzu's ideal of the measures he would adopt, should he ever be in control of a state. The restriction of activities, especially of commerce, between the individual communities, is simply incompatible with the medical conceptions in the *Huang-ti nei-ching,* in which the organism consists of centers of consumption and storage facilities, connected by a complicated system of transportation channels that support a lively exchange of materials absorbed from the outside and produced internally.

The *Huang-ti nei-ching* may thus be seen as reflecting various and quite different ideological currents. While the fundamental medical conceptions in most of the text appear to be related to the social and economic structures of the empire and the Legalist and Confucian ideals and values discussed in the previous chapter, significant traces of early Taoism are also evident in several sections of that scripture. In fact, the recent awareness, stimulated by evidence excavated from the Ma-wang-tui tombs, of a distinct Huang-Lao political philosophy may also improve our understanding of the sociopolitical affiliation of some of the thoughts expressed in the *Huang-ti nei-ching.*[13] To quote Tu Wei-ming:

> the tripartite division of Chinese thought prior to the age of Buddhist influence into Legalism, Taoism, and Confucianism may have been a convenient device in traditional Chinese historiography. But this simple image of neatly differentiated systems of ideas lacks explanatory value in analyzing the complex process of empire building in the first century of imperial China.[14]

Similarly, the contents of the *Huang-ti nei-ching*—which were conceptualized and compiled at the same time—should not simply be assigned, in a mutually exclusive manner, to Legalist, Taoist, or Confucian ideas. Just as "we may speculate that the union of two originally separate traditions of thought (i.e., Taoism and Legalism) was occasioned by the urgent task of empire building in the transitional period between Ch'in and Han,"[15] we may also assume that similar fusions of hitherto unrelated concepts were attempted to improve understanding and management of the individual organism, that is, in medicine. The *Huang-ti nei-ching* texts reflect these tendencies faithfully.

4.4. TAOIST MACROBIOTICS AND THE LIBERATION OF THE INDIVIDUAL

The pronounced aversion of Chuang Chou to the apparently widespread techniques of prolonging physical life had scarcely any influence on the subsequent development of Taoism during the Ch'in and Han periods. The intellectual triumph over physical death through a belief in two forms of a single existence was displaced by intensive efforts aimed at avoiding, for an indefinite period, the demise of the material body. The goal of immortality for the physical form of existence thus marked the abandonment of belief in the continual, inexorable process of transformation that underlies the human form of existence. Taoist adepts, who strove to attain immortality, or at least, longevity, in a variety of ways, were thus concerned only with the existential problems of the individual; for the time being, they provided no theoretical impulses for a reorganization of collective existence. This change may have been the cause or the result of the largely insignificant influence Taoism exerted on the political organization of a unified China.

An early philosophical foundation for the new, individualistic objectives of late Taoism during the Han period is contained in the fragmentary work of Yang Chu, who lived during the fourth century B.C. Unlike Chuang Chou, Yang Chu acknowledged death as a final boundary beyond which only the "moldering bones" of man remained:

> One man dies at the age of ten, another at the age of one hundred. Perfect saints die, dangerous fools succumb. During life, they were sacred kings like Yao and Shun, after death merely moldering bones. In life they were monsters like the tyrants Chieh and Chou, after death merely decaying bones. As moldering bones, all men are equal; who can differentiate here? Let us therefore seize the moment of life—why concern ourselves with the time after death?[16]

An intensification of happiness during physical existence (for Yang Chu the only possibility) was still based on a belief in a fixed allotment of one hundred years maximum for a lifetime, but the text clearly foresees the ardor with which Taoist practitioners of the Han period clung to earthly life and sought to extend it indefinitely, or at least sought to live their available time with the greatest possible vigor. Older shamanistic notions of feathered men, able to ascend into the air, now merged with the doctrine of the desirable harmony of individual life with the macrocosmic laws, resulting in the concept of the "immortal" (*hsien*), who was able to control the transformation of his being into elementary "matter" to such a degree that he ascended to the gods in a mist or on clouds, assuming his place in the celestial community. The notion of these "celestial immortals" (*t'ien-hsien*) was supplemented by the concept of "terrestrial immortals" (*ti-hsien*), who had little desire to exchange the pleasures of an enduring, free, earthly life for some dubious order in the world beyond.[17]

The arduous and sacrifice-filled search for the correct methods to achieve immortality led in various directions. One impulse was provided by the basic elements, which according to early Chinese thought constituted the foundation of all material existence. The belief that physical life was determined by certain "influences of finest matter" (*ching-ch'i*) led to the development of certain techniques designed to absorb these influences in the degree required to prolong material existence. It is in this connection that breathing techniques can be viewed, whose macrobiotic conceptualization is already evident in a document dating from the sixth century B.C.[18] The *Huai-nan tzu* derives the following statement from yinyang dualism: "The finest matter influences emanating from fire form the sun. The finest matter influences emanating from water form the moon."[19] In accordance with this concept, men (yang) subjected their bodies to the effects of the sun (yang); women (yin) subjected their bodies to the influences of the moon (yin). Gymnastic techniques (*tao-yin*) were intended to ensure that the circulation of these influences and their assimilation through the skin remained free from all disturbances.

Another concept within the same current proposes that water is the actual basic element of physical existence. The most visible proof for this assumption may have been seen in the consistency of male semen (also ching—i.e., "essence" or "finest matter" of water), whose role in reproduction was apparently known. The *Kuan-tzu,* a work from the late Chou or early Han period, contains the following remarks:

> Human beings are made of water. The [seminal] essence of the man, and the influences of the woman unite, and water flows, forming a new shape.[20]
>
> The essence of water is thick, viscous and congealed. It confers continuity of living, and not death. Why do we call water the preparative element? Because the myriad things get their life from it. So those who know on what water depends can know the true way in which water is preparatory to all things. People ask what water is. It is the *origin of all things,* and the ancestral temple of all Life. Water produces the beautiful and the ugly, the virtuous and the wicked, the foolish and the clever.[21]
>
> Thus if water collects in the form of jade, the nine virtues of jade appear. If water congeals to form human beings, the nine orifices and five depots appear. These are [part of its] essence. Such essence, being thick and viscous, can continue living and not die.[22]

The notion of the "essence" of water congealing or solidifying first into jade and then into man in an ongoing vital process uninterrupted

by death or conclusion indicates an early, purely naturalistic interpretation of Chuang Chou's ideas of the continuity of existence. It is
obvious that these views were not based on a concept of energetics,
but rather on the characteristically Chinese notion of matter refined
to the point of formlessness, which, when it congeals or solidifies again,
can assume any form. Out of these beliefs arose the conviction that
the life of a man could be prolonged indefinitely through the greatest
possible production of semen, which was then to be retained in the
organism. This objective, in conjunction with the incorporation of
sexual life into seasonal and daily rhythms as well as into the context
of other cosmic factors, constitutes the substance of Taoist sexual
techniques. They also served, as did all other techniques of longevity,
for the treatment of illness, and detailed instructions concerning positions, frequency, and intensity of therapeutic sexual encounters were
developed.[23] In this system, women were generally assigned the sole
role of a necessary supplier of the second component requisite for the
formation of life, that is, the yin influences, which they produced
during sexual intercourse. Accordingly, instructions dealing with longevity advised men to have relationships with as many women as
possible in succession at carefully calculated favorable times. In the
process, the goal was to prevent the male orgasm as long as possible,
assimilating instead the yin influences of the female partner.

4.5. THE ORIGINS AND EARLY DEVELOPMENT OF PRAGMATIC DRUG THERAPY

A second fundamental approach to achieving immortality rested on
supplying the body with substances which were, according to some
sort of evidence, effective in this regard. This approach is far more
significant for the development of healing in China than the techniques
discussed in the preceding section. Here, too, two currents must be
distinguished. The first of these found expression in the view that
certain substances or precious metals contained the materialized principle of immortality. In the case of gold, for example, a recognition
of its "incorruptibility" and permanence may have merged with macrobiotic considerations, for gold was yellow, and thus assigned to the
earth and the center. Another substance that attracted early attention
was mercuric sulfide (cinnabar), which in its pure form—due to its
insolubility—is the sole nontoxic mercury compound. Efforts to produce gold artificially, as well as the preparation of other substances

promising immortality, may have made China the birthplace of alchemy.[24] Some of the drugs subsequently developed in Chinese medicine resulted from the experiments with minerals by Taoist adepts
and from the doctrine of transformations and abrupt changes to which
these substances could be subjected.

The second current involved with supplying life-prolonging substances to the body was concerned with plants and, consequently, with
a search for the "herb of immortality" (*pu-szu chih ts'ao*). The use of
plants and other natural substances to cure illnesses is well documented
in sources of the latter half of the first millennium B.C. I have suggested
elsewhere, based on an analysis of the pharmaceutical contents of the
prescription manual *Wu-shih-erh ping fang* from the Ma-wang-tui
grave of 168 B.C., that Chinese materia medica emerged from two
different origins.[25] One of these appears to have consisted in attempts
to treat external affliction, that is, wounds, lesions, or burns, by an
external application of natural substances. The second origin of Chinese
materia medica may have consisted in experiences with the oral inges-
tion of plant, animal, or mineral substances, whatever the actual reasons for their consumption may have been. The imaginative impulse
that caused practitioners of longevity to turn their attention to the
plant world, though, may have originated from reports, transmitted
to China sometime during the fourth or third centuries B.C. from
Indian culture, of a plant that when ingested resulted in immortality,
enabled contacts with the gods, and even raised the dead. Only the
unexpected appearance of fantastic supporting evidence from a foreign
civilization can explain the sudden, intensive efforts of Ch'in Shih
Huang-ti, China's first emperor, to obtain this extremely promising
plant. Apparently these reports, as first Wasson and then Needham
have convincingly demonstrated, concerned the *soma,* toadstool, which
played such an important role in early Indian religion.[26] The receptive
Chinese were never able to view the actual object of these reports.
Under mysterious circumstances, Ch'in Shih Huang-ti was sent by his
advisers into the mountains to find the herb *chih,* which no one had
ever seen. When these efforts produced no tangible result, the emperor
heeded the strange requests of a man named Hsü Fu, sending him
with a large number of virginal boys and girls on a sea voyage to bring
back the coveted substance from a distant land of immortals in the
East. Following the purported return and second, better-equipped
journey, nothing more was ever heard of the enterprise.[27] Such efforts
died down somewhat following the upheavals accompanying the fall
of the Ch'in and the founding of the Han dynasty, and Emperor Wu

was the first to have ample opportunity to heed similar advice; he opened his court to numerous established magicians (wu) and more recent "prescription scholars" (fang-shih),[28] who also exerted considerable influence. All of these groups can be roughly classified under the ideologically all-encompassing concept of Taoism.

During the reign of Emperor Wu, a man died whose open-mindedness toward the observance and investigation of nature assured him a permanent place in the early history of Chinese science. Liu An (179–122 B.C.), also known as Huai-nan tzu, was the son of a prince and himself a Taoist-oriented philosopher. He surrounded himself with a large circle of naturalists who devoted themselves to the multivarious activities that promised longevity. Because of his great desire for education, unusual for his social status, orthodox Confucians called Liu An "knowledgeable in heterodox (hsieh) doctrines."[29] A work entitled Huai-nan tzu, whose authors are to be found among Liu's followers, contains the first incorporation of Chinese medicinal herbs into a therapeutic tradition and, at the same time, the inevitable mythicizing of their origin in the initial deeds of a prehistoric cultural hero. One passage reads as follows:

> In ancient times the people subsisted on herbs and drank water. They collected the fruits from the trees and ate the flesh of the clams. They frequently suffered from illnesses and poisonings. Then Shen-nung taught the people for the first time to sow the five kinds of grain, to observe whether the land was dry or moist, fertile or stony, whether the land lay high or low. He tried the tastes of all herbs and [investigated] the water sources to see if they were sweet or bitter. In this way he taught the people what they should avoid and where they could seek help. At that time [Shen-nung] found on a single day 70 [herbs, waters, etc.] that were medically effective.[30]

Shen-nung, the "Divine Husbandman," is a legendary personality, hailed by a rather significant philosophical school, the Agrarian school (nung-chia), as late as the second century B.C.[31] It is possible that Shen-nung was first elevated to this rank by the Taoists; at any rate, he is also known under the designation Yen-ti, the Fire Emperor. The bibliographical section of the official history of the Western Han dynasty (206 B.C.–A.D. 8) already included the title Shen-nung Huang-ti shih-chin (literally "The Interdictions of Shen-nung and Huang-ti concerning Food"), an apparent dietetic manual. The actual work, however, has been lost. Several centuries later, during the Chin period (A.D. 265–420), several surviving medical and Taoist texts mention a "Classic of Shen-nung" (*Shen-nung ching*), possibly the same "Shen-nung's Classic on Drugs" (*Shen-nung pen-ts'ao ching*) first designated with certainty in the literature registry of the Sui (589–618) and T'ang (618–906) dynasties. The identification of Shen-nung as the founder of drug knowledge is thus reflected in the title of the original work of Chinese pharmaceutical literature, whose first authentic compilation was prepared by the renowned Taoist naturalist T'ao Hung-ching (452–536). In the centuries following Liu An, and even beyond Tao Hung-ching, interest in the further development of drug knowledge, as well as in the writings on drugs, is promoted primarily by Taoist-motivated persons, who at times belonged to the highest levels of government, including the emperor. The reserve of the Confucians toward this branch of knowledge is easily explained by the frequently cited aversion of this group, on the one hand, to manual labor, for drug therapy also encompassed knowledge regarding the collection and preparation of plant, animal, and mineral substances and, on the other hand, to the entire study of nature. But, in addition, a totally different reason may have formed the basis of the Confucian aversion to drug therapy.

Confucianism advocated the strict classification of each individual member of society into a rigid and normative social structure, and the Confucian world view linked the preservation of individual health with adherence to certain sociopolitically motivated codes of conduct. In opposition to this view, the Taoists strove for a liberation of the individual from such social obligations. Drug therapy, which promised each individual good health and possible longevity without aging, independent of adherence to social norms, must have seemed to them a much more attractive field of study than it did to their ideological opponents. An attempt to expand the medical theories of the medicine of systematic correspondences, which at first had no connection with pharmaceutics, to the use of drugs, was therefore made only at a time, during the eleventh century, when Confucianism and Taoism had temporarily come closer conceptually, at least on a restricted level. I will return to this development, which became known as Chin-Yüan medicine and which was closely associated with the rise of so-called Neo-Confucianism, at a later point.

The pharmaceutical tradition of the *Shen-nung pen-ts'ao ching* and subsequent works reveals, in comparison with the medicotheoretical tradition of the *Huang-ti nei-ching,* certain characteristic differences, which once again demonstrate that these two fields of knowledge cannot simply be subsumed under the general heading of Taoism. The most striking indication of a conceptual dichotomy is already evident in the fact that drug knowledge, during the first millennium, remained almost completely unaffected by theories of systematic correspondence. The *Shen-nung pen-ts'ao* does contain a reference to a sort of primitive categorizing such that all drugs can be differentiated according to whether they belong to yin or yang, but beyond that, there is no integration of, for instance, the effects of drugs into notions of systematic correspondence regarding the physiology of the organism. With the exception of a single description of a medicinal plant, the *Shen-nung pen-ts'ao ching* lacks any consideration of the doctrine of the Five Phases. Only the five varieties of the imaginary plant chih, the herb of immortality which Ch'in Shih Huang-ti had unsuccessfully sought, was placed in this theoretical framework.

A second significant deviation of this tradition of drug therapy from the medicine of systematic correspondences lies in the antithetical classification of drug effects into hierarchical positions that were borrowed from human society. In the *Huang-ti nei-ching,* those drugs in a prescription that are supposed to develop the actual active therapeutic effect are defined as "rulers" (*chün*). In addition, there are "minister" (*ch'en*), "assistant" (*tso*), and "aide" (shih) drugs, which were assigned only supporting roles. In contrast, the *Shen-nung pen-ts'ao ching* divided all drugs into three groups. The first and most important group was assigned the task of prolonging life, that is, the transformation of the body into the immortal condition of ethereal matter. These drugs are designated "rulers" (*chün*) in the *Shen-nung pen-ts'ao ching;* they do not contain any "poison," or—as we should translate in a technical context—"medicinal effectivity." The third and lowest class of drugs was associated with the function of combating acute illness; drugs in this category were termed "assistants" (tso) and "aides" (shih). The symbolic identification of drugs responsible for combating acute illness in one case as "rulers" and in another as "assistants" and "aides" indicates two opposing sociopolitical assumptions. Symbolically, illness in the individual corresponds to a crisis in society. The *Huang-ti nei-ching* reflects a world view that considered the most important task of the ruler to be to find solutions to such social crises; subordinate ministers, assistants, and aides supported the ruler in this function. In contrast, the true ruler envisioned in the *Shen-nung pen-ts'ao ching* is not concerned with authoritarian intervention in the lives of the people in order to eliminate such social crises, but rather strives to bring harmony into the entire system: he does not initiate "poisonous influences on the lives of men," that is, punishment and other legal measures for direct elimination of acute crises. The difference between Confucian and Taoist social theory articulated in these two symbolic terminologies represents a further subtle parallel in therapeutic concepts.

In concluding, we should recall that Taoism supported, over two thousand years of Chinese history, two major therapeutic tendencies, namely demonic medicine and pragmatic materia medica. The notions underlying the belief in the illness-causing nature of demons and in the illness-preventing and curative properties of drugs all contradicted, as I have pointed out repeatedly in the preceding chapters, the assumption that only a life-style in accordance with a specific moral could guarantee health. As shall be demonstrated in the following chapter, though, the multifaceted nature of Taoism harbored yet another therapeutic approach that stood in marked contrast to the two tendencies just mentioned. The rise of a Taoist "church," and its temporal acquisition of actual political power, brought forth a system of health care that shared a fundamental aspect with the medicine of systematic correspondence, that is, its close links with a specific set of moral norms.

5. Religious Healing: The Foundation of Theocratic Rule

Chinese primary sources and Western secondary literature dealing with the history of the numerous imperial dynasties and other short-lived or more durable small and large states seldom even mention prevailing medical concepts and practices. The present study, which attempts an integral historical approach combining general cultural concerns, in particular the sociopolitical developments, with the more specialized field of medical thought, thus represents a completely new approach to Chinese history. There is, however, an extremely important exception. During the second century A.D., the so-called revolt of the Yellow Turbans broke out in China; almost simultaneously, but without direct connection, a small renegade state was established in the western part of the country. Both of these occurrences, which otherwise were in no way unusual, achieved historical significance because they were associated with attempts to establish theocratic ruling structures based on a religious organization. Among the numerous studies and histories dealing with the sociopolitical events of this period, we know of none that does not include an analysis or presentation of the prevailing health care concepts. Indeed, the close relationship between sociopolitical ideals and therapeutic thought throughout the entire history of Chinese culture has never been so apparent as during this brief period spanning several decades during the second century. The art of healing constituted both a foundation and an integral component of the attainment and exercise of power and was understood and described as such by all historians of this period.[1]

5.1. SOCIAL CONDITIONS DURING THE LATER HAN

In A.D. 184 members of the movement "The Way of Great Peace" (*t'ai-p'ing tao*) staged the so-called Yellow Turban Revolt. As Michaud has convincingly demonstrated, it is scarcely possible to identify any specific underlying cause for this rebellion. It appears that a number of unfavorable factors during the second Han dynasty (A.D. 25–220) ultimately created a political climate that required only determined leaders to ignite the flames of rebellion. Internal political conditions, foreign policy concerns, natural catastrophes, and mass epidemics undoubtedly smoothed the way.

Only several decades after the founding of the second Han dynasty, the vast empire was no longer ruled by an adult monarch, but by a series of boys who, completely unequal to the task, became pawns of their advisers in the intrigues of various groups within the imperial family. Prince Chao was the first of these child emperors, ascending the throne in A.D. 89 at the age of ten. Until the collapse of the dynasty more than 130 years later, none of the rulers was older than fifteen at the time of accession, with the youngest being installed at age two or three. Occasionally during the periods of minority, the regency was assumed by the widow of the father or preceding emperor, and some of the youthful rulers, to counterbalance this familial authority, took the castrated palace servants into their confidence. Initially, the eunuchs usually lacked a decent education and were thus totally unprepared for conducting state business. Their natural opponents therefore were the Confucian officials, who were thoroughly educated administrative experts. Despite this animosity, the eunuchs were able to strengthen their influence to such an extent that, after a final attempt to reverse this development to their own advantage, the Confucians were outlawed as a "forbidden party" in 168 and persecuted throughout the empire like common criminals. The eunuchs also removed qualified officials from the highest administrative positions, establishing in A.D. 178 their own training centers for favorites, whom, despite their continued lack of ability, the emperor then appointed to the vacated positions. The eunuchs appear to have used their new-found power primarily to squeeze enormous wealth from the population for their own personal gain. Thus, five leading members of this group, for their assistance in exterminating the Liang family in A.D. 159, which had grown too powerful for one of the emperors, each received the income of 13,000 to 20,000 families plus a total sum of 56 million cash, an amount whose true significance can be appreciated by realizing that this sum equaled the large state expenditures during the decades of struggle with the neighboring Ch'iang. Moreover, it is probable that this one-time, enormous payment represented only a fraction of the wealth amassed by the eunuchs, which ultimately had to be taken from the people in the form of heavy taxes.[2]

The wars with the Ch'iang, particularly in the years from 107 to 118, 134 to 145, and 159 to 169, when invasions of Chinese territory entailed considerable defensive measures, placed an additional burden on the Chinese economy. The outlying provinces, which bore the brunt of the conflict, contained no less than a fourth of the entire Chinese population. Increased taxes in the areas not directly affected by the fighting were required to compensate for lost revenue in the remote regions.[3]

Finally, it is necessary to mention the great number of natural catastrophes—droughts, earthquakes, torrential rains, floods, hailstorms, locust plagues, and epidemics—which placed even more hardship upon the people. Chinese sources record only a total of ten years during the two centuries preceding the Yellow Turban Revolt that were purportedly free of such disasters. A word of caution is advised here, however, since the political significance of such obvious signs of celestial displeasure concerning the reign of the emperor may have resulted in the possible omission of some catastrophes or, conversely, the exaggeration of what was in actuality an insignificant event.[4]

An indication of the growing unrest and disorder in the empire was the unusual growth, evident by A.D. 103, of the unregistered itinerant population. Official attempts to settle these groups and incorporate them into the economic system met with varied success; after A.D. 170, authorities seemed to have lost all control over these developments. In the capital, officials were too concerned with struggles between various cliques, and the number of the migrant masses soared. The amount of cultivated land decreased as innumerable peasants fled the intolerable conditions imposed by the large landowners; famine and the formation of numerous local gangs ensued. The condition of the government at this time is evident in the creation of a department in A.D. 179 in which public offices were offered for sale.[5]

All these events contributed to a situation in which large segments of the population had apparently lost confidence in the prevailing form of government and were ready to embrace a new leadership which, on the basis of a system of healing, promised a better future. Chang Chüeh and his "Way of Great Peace" provided the nucleus for open rebellion.

5.2. *T'AI P'ING* IDEOLOGY AND THE
YELLOW TURBAN REVOLT

Chang Chüeh was born in Chü-lu, located in what is today Hopei. His activities remained centered in this area and the surrounding provinces of eastern China, although the effects were visible in nearly all other portions of the country. The doctrine with which Chang Chüeh was able to attract the masses from ca. 173 to 184 was drawn from various sources. The most important concepts of the ideology were taken from a partly written tradition that believed it had discovered how society could find the "Way of Great Peace." Proponents, so tradition indicates,[6] had already attempted, in 300 B.C., 6 B.C., and once more during the reign of Emperor Shun-ti (A.D. 126–144), to present their ideas in the form of a "Classic of Great Peace" (*T'ai-p'ing ching*) to the ruling parties, but their views on social reorganization were repeatedly perceived as dangerous to state authority and branded as heresy.

T'ai-p'ing ideology rests on a belief in the

cyclical recurrence of immense world catastrophes, which are survived only by a small, select group of men. It reveals how man can withstand these periodic cataclysms and join the chosen few who survive. The critical point is preceded by a period of increasing floods, droughts, failed harvests, political disruptions, wars, and especially pestilence, as was the case near the end of the second Han Dynasty.[7]

A "divine man of the great Tao," it was believed, had revealed to mankind the possibilities of a code of conduct favorable for survival and had also presented specific measures to be enacted by the government. The ethics of government, according to these precepts, must concentrate on a modest and economical court, support of the poor and indigent, care of the elderly, and the reduction of taxes and penalties.[8] Those who followed the ethic of the "divine man of the Great Tao," were guided safe and sound through the collapse by sacred emissaries and led into the ensuing new age of great peace.

Chang Chüeh had apparently come into possession of a copy of the *T'ai-p'ing ching* that purportedly had been given by Lao-tzu himself to the Taoist Yü Chi, also active in the second century. The version of the *T'ai-p'ing ching* that has survived in the Taoist canon, which is not necessarily identical to the one of Chang Chüeh, contains a commentary dealing with this occurrence, and indicates that the purpose of the work was, on the one hand, to reveal instructions concerning the achievement of physical immortality, and rules regarding the attainment of harmony in society, on the other hand.[9] Nowhere else do we find such a clear admission of the complete integration of medical and political concepts.

Around the year 173, Chang Chüeh began to preach this doctrine among the population. His success, particularly among the nonregistered migrants, was extremely impressive. The official history of the period mentions hundreds of thousands of followers; when Chang Chüeh called public gatherings, the streets were blocked by the enormous crowds. The medical portion of his doctrine had three components. Chang Chüeh stood in the tradition of demonic medicine, which, with the aid of oral, written, and gesticulated spells and interdictions, attempted to resist harmful demons or expel those that had already invaded the body. Chang utilized a bamboo staff containing the magic efficacious number of nine knots, in conjunction with specific gestures, to enact a spell. In addition, Chang had the masses confess their sins during impressive rituals, in order to induce the "divine man of the Great Tao," who watches over longevity and the approaching epoch of Great Peace, to prolong the time allotted to individuals, a period easily diminished when the *t'ai-p'ing* was violated. Finally, Chang Chüeh utilized written characters, in which certain cosmic relationships were expressed. These characters therefore possessed the power to eliminate pathological disturbances that resulted in the physical microcosm losing its place within the macrocosm of universal actions, which itself was brought about by sinful conduct. Chang Chüeh wrote down for his followers the various necessary character combinations; the consumption of the ashes of characters, which followed the purification achieved through public confession, provided the desired protection and healing.

Chang Chüeh soon was unable to handle by himself the great influx of devotees from wide areas of the country. He then dispatched, again in accordance with the significant number nine, eight disciples, whom he had initiated into the secrets of his teachings. In addition, a group of four military commanders and deputy commanders was appointed to each of the ideological leaders, including Chang Chüeh, and the masses were assigned in groups of thousands and ten-thousands to the resulting thirty-six organizational units.

The year 184 marked a significant phase. In this year the Chinese calendar began a new sixty-year cycle, and the leaders of the t'ai-p'ing movement promised the downfall of the existing order and the establishment of a new rule for this period. The rebellion of all sympathizers, however, intended for 184, was betrayed by an insider shortly before the planned surprise attack; the central government finally emerged victorious from the fierce fighting, which left at least 241,000 rebels dead.[10]

5.3. PHYSICAL EXISTENCE: TENSIONS BETWEEN DAILY LIFE AND THE ETHOS OF NATURE

In the cult of Chang Chüeh, the religious medicine that concentrated on a recognition and confession of past misconduct, could only, albeit unsuccessfully, assume the function of achieving power; the exercise of power was denied to Chang following the unfortunate collapse of the rebellion. Only a few years later, however, a small state was established in the western part of the empire, in which the same principle—linking sin and illness—produced a form of government, over a period of three decades, which differed greatly from the Confucian social system. Even more clearly than the views of Chang Chüeh, the ideology adopted by the founder of this state, Chang Lu, was founded on non-Confucian social philosophies. Moist, Buddhist, and Taoist ideas influenced a regime, in which a religious leader, on the basis of "communality," supervised the lives of subjects that were free of sins and, consequently, illness.[11] The three forces of Heaven, Earth, and Water were accorded the highest existential authority; in addition, the presence and actions of evil demons were to be combatted through a suitable code of conduct. The *T'ai-p'ing ching,* which formed the basis of Chang Chüeh's teachings, achieved a certain renown in the new state, but it appears that another work, an individualistic annotated version of the *Tao-te ching,* fragments of which have survived under the title *Lao-tzu Hsiang-erh chu,* played a much more significant role.[12]

We have already encountered the belief in a spectral world that punishes human misconduct in the ancestor therapy of the Shang; deceased ancestors exhibited their displeasure with living descendants by means of illness-causing curses. Such views are recorded explicitly for the first time in the work of Mo Ti (479?–381 B.C.), a philosopher living during the highly unstable period of the Warring States, who, in violent words, reproached those of his contemporaries who believed they could deny the existence of spirits and demons. Mo Ti had reached the conclusion that only the fear of retribution by such forces could induce society to adhere to certain virtues and behavioral norms; he also believed to have discovered the underlying cause of the chaos of his time:

Master Mo Ti said: Since the sacred kings of the three dynasties of antiquity are no longer living, and the world has renounced their principles, feudal lords consider force to be the correct basis for all actions. Between prince and subject, superior and subordinate, goodwill and loyalty no longer prevail; between father and son, between younger and elder brother, kindness and piety, fraternity, respect, virtuousness, and harmony no longer exist. The leaders of the state no longer strive to govern and the simple folk do not attempt to fulfill their obligations. The people are evil, violent, thieving, and rebellious; thieves and robbers attack innocent men on the roads and byways with weapons, poison, water, and fire, seizing wagons, horses, clothes, and furs, in order to enrich themselves. All of this has the same cause, and brings the empire into disorder. What lies behind these conditions? All now doubt the existence of spirits and do not perceive that spirits have the power to reward the industrious and punish the evil. If all men of the empire could be convinced that spirits are capable of rewarding the industrious, and punishing the evil, how could the empire be disrupted?[13]

Therefore Master Mo Ti said: if the fact that spirits reward the good and punish the bad can be made the foundation of the state and be explained to the people, then this is a way to preserve order in the country and to benefit the population. If then integrity and selflessness no longer prevail among the officials, and if men and women are no longer separated, this would be seen by the spirits. When the people are depressed and corrupt, and rise in rebellion, when thieves and robbers lie in wait for innocent men on the roads and byways with weapons, poison, water, and fire, and steal wagons, horses, clothing, and furs in order to enrich themselves, this, too, the spirits would see. For these reasons the officials will not dare to be corrupt and self-seeking; when they encounter the good, they will not dare fail to reward them, and when they encounter the bad, they will not dare fail to punish them. And the fact that the people are depraved and corrupt, rebellious and hostile, that thieves and robbers attack innocent people on the highways and paths with weapons, poison, water, and fire, stealing wagons, horses, clothing, and furs, in order to enrich themselves, all this shall stop from that point on. One cannot escape the alert eye of the spirits in dark valleys or vast marshes, in the mountains, forests, or deep ravines, for the eyes of the spirits will still see him. One cannot avoid the punishment of the spirits through wealth, nobility, numerical superiority, arms, or weapons, for these will not hold off retribution by the spirits.[14]

Therefore Master Mo Ti said: If kings, princes, high officials, scholars, and noblemen today truly desire to make the empire more beneficial and prevent any harm, then they must acknowledge the existence of spirits and demons and honor them accordingly, for this is the way of exemplary kings.[15]

The specific forms of punishment meted out by the spectral world, which Mo Ti so forcefully stresses, are also described. Several examples are provided, particularly how men unjustly executed return to take revenge upon those responsible. Mo Ti likewise describes the rewards of a virtuous life: attentive gods prolong the lives of those who are virtuous.

These notions were not restricted to the Moists; they were also cultivated in Taoist circles, and it is possible that these groups first associated such ideas explicitly with the origins of illness. In this connection, the *T'ai-p'ing ching* remarks:

> Heaven knows of all failings, whether grave or minor. For each year of life it has accounts, in which all good and evil actions are recorded. Each individual day and month are examined, and in accordance with the evaluation, units [of three days] are deducted [from the originally fixed life span], and the length of life is decreased.[16]

At the beginning of the fourth century, the Taoist and natural philosopher Ko Hung recorded several concepts that had possibly already influenced Chang Chüeh and Chang Lu:

> In the *I-ching,* section "Nei-chieh," and in the Classic of Ch'ih Sung-tzu, as well as in the *Ho-t'u chi-ming fu,* it is written: "In heaven and on earth there are spirits who observe misconduct. According to the severity of the sins committed by man, several years are deducted from their life span. A decrease in the originally alloted lifetime causes the victim to fall into poverty and illness; if the originally alloted time is exhausted, he dies!"[17]

> There are three beings in the body. They are actually present, even though they are formless. They belong in fact to the group of souls, demons, and spirits. Their primary objective is to bring man an early death, for this enables them to then function as demons, move around freely, and treat themselves to the offerings presented by men. For this reason, they ascend each *keng-shen* day to the ruler of all fates in heaven and report the failings of men. In addition, on the last night of each month, the god of the kitchen ascends to heaven, in order to report the evil deeds of men. For grave [sins] a year of 300 days is deducted [from the originally alloted life span]; for minor failings, the life span is decreased only by a unit of three days.[18]

Finally, the Hsiang-erh commentary on the *Tao-te ching,* which supposedly played such a central role in the Chang Lu state, linked the concepts of a connection between sins and life span with notions of a life based on the *Tao* and belief in the influences on men by ch'i, which transforms itself in the organism into the life-giving essence ching, one of whose manifestations was male semen. Again and again, the Hsiang-erh commentary stresses the senselessness and foolishness of the widespread tricks for prolonging life, in particular the sexual techniques which attempted to protect against the loss of semen by returning this precious substance to the brain. The numerous passages dealing with this problem underscore the intention of shaking the faith in mechanistic, and therefore amoral, longevity practices, and drawing the attention of the reader instead to the inseparable link between adherence to an ethic of the true Tao, on the one hand, and the enjoyment of the longest possible life free from illness, on the other hand:

> Men who conduct their lives in accordance with the doctrine of Tao accumulate essence and their spirit realizes its full potential. Unfortunately, these days several tricks masquerade under the name of "Tao." In following the writings of the Yellow Emperor, the mystical maiden, Kung-tzu, and Jung Ch'eng, some men spend their lives in incessant pursuit of the female sex, hoping to strengthen their mental faculties through the return of the [seminal] essence. For these people, mind and spirit no longer form a whole; in reality, they lose that which they thought to preserve. . . .
>
> The corporeal soul is white and therefore the [semen] essence is white; the primordial influence [to which man owes his life] has the same color. The body is a wagon loaded with [semen] essence. If this essence flows out, more must be loaded to reestablish the correct proportion. When the spirit has realized its full potential, the essences flow into the body until the correct level has been reached again. One now desires to maintain continually the achieved level [of essence] and not lose the unity [of mind and spirit]. If this unity is attained, it signifies the [complete harmony of personal existence with the] Tao. But how is the presence of this harmony in the body to be understood? How can this unity be preserved in the body? It is not present in the body from the very beginning, and this is why the widespread tricks that are concerned with the body do not [conform to the] true Tao. The harmony comes from beyond heaven and earth, entering from there the region between heaven and earth. When it then enters the body, it does not occupy one specific spot, but fills the entire space enclosed by the skin. He who today conducts his life in accordance with the ethical precepts of the Tao, he who heeds this ethic and does not violate it, shall preserve harmony. He who does not conform to this ethic shall lose harmony.[19]

In subsequent sections, to be cited below, the commentary discusses the accounting procedures of the celestial authorities, consisting of left (positive) and right (negative) halves. At birth, all men receive a specific, fixed life span that is recorded on the right half of the account. In addition, each person receives the same period of time credited to a celestial account on the left side. Through exemplary conduct, the balance on the left side can be withdrawn and transformed into earthly existence. Violations of the Tao ethic, conversely, result not only in a blocking of the left account but also in a reduction of the amount recorded on the right side, the time remaining in the allotted life span:

> He who strives to achieve the longevity of the immortals and the good fortune of heaven, must devote himself with confidence to the Tao. He must follow the ethical precepts and must not betray his faith [through contrary behavior]. He must not make even two mistakes, for all sins are recorded in a list by the officials in heaven, until [the account] on the right side is exhausted and [no years] remain in the life span.[20]
>
> The immortals of antiquity preserved the abundance of their essence, thereby maintaining their life. The men of today lose their essence and consequently must die. This is truly the case! Can life today be extended simply by accumulating essence upon essence? By no means! Every aspect of life must contribute to [the goal of longevity]. Essence is only one of the many emanations of the Tao. They enter man and form the basis [of his existence], but half is withheld from him from the very beginning. If one desires to amass essence [in the body], he must devote his entire life to carrying out all kinds of good deeds. One must conform to the Five Phases and reject any emotional stimulation, be it joy or anger. The left half of the account [of the life span] maintained by the celestial officials will then show available credit, and one is protected against the loss of [vital] essence. When evil men desire to amass essence, all their efforts are in vain, and they must ultimately lose their lives, for all their essence [despite sexual techniques] flows inexorably away. One should carry out his good deeds with a virtuous attitude and, appealing to the three powers of the Hall of Light (*ming-t'ang*), confess all evil and injurious actions [which one has caused], in order to achieve the correct measure of finest emanations of the Tao. The vital essence can be compared to the water in a pond, the body to the dam that surrounds this water, and the correct life to the source [of the water]. When all three components are in their ideal state, the pond is filled to the rim. If a person places no special value on good deeds, the dam is missing and water flows away uncontrolled. If one has accumulated no beneficial works during his life, the source is obstructed, and the water unavoidably dries up. [Or it happens that] the waters burst forth like the violent torrents into the wilderness and flow away, even though a dam is present, so that the source is not obstructed, but [the pond] is nevertheless empty. The walls of the dam (?) finally burst from dryness and—at the same time—all kinds of illnesses arise. If one is incautious regarding the three [components: water = vital essence; dam = body; source = correct life], the pond becomes merely a dry hole.[21]

We know of no older text in which the naturalistic concepts of "essence" (ching) and finest matter influences (ch'i), which determine physical existence, are so obviously linked with the ethics of Tao. The transformation of the account on the left side into actual years of life and, conversely, the affliction or even curtailment of physical existence are the result of the quantity of influences that the Tao pours into man from diverse sources. A harmonious proportion of influences makes possible the continued necessary formation of "essence," from which the body takes its life; an imbalance or loss among the influences is accompanied by illness or even death. The rather cynical-sounding pronouncement in the *T'ai-p'ing ching*—"Fear is the basis of life"—[22] blends well into this natural ethos.

5.4. THE FIVE-PECKS-OF-RICE MOVEMENT AND THE STATE OF CHANG LU

When the ideas outlined in the preceding paragraph found their theoretical and practical application in the philosophy and government of a renegade state in western China in A.D. 186, it was scarcely possible to ascertain which individuals had contributed concepts to the movement. It appears that two separate family traditions, both concerned with healing, developed in the same general area. Chang Hsiu, the leader of one of these traditions, required from the families of those he had healed the continued yearly payment of five pecks of rice, thus the name of the movement (*wu tou mi tao*). Possibly encouraged by the Yellow Turban Revolt in eastern China, Chang Hsiu and his followers initiated a revolt in A.D. 184. Since none of the Chinese sources mentions suppression of this uprising,[23] it seems likely that Chang Hsiu was able to establish his own political entity, which was even tolerated to a certain degree by the governor of the neighboring province I.

The second of these traditions arose at about the same time, with the appearance of Chang Lu. Chang Lu declared himself the grandson of Chang Tao-ling, a local magician who up to that time had probably had only a very limited following and who had purportedly introduced written spells. According to a report in the possibly oldest biography of Chang Tao-ling, written by Ko Hung in the early fourth century, Lao-tzu himself is supposed to have procured him a "contract with innumerable spirits in the world."

As a result, he was able to heal illnesses and the number of his disciples increased so greatly, that he organized them into communities watched over by *chi-chiu* ("libationers"). At the same time, he established regulations and assessed natural levies in the form of millet, silk, utensils, paper, brushes, and firewood. He had his followers improve the roads. Anyone who refused, he punished with illness. He despised the system of punishment and taught the people modesty and shame. He had all sick people make a complete confession of all previous failings. Then a written contract with the spirits was drawn up, in which the patient pledged his life never to sin again. Thereupon the [notorious] criminals improved their lives and became good.[24]

As Eichhorn has already recognized, the information on Chang Tao-ling must doubtless be seen as a projection of the state later founded by his purported grandson, Chang Lu.[25]

Apparently authentic sources report that the mother of Chang Lu was also a practitioner of demonic medicine. By means of these abilities and her supposed beauty, she gained access to Liu Yen, the governor of I province, who awarded her son a military title. In addition, Liu commissioned Chang Lu and Chang Hsiu to eliminate the governor of the neighboring territory, Hang-chung. It is possible that Chang Lu became acquainted at this opportunity with the organization of the followers of his comrade, for he killed Chang Hsiu shortly after the successful conclusion of their mission, took over his cult, and proclaimed his own state in the strategically important and easily defended area of Han-ching. After he had the local representatives of the central government killed, Chang began a thirty-year reign (A.D. 186–216), during which the principles of religious medicine and the concept of "civic spirit" (*kung*) formed the ideological foundation of individual and collective action.

> The entire system of Chang Lu was built upon a fear of the power of evil spirits and demons, who threatened human society from all sides and constantly strove to cause injury or even death. A comprehensive contract provided the supreme leader of the community with an instrument for protecting those who professed their loyalty to him from the evil influences of spirits and demons. He was the guarantor of the life and prosperity of his subjects, who lived under the constant threat of evil forces. This meant that unbelief and skepticism regarding the power of the spirits and demons were considered an attack on the basic authority of the state itself.[26]

In comparison with demonic medicine, which, as we have already seen, was only an amoral, individualistic system of reference between individual men and individual demons, religious medicine contains the new element of a churchlike organization, which establishes norms for individual conduct in the collective and thus confronts demons as a representative of this collective.

As an alternative to the traditional civil service of the Han dynasty, Chang Lu created a new hierarchy, which stretched from the "warriors against demons" (*kuei-tsu*) and "soldiers against immorality" (*chien-ling*), who were the lowest officials under the "libationers" (*chi-chiu*) mentioned in the biography of Chang Tao-ling, up to the "district governors, grand libationers" (*chih-t'ou ta chi-chiu*) and ultimately the "master of masters" (*shih-chün*), Chang Lu himself. All of these officials were charged with supervising various-sized groups of the population. The objective of this tightly woven social control was to maintain an unquestioning belief in the magical powers of Chang Lu and, thus, enforce observance of social norms.

The so-called free hostels (*i-she*), presided over by the libationers, provided free lodging and meals to travelers. Moreover, each inhabitant of the state could partake of the food provided in front of the free hostels. Demons and spirits caused illness in anyone who abused these institutions. Secular authorities intervened only when someone had repeated a crime three times. Even then, the punishment, such as the obligation to repair one hundred feet of a street, was mostly symbolic in nature.

The sick were admitted to "chambers of silence" (*ching-shih*), where they had the necessary peace and leisure to reflect on the failings that underlay such bodily suffering. When the sins of the past were finally recognized, passages from the *Tao-te ching* were read aloud, prayers were directed to the spirits, and the three supreme powers—heaven, earth, and water—were placated by writing the misdeed on three pieces of paper, one of which was then placed at the top of a mountain, a second buried in the ground, and the third consigned to a river.[27] In addition, those who were cured in this manner, as had been the case under Chang Hsiu, were required to pay five pecks of rice or other crops to the libationers, who then added them to the supplies in the free hostels.

Not only were illnesses themselves treated but society was also admonished to carry out preventive measures. From time to time, the inhabitants would assemble for meditation, during which each individual would reflect upon his recent conduct so as to discover any unnoticed sins. If it then appeared necessary, on the basis of such self-contemplation, the individual could prevent punishment by spirits and thus physical illness by performing some voluntary community service, such as the collection of medicinal herbs.[28] This last aspect is significant, since it indicates that the use of medicinal plants was officially tolerated and, perhaps, even actively promoted.

Although, as Kaltenmark has shown, it is doubtful whether the entire *T'ai-p'ing ching* preserved in the *Tao-tsang* is identical with a text of the same title providing the ideological basis of Chang Lu's regime,[29] the *Tao-tsang* version, nevertheless, contains a rationale for the application of various therapeutic techniques in a religious context. After all, drugs, moxa, and needles appear to have been well-established curative means in the Chinese population by the time of the Han, and it might have been difficult for any group striving to gain political control over the masses by promising social and personal health to neglect these techniques entirely.

Herbal and animal substances were identified as being sent down to earth by celestial beings; it was believed that the bodies of birds contained some "divine celestial medicine," and that herbs and trees contained the tao and, consequently, the powers te resulting from a realization of the tao.[30] Even the application of such seemingly straightforward technical procedures as moxa-cauterization and acupuncture were legitimated on grounds of their moral nature, as the following excerpt from the *Tao-tsang* version of the *T'ai-p'ing ching* may indicate:

Cauterization and pricking are means to harmonize the 360 arteries, to provide passage for the *yin* and *yang* influences, and to eliminate suffering. The 360 arteries correspond to the 360 days of a year. Each day one of the arteries controls the affairs [of the organism]; their activities correspond to the four seasons and to the Five Phases. They come out to the body's surface, moving around it everywhere; above they unite at the top of the head, and internally they are tied to the depots; their depletion and repletion corresponds to the four seasons. If the movement [of the activities from one artery to the next] suffers from an illness, it does no longer correspond to the calendrical cycle. The sequence of the movement loses its order, resulting either in tie-ups or in injuries, [the movement] taking sometimes the proper, sometimes a contrary direction. This, then, must be treated. Cauterization is the essence of the Great-*yang*, it is the brilliance of public spirit and truth. For this reason it discovers licentiousness and expels suffering and evil. The needles are the essence of the Minor-*yin;* they are the light of the Great-white. For this reason one makes use of their righteousness in order to subjugate any rebellion. One hundred therapies will yield one hundred successes; ten therapies will yield ten successes. All this is made possible through the receipt of the arteries-prophecy-writings from the celestial scriptures.[31]

In the year 215 or 216, Han-ching was occupied by a general and troops of the central government. Initially, Chang Lu fled to friendly Tibetans but surrendered shortly thereafter. Thus ended, after some thirty years, the most successful attempt in the long history of China to establish a theocracy. But the underlying world view, and thus religious medicine, survived in esoteric circles, secret societies, and among the broad masses of the population. The idea of deities who in heaven, or in the human body itself, watch over earthly conduct and dispense appropriate rewards or punishment in such forms as good health and illness, assumed numerous credible forms and has remained an important aspect of Chinese medicine up to the present day.[32]

6. Buddhism and Indian Medicine

6.1. EARLY BUDDHISM IN CHINA

The Yellow Turban Revolt and the state of Chang Lu, as well as numerous less spectacular uprisings during the second century, signaled the approaching demise of the Later Han dynasty. Although these disturbances had no single underlying cause, the steady disintegration of internal administration played a significant role, culminating in the dissolution of the united empire in A.D. 220. The shadowy existence of the central government, reinforced by an underage ruler, undoubtedly provided the victorious generals with sufficient incentive to seize power for themselves. General Ts'ao Ts'ao, whose son Ts'ao P'ei administered the final blow to the Han dynasty, emerged triumphant from the civil wars, founding his own Wei dynasty (220–265) in the important regions of the north. Shortly thereafter, the Shu dynasty (221–265), centered in Szuchuan, was established in the southwestern portion, and the Wu dynasty (222–280) in the southeastern portion, of the former empire. This period, known as the Three Kingdoms, was succeeded by a brief interlude of unity under the short-lived Chin dynasty (280–316), which crumbled after only a few decades, primarily because of continuing conflicts with foreign invaders from the north and northeast. Some members of the ruling family were able to escape to the south and established there the Eastern Chin dynasty, which survived until 420. The so-called epoch of the Northern and Southern dynasties (*Nan pei ch'ao*), which continued from the beginning of the fourth century until the reunification of the empire under the Sui in 589, was distinguished, especially in the north, by unrest resembling that of the waning Chou period in the fourth and third centuries B.C. During the course of 170 years, twenty states—

ruled primarily by non-Chinese families of widely differing ethnic backgrounds—rose and fell in the north. During the same period, however, the south experienced only six dynasties and remained under Chinese control.[1]

Just as the two Han dynasties, following centuries of unrest, had established a totally new culture in China, the chaos that erupted following this period of "classical Chinese antiquity" also gave birth to a unified country, the cosmopolitan culture of which, though, was remarkably different from that of the largely independent and self-contained Han civilization. The unrest and social uncertainty of the transitional period once again shaped the intellectual outlook of all segments of the population. During the final century of the Late Han, the rural population had experienced increasing misery, as the formation of large estates and quasi-feudal conditions forced them from their lands and into a nomadic existence. These masses constituted a willing source of converts to religious Taoism, whose influence had by no means ended with the destruction of the state of Chang Lu; in the following centuries, Taoism provided the ideological basis not only for more or less secret movements but also for certain smaller states. Even the upper strata of Chinese society were affected by the intellectual consequences of the decline of the Han order. In the north, where Chinese officials were forced to administrate the governments of foreign rulers, the Confucian system of values lost almost all of its binding force. In the south, the inability of the system to protect China from barbarian invasion and the partition of the united empire may have raised doubts about the value of Confucianism as a social philosophy; here, too, non-Confucian currents, especially Buddhism and the strain of macrobiotic Taoism propounded by Ko Hung during the early fourth century, attracted great attention and a large following. As Franke and Trauzettel have pointed out, these trends were accompanied by an increased emphasis on the individual; there are numerous instances of pronounced social nonconformism. "State and Family were no longer the primary concern, but rather the autonomous 'I'."[2]

Historical conditions proved particularly favorable to Buddhist doctrine, which greatly influenced the further development of the above-mentioned tendencies. Buddhism had entered China through Central Asia in the first century. The earliest reliable indication of the existence of a Buddhist community dates from A.D. 65. It appears that the upper stratum of society was the first attracted to the new teaching. But by the fourth century at the latest, Buddhism had infiltrated all segments of the population. It was inevitable that such fundamental ideological upheavals also brought a new dimension to the treatment of illness, expanding the already existing spectrum of distinctly conceptualized therapy systems in China. The system of healing introduced by Buddhism differed, as we shall see, from purely Chinese systems in that, almost from its very arrival in China, it proved to be conceptually far more intricate. The integral tradition of Indian medicine, which combined secular elemental doctrine with aspects of demonology, mythology, and moral-macrocosmic concepts, entered China with traveling monks and the texts they brought with them. But like the medicine of systematic correspondences, for instance, Buddhist medicine also combined a primarily non-normative science, that is, the doctrine of Four Elements—which, at least superficially, resembled the Chinese doctrine of the Five Phases—with ideas that derived directly from the normative moral system of Buddhist religion. An understanding of Buddhist medical writings in China is impossible without a knowledge of the basic concepts of Buddhist religion.

The origins of Buddhism are traditionally associated with an Indian prince named Gautama Sakyamuni, who lived during the sixth and fifth centuries B.C. Raised in luxury and with all earthly benefits as the son of the ruler of a small kingdom at the foot of the Himalayas, the young prince nevertheless decided to leave his carefree existence to search for religious enlightenment. At the age of thirty-five he had a vision; for the rest of his life Gautama was known as Buddha and preached his insights to great numbers of disciples. Like Taoism (although not nearly so restricted geographically), the doctrine of Buddhism that developed from these beginnings, and which later spread throughout Asia, is a philosophy fragmented into numerous individual movements and frequently contradictory interpretations. These sects were (and still are) related only by their belief in *karma* and rebirth, two concepts adopted from previous Indian thought. Karma can be translated roughly as "deed" or "action." Every human action has an effect that produces happiness or suffering during a later existence. The accumulation and assessment of positive or negative karma proceeds under its own autonomous law; supervision by identifiable, personified metaphysical authorities is not required. Similar concepts are already present in the *Upanishads*. The new dimension introduced by Buddha to the karma concept is the moral foundation on which the evaluation of human action is carried out. Buddha taught that the performance of certain ritual (and frequently severely ascetic) measures was, in itself, neither appropriate nor necessary for the accumulation of positive karma; consequently, not only did human conduct have to follow ethical laws, but the actual performance of a good deed could be recognized only if it had been carried out with good intentions. It was thus possible to amass positive karma solely through good intentions, even if one had been unable to carry out the action itself.

Depending on the karma accumulated in the past, each individual must endure an endless cycle of innumerable reincarnations at various levels of existence. Two positive forms—god and man—are contrasted with three negative possibilities of existence—reincarnation as an animal, as a demon, and as the inhabitant of one of the numerous hells. One of Buddha's fundamental insights is the recognition that all life consists primarily of suffering. Birth, growing old, death, separation from loved ones, unfulfilled desires—all this is suffering and characterizes human existence from beginning to end. Only one who is able to escape the endless cycle of rebirth and death and enter an indescribable state or condition, in which there is no existence as we know it and consequently no pain, can achieve salvation. Mortals lack the words to describe this condition, *nirvana,* for man can only comprehend in categories of good and evil; any such dualism is absent in nirvana. Buddha therefore declined to communicate any further details about nirvana.

The long path that leads to enlightenment and, ultimately, salvation begins with an understanding of the Four Noble Truths, which Buddha revealed in his first sermon: (1) life is composed of suffering; (2) this suffering is caused by the urge to live and the craving for sensual pleasure; (3) a possibility exists to end this pain; (4) this possibility lies in the Eightfold Way—correct views, correct intentions, correct speech, correct behavior, correct living, correct effort, correct attitude, and correct concentration. Buddha summarized this ethos in the following imperative: "Do no evil; perform good deeds and purify the spirit!" Every action is evil, he explained, that harms others, harms oneself, or harms both others and oneself. Correct speech is the avoidance of lies, slander, and insults. Correct behavior is exemplified by one who does not kill, steal, and who lives a chaste life.

Gautama's teachings led first to the establishment of monastic communities, in which each member sought individual salvation. In Theravada or Hinayana Buddhism, as this early sect is called, the immediate goal is to become an Arhat, a "holy man" who has successfully discarded all passions and thus has achieved full control over his life. The Arhat can therefore look forward to an early transition to nirvana. The Theravada version of Buddhism is basically an antisocial philosophy. Only the monk (or nun), member of a monastic order, can attain salvation. The figure of the Arhat appears as a cold, passionless ideal who has eliminated all appetites and who, outside of human society, dedicates himself to a private religious life organized solely for personal benefit.[3] The prerequisite, then, was the renunciation of all ties to family and state. The accumulation of meritorious karma was restricted to those who had performed the appropriate good deeds; the possibility of a transferral of positive karma to less fortunate persons was not present in early Buddhism.

Even before these teachings reached China, a second sect, the Mahayana version, arose in Indian Buddhism. According to this new view, everyone, both monks and laymen, could seek and attain salvation. The religious ideal of this doctrine, a doctrine based on belief in and devotion to Buddha and love and compassion for all mankind, was the bodhisattva. The bodhisattva, a being already destined for salvation because of his inexhaustible wealth of positive karma, nevertheless postpones his transition to nirvana in order to assist those unfortunate souls unable to accumulate any positive karma for themselves. The bodhisattva has the power to allow the needy to share his karma. Of the numerous individuals from antiquity who were subsequently active as bodhisattvas, Avalokitesvara probably has the most significance for medical care. Avalokitesvara—known in Chinese Buddhism since the seventh century as the Goddess of Mercy, Kuan-yin—is constantly searching with a thousand eyes for sufferers, whose misery he is able to alleviate with a thousand hands. He reduces the pain of those individuals in the numerous hells, and on earth he protects man whenever possible from the dangers of water, fire, demons, and other enemies, as well as from illness. These notions of the activities of the bodhisattva were reflected in religious practice: during periods of extreme misery and indigence, the faithful prayed to these benefactors, seeking their assistance.

For centuries, educated Chinese considered the new doctrine, which had been brought to China over southern trade routes by Central Asian and Indian monks, to be only a new variant of religious Taoism. According to legend, Lao Tzu had disappeared in the west near the end of his life, giving credence to the notion that he subsequently reappeared there as Buddha. Chinese Taoists soon were assisting in the selection and translation of Buddhist texts, a process that had significant influence on the terminology of early Chinese Buddhist literature.

By about A.D. 100, there were already several regional strongholds of the new doctrine in China. In Lo-yang foreign monks organized the first center devoted to intensive translation. Foreigners active in Lo-yang included Parthians, Scythians, Sogdians, Indians, and other, unspecified Central Asians. Soon after the beginning of missionary activity, and still during the Han period, Buddhism in China experienced a first conceptual expansion. The original Indian concept of an endless chain of rebirths, occurring without a soul to provide successive existences with the appearance of individual continuity, was revised in China by the idea of an eternally indissoluble soul, which each time during the ongoing process of reincarnation was provided with a different mortal shell. Additional diverging interpretations of the original doctrine soon followed, each accompanied by the establishment of corresponding movements and sects and literary genres. Further details are available in the special literature on the subject and need not concern us here, since these developments are of minor significance for an understanding of Buddhist healing.

The political division of China into a northern half ruled by barbarians, on the one hand, and into various southern, Chinese-dominated dynasties, on the other hand, also split Buddhism. In some of the northern regions Buddhism took a form resembling state religion, characterized by chauvinistic attitudes that required action for the benefit of the state; in the south, the religion of Buddhism had a more fundamentally educational nature. Despite these diverse developments, it is important to remember that during this century, prior to the reunification of the empire near the end of the sixth century, Buddhism—to an even greater extent than religious Taoism—became an integral part of Chinese culture, affecting nearly all social strata.

6.2. INDIAN MEDICINE AND THE BUDDHIST LITERATURE OF CHINA

I have already pointed out that Buddhist healing, like the medicine of systematic correspondences, combined primarily non-normative insights of natural philosophy with normative conceptions generated by the moral prescripts of Buddhist religion. A comparison of the norms of the medicine of systematic correspondences with those reflected in Buddhist medical literature reveals an obvious parallel to the well-known saying of Hsiao Tzu-hsien (489–537) in his history of the

Southern Ch'i dynasty: "Confucius and Lao-tzu were mainly concerned with the order of this world; for Shakyamuni, the most important goal is to depart from this world!"[4]

The norms reflected by Buddhist medicine are directed exclusively toward the elimination of individual suffering; unlike the medicine of systematic correspondences, they contain no indications of an ideal earthly existence or harmonious society. This situation was not changed by the so-called altruism of Mahayana Buddhism, with its advocacy of compassion toward all mankind, or by the proscriptions against killing, theft, and other injurious actions that were derived from Hinayana doctrine. Each individual was simply confronted with a list of ethical commandments; compliance would eventually lead to release from the cycle of suffering caused by birth and death. Wolfgang Bauer has summarized these basic tenets in Buddhism:

> It is obvious that this intellectual climate was not propitious to the creation of models for an ideal social order. It was not worth the effort to construct emergency solutions for a world doomed to inevitable suffering, for they could not have the eternal validity indispensable to any ideal. What was the use of an exemplary political system or of a happy life in a setting where it was commonly held that the monk who had freed himself from the obligations and pleasures state and family might offer was closest to ultimate salvation? It was a world where, as stubborn Confucians often complained, fanaticism did not stop short of self-mutilation if this would ensure salvation. Thus hope turned from this calamitous vale of tears to the beyond.[5]

The strenuous efforts for deliverance from individual suffering, efforts which even encompassed tangible physical pain—in the case of illness—as well as the lack of normative structures that could have supported a specific social system, may have contributed to the ease with which Buddhist literature fused various secular and pre-Buddhist nonsecular systems of Indian medicine into a conglomerate of differing concepts. Numerous non-Buddhist texts in China, at least since the T'ang period (618–906), combine regulations and arguments adopted from many systems of ideas. It was not unusual for the same author to recommend several remedies for a specific ailment, some borrowed from pragmatic drug therapy, some from demonology, and some from the medicine of systematic correspondences, or even Buddhism. But authors of such compilations were practitioners concerned solely with providing a spectrum of possibly efficacious prescriptions. I have emphasized conceptual diversity in Buddhist literature because it is Buddha himself, the creator of the dogma, who is credited with therapeutic eclecticism. We know of nothing similar in any other advanced religion or philosophy. Christianity provides an instructive comparison. Jesus of Nazareth is portrayed in the New Testament as a proponent of a strict, narrowly conceived system of healing that assigns God the Father sole power over well-being and illness and allows not the slightest doubt that the future dominion of God on earth is both complete and unlimited. There was no place for a secular science that could have challenged this primacy; it was only much later, in part against fierce opposition by dogmatists, that such thoughts became part of the Christian world view.[6]

The ultimate goal of Buddhism—the termination of existential suffering for every individual—invites comparisons with the objectives of medicine. Buddha is frequently termed the "King of Physicians," the only possessor of the true remedy for the eternal cure of illness:

> The worldly medical man knows of no true remedies, those that can cure him from birth, growing old, illness, and death. He knows only the four elements that comprise the body, while Buddha—that supreme physician—incorporates six elements[7] and eighteen levels[8] into his deliberations and takes into account the passions; Buddha is therefore concerned with the entire phenomenon of suffering and liberates mankind from birth and death.[9]

The above-mentioned Four Noble Truths are often formulated in medical terminology reminiscent of the cycle of diagnosis, etiology, remedy, and therapy. The following passage from the *Samyuktagama*, for example, attributed to the Hinayana school, was recorded in a Chinese version at the beginning of the fifth century:

> A sutra spoken by Buddha: He is a great king of physicians who is able to realize the following principles; first, to understand the illness well, which means [to be able to differentiate] the various illnesses; second, to understand the origin of illness, whether it be caused by wind, phlegm, saliva, or various types of colds, whether the illness is acute or due to the season; third, to understand the antidotes, these are salves, cough remedies or emetics, laxatives, nose drops or aromatic medications; fourth, to be skilled in treating illnesses without fear of a relapse.[10]

In this connection, only nirvana is described as the attainment of absolute health; a Chinese formulation defines nirvana as *wu-ping*, that is, "the condition free from illness."[11]

The Hinayana and Mahayana doctrines differed greatly in their attitude toward medical practice. In older Hinayana writings, medicine had been considered a worldly science that monks were forbidden to learn. Members of the monastic community were expressly prohibited from earning their livelihood by the medical treatment of laymen. Buddha, however, upon finding a sick monk who had been ignored and neglected by fellow brothers striving for their own personal salvation, had admonished the latter to assist one another in such circumstances. Thus it became the duty of monks to preach to brothers who had fallen ill, to recite to them the precepts of ancient sages, and, if necessary, to summon Buddha himself to the sickbed for assistance. Only a monk, it was claimed, is competent to provide the necessary spiritual assistance—the recitations from doctrine, the encouragement of indifference and patience—the specific "remedies" an ill monk requires above all else. Attendance by anyone other than a monk can only be a temporary measure, for religious support not only possesses moral value but also leads to physical recovery from illness. A sutra of the *Ekottaragama* records the five characteristics that indicate an incompetent monastic attendance: first, ignorance of effective remedies; second, signs of unwillingness and a lack of dedication; third, indulgence in expressions of disgust and insensitivity; fourth, attendance of the patient solely with the intention of being compensated for the care; and fifth, failure to preach to the patient or converse with him. The patients, too, were reminded of the five types of faulty behavior that impede recovery: first, indiscriminate eating and drinking; second, refusal to take nourishment at the prescribed times; third, refusal to take medications; fourth, indulgence in excessive grief, joy, or disgust; and fifth, insufficient compassion and attention from the other monks. Hinayana writings repeatedly emphasize that the treatment of monks and nuns must be carried out in complete secrecy; any contact with the public must be strictly avoided. Violations of this rule were viewed as sins and entailed the appropriate consequences.[12]

The principle of universal sympathy and compassion toward all fellow men, developed by the Mahayana school, had a completely different effect on medical practice. Each person was reminded of his duty to care for and treat all who are sick, whether monk or layman. Medicine is one of the five secular sciences whose study is mandatory even for the bodhisattvas, and active medical treatment is expressly required. A short anecdote from the *Gandavyuha,* translated into Chinese toward the end of the seventh century and again at the end of the eighth century, illustrates the bodhisattva principle that only a sound body possesses the healthy spirit that enables the free pursuit of knowledge and enlightenment. The passage relates how the young Sudhana, in search of religious instruction, meets his friend Samantanetra. Samantanetra, an apothecary initiated into medical science by the bodhisattva Manjusri, advises Sudhana to study medicine. Astonished, Sudhana answers that he has come to discover which skills are required of a bodhisattva and asks why he should learn medicine. To this, the apothecary replies:

> Behold! What an eminent man! For a bodhisattva attempting to achieve enlightenment there is no greater obstacle than illness! When living beings are burdened with an ailing body, the spirit cannot be at peace. How can perfection be achieved under such circumstances? The bodhisattva who strives for enlightenment must therefore first heal the afflictions of the body.[13]

This explicit sanction of medical treatment was based on intricate conceptions of body structure, the causes of illness, and the measures required for the treatment of illness. According to the dominant natural-philosophical theory in Chinese Buddhist literature, the body was composed of four elements—earth, water, fire, and wind.[14] The *Ratnakuta,* translated into Chinese in the second century, offers the following commentary:

> 1. Earth comprises all that is solid in the human body. This includes hair, nails, teeth, skin, flesh, muscles, bones, spleen, kidneys, liver, lungs, intestines, feces, bladder, membranes, brain, etc.
> 2. Water comprises all that is fluid in the human body. This includes tears, perspiration, nasal mucus, saliva, pus, blood, marrow, milk, urine, etc.
> 3. Fire comprises all that is fiery or warm in the human body. This includes the entire digestive system.
> 4. Wind comprises all that is in motion in the human body. This includes the winds in the four limbs, in the five parts of the body, inhalation and exhalation, etc.[15]

Illness arises when one or more of these four elements is increased or decreased excessively. The resulting imbalance can cause 101 afflictions associated with each element, making a total of 404 possible illnesses.

The *tri-dosa* theory of Ayurveda medicine was also introduced to China from India, but it never achieved there the influence and respect it commands to this day in its native land. While the terms earth, fire, water, and wind were easily translated into Chinese, the three *dosa* apparently posed significant difficulties. No single definition exists in the Chinese Buddhist canon for the concepts wind, mucus, and bile, which had been equated with various terms in various Chinese texts.[16] The term *dosa* itself was translated by the Chinese *tu* "poison," which only vaguely conveys the original meaning of "deficiency, defect." The concept of the four "elements," which later was usually rendered as *ta* ("large") or *chung* ("seed, kind") for the Sanscrit *mahabhuta*, also underwent a shift in meaning when it was translated as *ping* ("illness") in a Chinese text from A.D. 230. It is possible that the notion of the four-part elementary composition of the body was so foreign to the Chinese, who—and here it is necessary to recall the initial interconnection of Buddhism and Taoism—adhered to the conception of finest matter *ching*, that the choice of *ping* was an attempt to establish a relationship with more familiar ideas of the causes of illness. The imprecision resulting from such terminology is evident in the following passage of the sutra "Ch'i-ch'u san-kuan ching," which was translated into Chinese as early as A.D. 151 by the Parthian An Shih-kao:

> I learned the following. Once, while staying in Sravasti, Buddha went for a walk in Jetavana Park. There he spoke to the monks: Shih-chien yu san ta ping. Jen-shen chung ko tzu yu. Ho teng wei san. I wei feng. Erh wei je. San wei han. Shih san ta ping.

Here the Chinese terms *ta* and *ping* are combined. Buddha's remarks could be translated as follows, in the manner that would certainly have been most obvious to an impartial Chinese reader:

> In this world there are three grave illnesses. All appear independently in the human body. What are they? The first is [caused by] wind; the second is [caused by] heat; the third is [caused by] cold.

If however, we recall that "mucus" in the tri-dosa doctrine was occasionally translated with *leng* ("cold") and "bile" with *je* ("heat"), it is possible to view this text as an erroneous interpretation of a tri-dosa statement that utilizes terminology from the four-elements doctrine. The passage could then be translated as follows:

> In this world there are three elements [= deficiencies, *dosa*]. All are present in the human body from the very beginning. What are they? The first is wind; the second is bile; the third is mucus.

The text then continues:

> Monks are familiar with three remedies for these three "grave illnesses"
> [or *dosa*]. If a monk is stricken with the "grave illness" of wind, hemp-
> oil or hemp-oil-like [medications] are essential remedies (*ta-yao*). If he
> has been stricken with the "grave illness" of heat, butter cheese or butter
> cheese-like [medicines] are important remedies. If he has been stricken
> with the "grave illness" of cold, honey or honey-like [medications] are
> important remedies. These are the three "grave illnesses" and the three
> essential remedies of the monks.
>
> Human beings suffer from three more afflictions, with which they grow
> up and live and which are detected by ethical measures. What are they?
> The first is desire; the second is anger; the third is ignorance. Monks
> are familiar with three important remedies for these three "grave ill-
> nesses." When a monk has been stricken by the "grave illness" of desire,
> the only significant medication is [the consumption of] his own excre-
> ment and meditation. He who is stricken by the "grave illness" of anger
> must practice universal compassion. Reflection on the ultimate origin
> and causality of all things is the essential medicine for one who has
> been stricken by the "grave illness" of ignorance. These are the three
> remedies for the three "grave illnesses" of monks. Thus spoke Buddha![17]

Toward the end of the sixth century, one author combined these
and other concepts into a six-part etiology, which differentiated among:

1. illnesses caused by disharmony among the four elements;
2. illnesses caused by imbalanced nutrition
3. illnesses caused by excessive meditation
4. illnesses caused by demons
5. illnesses brought about by evil gods (Mara)
6. illnesses caused by improper conduct during a previous existence.

Accordingly, there were various types of appropriate therapy. These
were, for illnesses from categories one and two: medicinal and dietetic
measures; for illnesses from category three: an improvement of ascetic
and meditative routine, as well as close regulation of breathing; for
illnesses from categories four and five: amulets, incantations, introspection; and for illnesses from category six: introspection, confession,
contrition, and penitence.[18]

The incantations (*dharanis*) recommended to combat demons, which
continually attack the viscera, and evil gods, which confound the
senses, appear in Chinese translation beginning in A.D. 230. Demon-

ological concepts and belief in gods that cause or cure illness have their origin in ancient Indian cultural elements. Buddhism integrated these features to a certain extent (gods and demons were also subject to the law of karma), just as Hinduism had incorporated them. These ideas experienced a late renaissance in tantric literature, which appeared in India in the sixth century, reaching China during the eighth century.

6.3. INDIAN CATARACT SURGERY IN CHINA

Aside from the already-mentioned etiological concepts and their related therapeutic practices, some pragmatic therapeutic techniques appear to have entered China from India during the first millennium A.D. Most conspicuous in Chinese medical literature is cataract surgery, which may have been introduced to China at some time between the seventh and the ninth century.

Cataract surgery could be called a "mechanical" therapeutic intervention based on the "mechanical" idea that a specific kind of impaired vision is the result of the movement of a certain substance into the eyes (with the movement of this substance having been stimulated by some external pathological influence). Such an idea differs from the understanding characterizing the medicine of systematic correspondence. The latter, in general, focuses on functions; it sees illnesses mainly as evidence of a malfunctioning of one or more of the recognized functional units constituting the organism. Hence the medicine of systematic correspondence seeks to alleviate illness by manipulating the functions of those basic units in the organism that are associated, through the chains of correspondence defined by the yinyang and Five Phases paradigms, with those sections of the body where an illness has become manifest. This approach to therapy did not stimulate the development of surgery; on the contrary, by adding needed influences from outside (for instance, by means of drugs or food) or by affecting the internal course and generation of influences through certain external stimuli (such as needles), the medicine of systematic correspondence sought to redirect all the functional units of the organism to their normal, or ideal, level of activity.

Ophthalmology may serve as an example. Chinese medical texts based on the concepts of systematic correspondence saw vision and the eyes as intimately tied to the functioning of the liver. An impaired functioning of the liver, then, may lead to impaired vision. Hence one must treat the liver in order to cure the eye. To apply surgery (which, in this understanding, could be directed against nothing but a secondary symptom) at the eyes lay beyond the imagination of the adherents of the medicine of systematic correspondence. As becomes apparent from a survey of Chinese ophthalmological literature, the idea of treating certain ailments of the eyes surgically was introduced to China solely through Indian mediation. It remains unclear, though, whether a conceptual bridge existed that reached from the earliest references to cataract surgery in Greek sources of the second century B.C. via such references in the Indian medical classic Susruta (first half of the first millennium A.D.) to the first known references to cataract surgery in China only a few centuries later.

In chapter 21 of his voluminous collection of prescriptions *Wai-t'ai pi-yao* (compiled A.D. 752), Wang Tao introduced a Taoist named Hsieh who allegedly had received ophthalmological instructions from a foreigner from a Western country, which was identified as *T'ien-chu*, India. This Taoist Hsieh explains in a number of essays the nature and the structure of the eyes, basing his arguments partially on the Buddhist four-elements theory as it was introduced to China about six centuries ago through the *Ratnakuta-sutra* (see above p. 141). Here, possibly for the first time, references may be found to cataract surgery in Chinese literature. Hsieh describes the "screen" to be

> of greenish-white color. One cannot distinguish [individual] items, but one knows whether it is light or dark and whether any of the three sources of light are present. One knows day and night. In such cases a downflow of brain causes the green-blindness of the eyes. Before one suffers from this affliction, he suddenly has a feeling as if he saw black spots such as flying flies in front of his eyes. [Once the screen has formed,] it is appropriate to apply the metal-comb to resolve [this problem]. Once [the eyes] have been needled, they are clear again, as if the clouds had opened and the bright sun appeared.[19]

In a subsequent paragraph, Hsieh points out that the screen, which is believed to be caused by the joint influence of heat and wind into a situation of deficiency, can be "removed through cutting [the eye] with a sickle" (*kou-ko ch'u chih*).[20] Details of the actual operation are not given. All the many suggestions, added by Wang Tao to these introductory remarks, for the procedure to cure "screen-ailments" of the eyes, belong to conventional treatment by means of drugs directed at the basic functional units of the organism.

The term *comb,* though, appears again in the context of ophthalmological surgery in a poem composed by Liu Yü-hsi (772–842), obviously expressing his own or somebody else's gratitude and surprise about a successful operation. The poem, entitled "The Brahman-Priest Physician Who Bestowed Eyes" reads:

> Three autumns [ago] injury harmed my vision.
> I wept all day; my journey had come to an end.
> With both my eyes dark henceforth,
> I was an old man in the middle of my life.
> I gazed at vermillion, gradually it turned to jade-green.
> I was afraid of the sun; no longer could I endure the wind.
> This master knows an art to comb it out entirely!
> How did he lift the covering?[21]

Which specific ailment was cured here cannot be determined with certainty. However, the use of the term "to comb" to illustrate the removal of a "covering" may refer to cataract surgery. This interpretation receives some justification by the fact that no other form of eye surgery has ever been documented in traditional Chinese medical literature. Perhaps we may conclude from the question in the final line of Liu Yü-hsi's poem that ophthalmological surgery—probably cataract surgery—was practiced in China in the ninth century but had not yet become integrated into Chinese medical knowledge and skills: it remained a domain of Indian priest-physicians.

The *Ishimpō,* a collection of medical lore practiced in China compiled by the Japanese Tamba Yasuyori in 984, refers to a specific text as a source offering instructions on cataract surgery.[22] It quotes a *Yen-lun,* believed to be the *Lung-shu yen-lun.* Lung-shu is the Chinese adaptation of the Indian name Nagarjuna. Nagarjuna (fl. second century A.D.) was the founder of a specific Mahayana school, and legend has identified him as a great healer.[23] The bibliography of the Sui dynasty, among its eleven titles referring to Indian medical lore, lists three texts ascribed to Nagarjuna, but the *Lung-shu yen-lun* is not included. A book of this title appears only in Sung bibliographies and seems to have been lost in China afterward. It is not clear whether a printed copy discovered in Korea and a Japanese manuscript of the same title and extant today are identical with the original.[24]

Quoting the (*Lung-shu*) *yen-lun,* the *Ishimpō* discusses various pathological states of the eyes to be treated with different needle- or sickle-shaped instruments employed to incise the eyes. The text provides some details on the operations to be performed but does not describe the entire process.

Another text to be considered here is the *Sheng-chi tsung-lu* of 1117, a comprehensive collection of prescriptions compiled on order of Emperor Hui-tsung (ruled 1101–1126). In chapter 111 it is stated again that the "screen" is formed by brain fat flowing downward.[25] In a subsequent paragraph, the reader is referred to a work named *Lung-mu lun* for details of cataract surgery. The *Lung-mu lun,* whose title once more refers to the Nagarjuna-Bodhisattva, was mentioned in a Ming bibliography in the ophthalmological section; it may not have been compiled prior to the Sung or Yüan dynasty.[26]

Finally, I wish to quote a few paragraphs from the *Yen-k'o ta-ch'üan,* an ophthalmological compendium published by Fu Jen-yü in 1644, a late source presenting cataract surgery in a Buddhist context. Fu Jen-yü spoke of "poking" (*po*) when he referred to the pushing downward of the cataract with a needle:

Prior to the poking one asks the patient to wash his eyes with icy water until the passage of blood and influences is interrupted. [Then] both [of the patient's] hands grasp a paper ball. [The patient] should sit upright on a chair. One employs two men to firmly hold the [patient's] head. The physician uses first the thumb and the index finger of his left hand to open the skin of eyes, and he firmly presses down the black pupil so that it cannot move. Then he takes with his right hand a metal needle. If the right eye is to be poked, the patient is asked to look to the right. This is of advantage for the insertion of the needle because the bridge of the nose will not obstruct the [physician's] hand. In the middle between the black pupil on the one side and the large corner of the eye on the other side the needle is slowly inserted. After that the needle is tilted toward its head until [its end] reaches the place of the affliction. There the brain-fat is poked downward. Again [the needle] is moved upward and another time [the brain-fat] is poked downward. Now the patient is asked whether he can see the movement of a finger or a greenish or white color and he will distinguish these clearly. Following this the brain-fat is brought to the large corner of the eye while a hole is opened to let the fat flow into the water until the entire place is free of it. Subsequently the needle is slowly removed. It should not be removed [too] early because there is a risk that the brain-fat returns to its original position. If the left eye is to be poked, [the patient] looks toward the left pointed corner of the eye.[27]

Whenever one applies the needle [in cataract surgery], he faces the spirits and offers a sacrifice to the Buddha on new moon or full moon. He declares his native village and his name, then he speaks the incantation [see below] with reverence. The use of the needle should also happen on new moon or full moon. The incantation should be spoken seven times. One talisman should be written, to be attached to the needle. Prior to using [the needle] one must fast. Also, incense and candles are to be offered. Then another talisman has to be written to

take hold of the divine light of the sun and to join it with the eyesight
[of the patient]. In addition, the following incantation has to be spoken:
"Save from bitterness; save from distress! I trust in you[28] Kuan-yin
Bodhisattva." Then the needle will turn by itself and he who uses the
needle will have both his heart and his gall[29] opened widely and he will
be free of any fear. After the "three sources of light" talisman has been
written one inserts the needle. It should be a clear day. Wait for a *k'ai,
ch'eng, ch'u,* or *shou* day; avoid a *tzu* day.[30]

The incantation reads:
Clear, pure eyes, purple gold lanterns.
Wine, wine, water.
Leave the yellow sand, fill depots and channels.
The Dragon King [Nagaraja] has
a thousand hands and a thousand eyes.
[to his left] Manjusri [the guardian of wisdom] the great
    officer rides on a lion;
[to his right] Samantabhadra Bodhisattva [the guardian of
    law] rides on an elephant.
The King says: Divine night conceals clouds and membranes.
The screen dissolves entirely and vanishes.
Strength over strength; happiness over happiness!
On high the assembly of *bala* [strength]
exerts the very best benefits;
in the eyes, everywhere is light obtained, and brilliance.[31]

The text continues with instructions on how to bandage the eye
after surgery and how to treat postoperative pain. Illustrations of the
two talismans to be written are also provided.

6.4. THE CHINESE RECEPTION OF
INDIAN BUDDHIST MEDICINE

Buddhist monks offered medical treatment to the inhabitants of their
host country for a great variety of reasons. In addition to the ethical
obligation to provide assistance to all men, the missionary value of
such action was recognized early and is mentioned as a reason for
therapeutic activity. Fo-t'u-teng (fl. 310–349), for instance, realized
that the tenets of his religion were too profound for the rulers in the
small state of Shih Lo (later Chao) to appreciate fully. He therefore
repeatedly demonstrated his knowledge and the value of his teaching
through various magical and clairvoyant activities, including raising
of the dead, rain spells, and divination.[32]

At the institutional level, Buddhists participated in various charitable actions and organizations. As a result of their influence, the alien dynasty of the Northern Wei, which had converted to Buddhism, established grain reserves to relieve the suffering of the population. It was not unusual for convents and monasteries to incorporate dispensaries for the treatment of lay patients. At the instigation of the empress Wu, a supporter of Buddhism at the time, these "hospitals" were even assigned to a special department during the governmental period *ch'ang-an* (701–705). Although frightened civil servants—citing Confucius who had criticized his pupil Tzu-lu for wanting to use his possessions for the benefit of the poor in the Wei state—attempted to rescind such official protection, the hospitals even survived for a time the extensive wave of secularization in A.D. 845. None of these activities, however, left a lasting impression on the Chinese public health system. The same is true for the "charitable apothecaries" (*hui-min yao-chü*) established by the state during the Sung (960–1279), a scandal-ridden and limited program that never achieved more than a brief significance. With the decline of Buddhism to a folk religion during subsequent centuries, official interest in such charitable organizations also seems to have died out. Not until the widespread appearance of Christianity during the nineteenth century did the integration of missionary and medical activities by a foreign religion reemerge in China, accompanied once again by the establishment of significant numbers of hospitals.

Medical concepts introduced to China by Buddhist literature followed a similar course. T'ao Hung-ching (452–536), the renowned Taoist and author of medical works, wrote a supplement to the prescription collection *Chou-hou fang* of Ko Hung (281–341) entitled *Chou-hou-pai-i fang* (Prescription Handbook Enlarged by 101 Prescriptions). In a preface dated 500—the only portion of the work that has survived—the author acknowledges Buddhist influence.[33] Additional evidence is provided by the "Indian" titles in the bibliography of the Sui dynasty (589–618), compiled in 636. Some of the therapeutic works listed contain the character *Po-lo-men* in their title, which most likely stands for "Brahman." Among the texts, for instance, is one entitled *Po-lo-men yao-fang* (Medicinal Prescriptions of the Brahmans). But as little survives from this work as from another long-lost title that indicates a knowledge of "Western," that is, Indian medical men: *Hsi-yü ming-i so-chi yao-fang* (Important Prescriptions Collected by Renowned Physicians of Western Lands).[34] Only purely religious elements of Indian healing gained a foothold in China, developing into an important component of the total spectrum of available medical care. Even today, Buddhists continue to pray for release from bodily suffering to the goddess Kuan-yin, the Chinese form adapted from the originally male bodhisattva Avalokitesvara. Buddhist oracular medicine is still prevalent wherever Buddhist doctrine is able to develop unimpeded. Receptacles in the temples contain numbered wooden slips, which the faithful draw out after an appropriate prayer. The number drawn refers to a prescription—kept in the temple—that is to be followed as a direction of the bodhisattva.

Of the six-part etiology reproduced above, only illnesses caused by disharmony among the four elements, excessive meditation, and improper conduct during a previous existence were completely new. While it is not difficult to understand that meditation- and karma-etiology remained restricted almost exclusively to Buddhist writings, it may at first seem surprising that even the doctrine of the four elements did not play a significant role in the medicotheoretical discussion in China. The only author influenced by such concepts was Sun Ssu-miao. He is repeatedly cited in Western secondary sources as an example of the purported Buddhist influence on Chinese medicine. But no mention is made of the fact that Sun Ssu-miao had no followers in this respect. Wang Tao simply quoted an obscure Taoist when he presented the four-elements theory. In subsequent centuries, Buddhist concepts of retribution appear only in discussions of medical-ethical problems;[35] occasionally, an author added a Buddhist incantation to his collection of prescriptions. The four-element theory—from my point of view the most significant—had, as far as can be determined from available sources, only a negligible impact on the secular-medical literature of China. We can only guess as to why this completely unknown doctrine, which claimed that the body was composed of different material elements, met with such a lack of interest in China. Perhaps the cultural gap was simply too great, or the attempts to bridge that gap too cursory, for genuine reception to have taken place. Sun Ssu-miao's text, reproduced below, tends to support this conclusion. In the first sentence the concept of the four elements is introduced with desirable clarity, indicating that a faithful presentation of the doctrine is to follow. But Sun Ssu-miao immediately incorporates the foreign concepts into Chinese notions of the influences to which all men are subject, thereby removing any attraction these ideas may have had as an alternative. Moreover, the author also included the five phases in his short presentation:

> As it is written in the commentaries of the Buddhist sutras, man is composed of earth, water, fire, and wind. Whenever the influence of fire in man is not in perfect harmony [with the other influences], vapor

and heat arise in the body. Whenever the influence of wind is out of balance, the entire body is extended and all pores are blocked. Whenever the influence of water is out of balance, the body swells up and breathing becomes heavy, gasping and raw. Whenever the influence of earth is out of balance, the four limbs are immobile; the voice is silent. When fire disappears, the body becomes cold. When the wind subsides, the [flow of] influences is interrupted. When the water dries up, so too does the blood. When earth is dispersed, the body bursts. Yet ignorant physicians do not take into account the pulse and treat illnesses in a completely incorrect manner. Thus, they cause the five phases to destroy one another in the depots and interrupt [the circulation of the influences]. This is the same as pouring oil on a burning fire [that one wishes to extinguish]! Great care must be taken! When all four influences are in balance, then all four spirits are also in harmony. If one influence is out of balance [with the others], 101 illnesses are caused. If all four spirits are disturbed, 404 illnesses arise at the same time. It is also said that there are 101 illnesses that disappear without treatment, 101 illnesses that require treatment to be cured, 101 illnesses that are difficult to cure even with treatment, and, finally, 101 illnesses that are fatal and are not treated.[36]

In a later chapter Sun Ssu-miao returned to the existence of 404 afflictions. In his efforts to reconcile this concept with the Chinese cycle of five, he does not hesitate to incorporate a mathematical inaccuracy:

There are four types of illness. These are: first, paralysis caused by cold; second, illness caused by [malignant or unbalanced] influences; third, malignant winds; fourth, poisoning by heat or hot poisons. When the patient has calmed down and has returned the influences to a state of harmony through the methods described here, none of the illnesses will remain uncured. All possible illnesses are connected with one of the five depots. In each depot, 81 kinds of illness are caused by cold, heat, wind, and influences. This makes a total of 404 illnesses. He who wishes to be knowledgeable must understand these relationships.[37]

Sun Ssu-miao's interest in the four-element doctrine remained an insignificant footnote in the history of Chinese medicine. The same is true for the possibly legendary figure of Hua T'o (110–207), whose successes in surgical practice are reminiscent of similar reports of achievements by the Indian physician Jivaka.[38] He, too, had no successor to carry on his art; the frequent references in Chinese and Western secondary literature to Hua T'o as an early example of surgery and anesthesiology present a distorted picture of the actual significance of such practices in China.

A careful survey of the vast body of Chinese medical literature not yet sufficiently scrutinized may, of course, bring to light further individual initiatives to develop surgery; petty surgery was prescribed in the Ma-wang-tui texts of the second century B.C. already, and throughout the centuries of the imperial era castration of eunuchs was a common practice. The question to be asked, in any comparative history of science that goes beyond pointing out such incidents, is why such initiatives remained without cultural success, why such isolated traditions did not develop into full-scale surgical medicine. It is too simple to blame some Confucian dogma concerning the invulnerability of the human body as a reason for an apparent cultural lack of interest in such practices.

The Christian doctrine in the early Middle Ages opposed surgery as fiercely as Confucianism did; Christian dogmatists may even have been more violent in their attempts to oppress this branch of science. And yet in Europe some social groups pursued their interests consequently, withstanding and overcoming all adverse pressures in the long run. China had an equally heterogeneous society since the Chou dynasty, and it had a number of social groups unaffected by the Confucian teachings. But the seeds of surgery, sown by some individuals or necessitated through certain social practices, did not fall on fertile grounds. The history of cataract surgery is a vivid example. A tradition of cataract surgery was indicated in the preceding paragraph; it could be further substantiated by quotations from other sources. This tradition, though, remained an isolated event. It stimulated the development of neither general nor ophthalmological surgery in theory or practice. It would be difficult to deny a need. When Peter Parker opened his clinic in Canton early in the nineteenth century, cataract patients flocked to him by the thousands. Why then, one might ask again, did Chinese cataract surgery, introduced from abroad more than a thousand years ago, not become a common practice in China, available everywhere, improved over the centuries through continuous research, and practiced by skillful physicians? An answer has yet to be found.

To summarize, the arrival of Buddhism offered China, through certain concepts of Indian medicine, an opportunity to become familiar with the analytic views of the body and the world that ultimately, in the Occident, led to modern science. But for various reasons, conditions were unfavorable for the reception of these ideas. Attempts in China to awaken an understanding for the Indian doctrine of the elementary structure of the organism were evidently much too superficial, and, consequently, the analytical beginnings remained unshakably rooted in categories of correspondence and wholeness. An important aspect inherent to Buddhism should not be overlooked as a possible cause for the failure of Indian concepts in China, namely its therapeutic tolerance. In contrast to numerous other world views that supported a specific medical system because it manifested the same sociopolitical values proclaimed for the social sphere, the Buddhists were completely unconcerned about which medical practices relieved their physical suffering. Success—the release from suffering— was the decisive criterion and not, as in other systems, the specific methods that led to this success.

7. Sung Neo-Confucianism and Medical Thought: Progress with an Eye to the Past

The year A.D. 500 marked the approximate conclusion of an epoch in China during which all dimensions that were to characterize Chinese medicine until the appearance of Western science had been created. This is not to say, however, that Chinese medicine did not progress or change during subsequent centuries. Numerous new physiological and therapeutic discoveries are contained in medical literature of the late first and second millennia. But the appearance of Buddhist medical concepts established the general boundaries that determined all medical thought of the following 1,500 years. And these boundaries were by no means narrow. Once established, the basic framework of distinctly conceptualized therapy systems permitted diverse constructs that served not only to expand traditional ideas in various directions but also, as I shall demonstrate, to integrate different elements of this complex and heterogeneous edifice. After the age of classical antiquity, political developments in China were marked, often enough, by periods of ruthless civil wars within individual regions, serious revolts, and interludes of unity that fostered intellectual creativity; these were followed, in turn, by disintegration of the empire and lengthy periods of rule by foreign, non-Chinese conquerors. Up to the time of the final collapse of the empire at the beginning of the twentieth century, however, none of these convulsions proved sufficiently far-reaching to stimulate intellectual fermentation similar to the process observable in the centuries preceding and following the first unification, during the genesis of Chinese civilization.

The following two chapters will demonstrate how medical scholars, influenced by social and political developments during the centuries

154

preceding the collapse of Confucian social structures, sought new solutions to the unending problems of illness and early death within the confines of existing medical thought.

7.1. A SURVEY OF POLITICAL AND INTELLECTUAL DEVELOPMENTS BETWEEN THE SIXTH AND THIRTEENTH CENTURIES

7.1.1. The Sui and T'ang Epochs

Except for the brief unification of Chinese territory under the Chin (286–316), nearly four centuries elapsed between the conclusion of the Han dynasty and a new, lasting period of unity; the magnificent T'ang period (618–906) was preceded by the short-lived Sui dynasty (581–618). The most remarkable characteristic of the T'ang period is to be found in its cultural cosmopolitanism; unlike the Han dynasty, the Chinese empire now stood in lively intellectual and economic contact with all accessible centers of foreign civilizations. The philosophical spectrum of the epoch was marked by the simultaneous but varied influences of Confucianism, Buddhism, and Taoism. Although the Chin dynasty of the Ssu-ma clan is considered to have viewed Confucianism with favor, and although the Taoists were favored by the rulers of the Toba Empire, for example, during the Wei dynasty (386–543) as well as during the T'ang period itself, it appears that from the first half of the eighth century on, in the scope and diversity of its consequences, Buddhism achieved an increasingly preeminent position in comparison with the two competing doctrines. Utterly insignificant and mistaken as an exotic appendage of Taoism as late as the Han period, the doctrine from India had, by the conclusion of the division of China into northern and southern dynasties, already surpassed the adherents of Lao-tzu in its appeal to the broad masses. During the Chin period (ca. A.D. 316), the number of Buddhists was approximately 4,000; under the Sui, millions had professed their faith in this religion. Two geographically and chronologically very limited secularization campaigns in the years 446 and 576–577 represented only temporary setbacks in the stormy rise of Buddhism. The underlying causes of this phenomenon must be sought both within and outside the religion itself. I have already noted the doubts about Confucianism as a social philosophy, expressed by certain thinkers after the disintegration of the first united empire. Confucianism had been unable to maintain its position of ideological leadership, and a portion of the Chinese intellectual elite became interested in the new doctrine that promised an alternative ethical approach. During the division of the empire, the influence of Buddhist monks and missionaries, particularly in the north, grew because their diverse abilities corresponded to the needs of the rulers. The performance of medical miracles was not the sole capability that demonstrated the value of their teachings to those who lacked sympathy for the philosophical concepts of the religion itself; rain making, a skill not to be underestimated in a primarily agricultural state economy, prediction of the outcome of the frequent military campaigns, and the divinatory investigations of ministers and purported friends, earned Buddhists the favor of the broad masses as well as of the rulers themselves. Not to be overlooked as well was the attraction the monasteries held for those refusing military service and those oppressed by heavy taxation. Both the rich and the poor made use of the monasteries. Buddhism created hopes for release from a bitter destiny. The concept of karma offered even those from the lowest station the eventual possibility of escape from earthly misery, if they followed a certain ethic. Finally, a need may have existed among the Chinese people for a metaphysical approach, that Confucianism, with its orientation on the ordering and harmonizing of earthly existence, could not fulfill. Perhaps it was the lack of warmhearted, sympathetic deities in indigenous Chinese doctrine, deities from whom those disappointed and embittered by human relationships could seek support and solace, that led the Chinese masses to place their faith in a foreign religion.[1]

It is therefore not surprising that the founder of the Sui dynasty—more for political reasons than because of personal conviction—saw in Buddhism the ability to provide the newly united empire with the necessary ideological cohesion. Nonetheless, the state was to last only a brief time, for in his efforts to bring North and South together, the emperor saddled the population with excessive burdens. The construction of three capital cities and of a canal to connect the sparsely settled but extremely fertile areas of the South with the more congested North, required the services of millions of conscripted laborers. Following several favorable campaigns against the Kitans in Manchuria and the western Turkic peoples, other less successful undertakings in Korea eventually overtaxed both the state treasury and the patience of the population. When the second Sui emperor sought to obligate the landed gentry to cover expenditures, he lost not only the sympathy of the masses but that of the aristocracy as well, and he was eventually assassinated in 618.[2]

Under the ensuing T'ang dynasty, the Chinese Empire reached a previously unknown geographical extent; administrative control encompassed—with decreasing intensity, of course, as the distance from the central capital increased—large portions of Central Asia and, at times, extended as far south as present-day Vietnam. The ruling family's name was Li, the same as that of the clan of Lao-tzu. This circumstance, coupled with repeated reports by Taoists of Lao-tzu's reappearance, proved beneficial to his supporters; with the exception of the extremely pro-Buddhist interregnum of the empress Wu (690–705), the Taoists enjoyed the favor of T'ang rulers. But this did not hinder administration officials from pursuing a tolerant policy toward other world views. The already established doctrines were joined by Nestorian Christianity, Islam, Manicheism, and other religions that attracted a significant following, primarily among the numerous foreigners.

As early as the Northern Chou dynasty (556–581) there had been public discussions concerning the relative importance of the three great doctrines. The emperor, having listened to the arguments of the participants, determined that Confucianism occupied the first place, followed by Taoism and Buddhism. Such debates were resumed under the T'ang, but for centuries the question was whether Buddhism or Taoism should be accorded priority; Confucianism was scarcely mentioned in this context.

Buddhist influence continued to grow under the T'ang, affecting more and more areas of public life. If, during the first centuries of its existence in China, the Indian doctrine had been largely dependent upon and overshadowed by Taoism, the relationship was now reversed to a certain extent. Increasingly, followers of Lao-tzu sought to conform to religious concepts and organizational forms cultivated in Buddhist monasteries. But the Buddhists no longer restricted their activities to the spiritual realm; beyond the purely religious life, they began to develop into an unmistakable factor in Chinese economic life. Monasteries frequently concealed significant accumulations of precious objects, which either had been donated by believers or entrusted for safekeeping by outsiders. Taking advantage of this wealth, monasteries began to function as credit institutions, increasing their income in part through usurious interest rates. The extensive landholdings of the monasteries were also partly a result of donations; in addition, monastery officials used profits to purchase additional land, which was worked by slaves, orphans, or even hired laborers. The monks and priests themselves (with the exception of a single sect) avoided such activity. Further profitable business ventures included the opening of numerous monasteries as hostels, as well as investments in water mills and oil presses, which were then leased out. As a result, the Chinese state lost enormous amounts of revenue, for most of the Buddhist income was tax free. When the third secularization campaign commenced in 845, this time encompassing the entire empire, it was less a result of ideological opposition than of the growing financial distress of the government. More than a quarter-million monks and nuns were returned to lay life; 100,000 slaves and more than double that number of workers were released from their obligations and, like their Buddhist masters, returned to a taxpaying status. Material possessions of bronze, iron, silver, gold, and jade were confiscated by the state. Followers of the other religions were not spared by these measures.

Initially, Confucian representatives played only a passive, restrained role in these developments. Even during the period of fragmentation that prevailed between the Han and Sui dynasties, the administrations of most smaller and larger political entities were based on an educated civil service constituted along Confucian guidelines. Knowledge of the correct rituals never completely disappeared and was continually handed down within certain clans. A revival of interest in this social doctrine is evident not only during the Chin dynasty (280–316), but under the Sui as well, where a reorganization of court rites, for instance, was carried out under the direction of Confucian scholars. But representatives of this tradition could not fail to note that the Han preeminence of Confucianism would be not only temporarily impaired but also permanently lost if considerable efforts were not directed to revitalizing its universal value. The indications were indeed alarming. Official rituals already exhibited clear traces of Buddhist influences, particularly since the first emperor of the Liang dynasty (502–556) had proclaimed his complete allegiance to the Indian doctrine and prohibited all blood sacrifices.[3] Even the burning of incense had already been adopted into official state rites. More significant, however, was the fact that, primarily because of their ability to read and write, Buddhists had been able to enter the administrative bureaucracy as well, gradually undermining the Confucian monopoly on qualified candidates for civil service positions.[4] Open, massive opposition to the broad "foreignization" of Chinese society by Buddhism and its followers, however, did not break out until the T'ang period. The minister

Fu Yi (554–639), for instance, emphasized in a petition the subversive nature of Buddhism. He demonstrated, among other things, that the idea that man owes both well-being and misfortune to Buddha leads to disloyalty toward the emperor, and that monks and nuns conduct their lives totally at the expense of the rest of society. In 819, the scholar Han Yü (768–824) wrote a daring essay in which he rejected the ceremonial cult surrounding Buddha relics, pointing out the dangers of this non-Chinese doctrine. But he succeeded only in bringing about his own banishment. Of the other scholars who raised their voices in warning at this time, Li Ao (died 849) deserves special mention, for he wrote an allegorical treatise on the problem that proved prophetic for the future development of Confucianism. Perhaps to avoid the fate of Han Yü and others, Li Ao veiled his views in a description of a certain plant. The disguise was so effective that even some modern authors refer to Li Ao as a "botanist." Li Ao related the story of a sterile man completely given over to shortsighted pleasures, who one day discovers in the "wilderness" a plant with two intertwined offshoots. Surprised, he takes the plant with him, but no one can tell him what it is. Finally, he is told to take it as medicine. After following this advice he becomes fertile again and, after consuming more of the plant, is eventually able to recognize the correct way (tao) that all mankind must follow. Superficially at least, Li Ao brings his story into the sphere of the three great doctrines by including a Buddhist priest, an old man, whom we suspect to be a Taoist, as well as Confucian officials. At a more symbolic level, the sterile man represents the Confucianism of the time. In the wilderness, that is, outside of civilization, he encounters two intertwined offshoots, obvious symbols for Taoism and Buddhism. Only the consumption of a "carefully sifted powder" prepared from these two unknown plants is able to restore to the man fertility encompassing many generations. And only the "fertile man" can comprehend the true "Principles of Human Existence." Li Ao's portrayal sketches the fate of Confucianism. Either it must be supplemented by certain elements from the two competing ideologies that it was lacking, or the tradition of Confucianism would soon come to an end.[5] This challenge was met by philosophers of the Sung period, whose efforts led to the development known as Neo-Confucianism.

The T'ang dynasty is regarded as one of the golden ages of Chinese culture, an assessment based in part on the cosmopolitan nature of life in the flourishing cities, with their hundreds of thousands or millions of residents. Merchants from all countries bordering directly or indirectly on China brought with them exotic goods and returned home with Chinese cultural objects. As a result, music and the fine arts experienced important new impulses; society amused itself with novel games. Exotic fruits enriched the marketplace, and previously unknown drugs found their way into dispensaries.[6]

If we turn our attention to medical thought during this era, however, we discover that no significant new concepts were developed. At the beginning of the seventh century, Sun Ssu-miao, a scholar versed in all humanistic endeavors, compiled an extensive collection of pre-scriptions in which he combined, as already indicated, the concepts of systematic correspondence with Taoist techniques of demonic exorcism as well as with certain Buddhist notions. Other surviving prescription works from the T'ang period, such as the *Wai-t'ai pi-yao* by Wang Tao (ca. 725), have a similar character. For the first time, a state-approved work on drug therapy was compiled—the *Hsin-hsiu pen-ts'ao* of 659—an event that demonstrates the favorable attitude of the government toward Taoists, who were the primary figures in this branch of knowledge. Another Taoist, Wang Ping, prepared a new edition of the classic of systematic correspondence, the *Huang-ti nei-ching su-wen*, in the eighth century—one of the three surviving versions of the text. With the temporary displacement of Confucianism into the background, interest in this classic seems also to have diminished noticeably. It is therefore possible that the contradictory character of this work is due partly to Wang Ping's revision. Philological research in this question has established only the fact that Wang Ping is responsible for the addition of a cosmobiological element (Chinese: *wu-yün liu-ch'i*) to systematic correspondence, which can be found for the first time in the T'ang version of the *Su-wen*. Surviving tables of contents from earlier versions of the classic do not yet indicate these concepts.[7] The cosmobiological impulse served to expand the already familiar and highly refined systematic lines of correspondence; the macrocosmic concepts of the sixty-year moon-sun cycle of the Chinese calendar could now be linked with illness and well-being by means of the concepts of yinyang and the Five Phases. Although this tendency is quite interesting—it was based on the observation of seasonally related illnesses and physiological rhythms, as well as on the recognition that the organism experiences certain generalizable cycles that parallel daily cycles—it remained undeveloped and, even today, is viewed by an apologist for healing based on systematic correspondence as "the weakest and a deservedly controversial element in the theoretical framework" of this system.[8]

It may seem surprising that such a cosmopolitan age as the T'ang dynasty, shaped by generations of peace and by contact with foreign modes of thought, contributed so little to the understanding of the causes, nature, and treatment of illness. An explanation of this phenomenon is proposed by Franke and Trauzettel, whose analysis of the T'ang dynasty is based on factors other than medical concepts of the period:

> No new social class entered the historical arena, no revolution toppled old barriers, no new ideas or images reveal previously concealed impulses. On the contrary, we can discern only gradual changes, a constant progression of that which was already present, with no distinction as to whether it was of foreign or Chinese origin.[9]

The field of medical thought was no exception.

The decline of the T'ang dynasty began with the revolt of a military governor in 755, a consequence of the virtually unlimited civil and military power granted to commanders of the extensive border troops. The foreign troops, which the central government was forced to call in for support, were themselves a source of additional unrest after the uprising had been crushed. The clash between scholar-officials and the eunuchs, which had played such a crucial role during the Later Han, once again developed in the civil service. Growing corruption, disintegrating administrative control, increasing misery among the peasants following the ruthless appropriation of land by powerful landowners, and finally, after several isolated hunger revolts, the great uprising of 875, led first to a shadowy existence for the last emperors and, ultimately, in 906, to the final collapse of the dynasty.

7.1.2. The Sung Epoch

The ensuing struggle for control of China continued for some fifty years; in the North, five states rose and fell in rapid succession; in the South, a total of ten dynasties were founded before an army general from the North was proclaimed emperor of a new Sung dynasty by his troops in 960 and, in the following years, was finally able to suppress any remaining opposition. Once again, China was under the control of a single central government, but the circumstances were different from those in the T'ang period. The empire was now surrounded by powerful hostile states, some of which held Chinese territory. From the very beginning, Sung policies were aimed at maintaining a nonbelligerent stance toward these neighbors; high yearly expenditures stretching over many decades were successfully directed to this goal. Although the even higher costs of war were thus largely avoided, the drain of both material and financial resources, as well as the enormous expense involved in maintaining large standing armies, nonetheless constituted an oppressive burden. In addition, the virtually permanent scarcity of money was further exacerbated by a foreign trade deficit. To solve these difficulties, paper notes were circulated, a process which itself only fueled inflation. The avoidance of taxes, primarily under the auspices of a revived Buddhism, also contributed to the economic distress.

Not only the conditions on the borders were different, however. Chinese society itself had undergone fundamental changes. In connection with the following discussion of Sung medical thought, it is especially important to note the social and economic differentiation that increasingly characterized public life. The growth of the cities continued undiminished; the exodus of peasants from rural areas and an immense migration to the South contributed to this development. In the cities, professional life became more and more specialized; the government itself—probably unintentionally—fostered this trend by requiring the organization of individual enterprises into guilds, thereby facilitating supervision of such groups. Through the introduction of new or improved techniques, both agriculture and the processing industries experienced an upswing. Consequently, large areas became dependent upon a particular economic product, and clear regional distinctions developed, so that increased mutual economic interdependence began to replace the earlier economic self-sufficiency of individual regions.[10] The continuing specialization even found its way into state examinations and therefore into the training of civil servants, which up to that time had been marked largely by the Confucian ideal of a comprehensive classical education. When Wang An-shih began his reform of the examination system in the eleventh century, his intention was to reorganize it more specifically in terms of such specialties as law, finance, military, geography, and even medicine.[11]

The reorganization of Chinese society during the Sung period thus brought about a development in two directions that are only seemingly contradictory. On the one hand, we find a tendency to restrict both individual and regional competencies and concomitant increased interest in fine details. On the other hand, whether consciously or subconsciously, there was the feeling of an increased dependence upon an expansive, larger whole, to which the individual parts, with their highly specific functions, made a vital contribution. Such a sweeping reorganization could scarcely leave unaffected the philosophy of the era; it provided the basis out of which Confucianism was eventually able to add essential elements to its already traditional synthetic-integral social doctrine and, at the same time, adopt an analytic approach, concerned with the essence of individual phenomena, that it previously had never possessed to this degree. Such an intellectual climate, in turn, required its own foundation, namely, the refinement of technical and other detailed knowledge. The Sung period thus constitutes one of the pinnacles of technological and scientific progress in Chinese history.

In this context the reemergence of Taoism during the Sung era becomes comprehensible. For more than a millennium, its followers had been occupied with the detailed analysis and observation of natural laws; many of the insights that now proved useful were derived from the discoveries and preliminary work of Taoist researchers. An example of this was the invention of gunpowder, which became a part of the Chinese arsenal during the Sung period. To be sure, a primary concern of Taoist efforts remained the desire to prolong life through such measures as the taking of certain substances either produced through technical processes or found in nature itself. Although it would be going too far to see in the therapy utilizing crystalline products distilled from urine, which developed during the course of such efforts, a forerunner of modern hormone therapy[12] (particularly since the conceptual framework was totally different), this example nonetheless illustrates the breadth of activities at the time. It should not be overlooked, of course, that Sung Taoism, especially the *cheng-i* school, was also deeply involved in techniques of demonic exorcism. The fundamental significance of Taoist ideology during the Sung period was reflected in its growing role in the official state cult.

Buddhism followed a totally different course during the same period. It had largely recovered, at least superficially, since the secularization of 845, but the spiritual force of the doctrine appeared to have been broken. This despite the fact that the first Sung emperor immediately ordered the ordination of 8,000 monks on the occasion of his birthday, sent out missions to the West, and even established another Bureau of Translation. The emperor himself took Buddhist vows and ordered the first publication of the Buddhist literary canon. Later Sung emperors looked upon Buddhism and its adherents with equal favor; in the year 1221, nearly 400,000 monks, more than 60,000 nuns, and some 40,000 temples were counted.[13] The economic involvement of the monasteries surpassed even that of the T'ang period. But of the numerous schools active in that earlier epoch, only two maintained their old significance under the Sung; both, moreover, were not greatly concerned with the interpretation of Buddhist literature or with the refinement of rituals, and thus contributed very little to the debate among Chinese intellectuals. The decline of Buddhism was accelerated by one measure of the government that promised financial benefit, but which in the long run only exacerbated the problems. It had been customary that the ordination of monks and nuns, and the accompanying series of privileges, including the tax-exempt status, were sanctioned and therefore legalized by a certificate, attesting to the fact that the bearer had passed the necessary examinations in Buddhist doctrine. As a result of its fiscal difficulties, the Sung administration began to offer these certificates for sale. In this way great numbers of people with absolutely no spiritual link to Buddhism entered the monasteries, and the standing of monks and nuns diminished rapidly.

Yet another reason behind Buddhism's declining appeal for Chinese thinkers was the success of certain philosophers in developing an alternative attractive enough to claim the attention of the intellectual elite. Impressed by the successes of Taoism and Buddhism, various thinkers had identified the essential features lacking in Confucianism, gradually offering new ideas that were eventually synthesized in the philosophy of Chu Hsi (1130–1200). In the T'ang "botanical" allegory cited earlier, Li Ao had not only demonstrated that Confucianism required elaboration to survive, he had, in another passage, indicated those aspects he considered crucial for this objective:

> Although writings dealing with the Nature and with Destiny are still preserved, said Li Ao, none of the scholars understands them, and therefore they all plunge into Taoism or Buddhism. Ignorant people say that the followers of the Master (Confucius) are incapable of investigating the teachings on the Nature and Destiny, and everybody believes them.[14]

Knowledge concerning processes and phenomena in nature and an all-encompassing, macrocosmic ethic that linked human morality on a metaphysical plane with the entire universe were indeed the weak elements of Confucianism. In the eleventh and twelfth centuries, the conceptual impulses of the T'ang forerunners of Neo-Confucianism bore fruit. Unlike earlier attempts, criticism of Buddhism was no longer solely negative, but offered a genuine alternative to the Buddhist notion that the phenomenal world represented not reality but pure illusion, from which we can and must free ourselves. Chang Tsai (1020–1077) was the first to oppose this doctrine with the argument that material finest matter (ch'i) had existed from the very beginning of time. He claimed that all things were real, since they come into existence through the concentration of ch'i-influence, and end by returning into finest influence. The notion of the convergence and dissolution of matter based on the concept of finest influences was certainly not new. As we have seen, it was already in existence during the Han period, and it found renewed interest especially in T'ang Taoism.[15] Chang Tsai extended these concepts by combining them with the ethic of human relationships. Chang wrote:

> Since all things in the universe arise from the same ch'i, then the people of the world are our brothers: things are my companions. . . . All those who are exhausted and prone to illness, maimed and deformed, lonely and childless, widows and widowers, are our brothers and sisters who are in difficulties and have no one to appeal to. If one protects them at the proper time this is to show the reverence of a son. If one does one's work with joy and without grudge, this exemplifies the purity of filial piety. To do the contrary is to deviate from one's moral virtue and he who violates *jen* (benevolence or human-heartedness) is a robber.[16]

Recalling the restrictions that were placed on the original Confucian concept of correct human relations, we can clearly see here the desire of the author to claim for Confucianism the notion of charity toward one's fellow man, which previously had been limited to Buddhism. At the same time, Chang Tsai's deliberations contain a clear call to face all the realities of life, instead of avoiding the obligations of daily life by entering a monastery, for example.[17]

Ch'eng Hao (1032–1085) and Ch'eng Yi (1033–1107), two nephews of Chang Tsai, pursued a different course, arguing that a specific principle (li), which could be fathomed with the appropriate study, underlies all phenomena and existence.

Chu Hsi (1130–1200) was finally able to forge these disparate arguments into a system in which li constituted the immaterial organizational principle controlling all genesis, existence, and decay, and ch'i the material finest influence that brings genesis, existence, and decay to fruition. In addition, Chu combined the doctrines of li and ch'i with the cosmogony developed by another Sung philosopher— Chou Tun-i (1017–1073)—creating an organic model of the universe, in which each material phenomenon and each ethical category could be explained. For Confucians, the study of nature was now finally "legal"; the motto "achieve an understanding of things by investigating them" (*ko-wu chih-chih*) spread like a veritable signal of freedom. Chu Hsi's construct conferred upon human existence a meaning within a metaphysical system without recourse to the deities, spirits, and demons of competing doctrine. Chu Hsi demonstrated that the evolution of the universe in accord with an all-embracing organizational principle is accompanied at the appropriate time by the genesis of certain conceptions of morality and virtuous conduct; the necessity for some being situated beyond space and time, who controls the destiny of man and watches over his adherence to certain moral values, simply did not exist in this conceptual system.[18]

To summarize this brief survey of Neo-Confucianism: Chu Hsi and his predecessors offered a comprehensive, naturalistic, and organic world view that reinterpreted and expanded traditional Confucianism in a twofold process. On the one hand, Neo-Confucianism adopted concepts that previously had belonged within the purview of Taoism, so that in fact it is possible to speak of partial syncretism. On the other hand, totally new concepts were developed that were directly opposed to comparable ideas within Buddhist doctrine, so that although the latter did not have to be integrated into Chinese thought, their function had nonetheless been fulfilled. This differentiated development of Confucianism soon radiated a great intellectual vigor and appeal. The study of the classics once more became a vital topic. The impulse to investigate carefully individual phenomena of nature and in so doing to understand one's own position in the larger scheme of the universe, culminated in the scientific activities of the period that I have already mentioned.

7.2. CULTURAL AND SOCIAL TRENDS AS REFLECTED IN MEDICAL THOUGHT

For approximately 1,000 years, until the Sung period, Chinese medical thought, as far as surviving literature indicates, developed along the lines established by the compilation of the *Huang-ti nei-ching* and the *Shen-nung pen-ts'ao ching*. I have already discussed the nature of the widespread activities of demonic medicine as well as Buddhist healing during the first millennium A.D. The pluralism of healing systems is evident not only in medical literature itself, but also, for instance, in the official list of medical specialties and examination subjects compiled during the Sung period. Taoist and Buddhist exorcistic techniques were just as much a part of the reservoir of recognized and required knowledge as the ability to prepare prescriptions or apply needles according to the rules of systematic correspondence. While the tradition of systematic correspondence, including the integrated therapeutic technique of acupuncture, underwent what could be termed a "development" over the centuries only in terms of minor details, the literature of practical drug therapy, which remained virtually untouched by the concepts of systematic correspondence through the end of the Northern Sung (960–1126), is marked by an intensive progression. Not only was the number of available medicinal plants, animals, and minerals continually increased, but individual drug descriptions were regularly revised with new information on drug properties and errors of earlier authors corrected. If we compare the earliest drug work whose author can be identified—the *Pen-ts'ao ching chi chu*, written by T'ao Hung-ching about A.D. 500—with the extensive compendia of the Sung period, this advance in knowledge is immediately evident.[19] There is no doubt that the productive development of pharmaceutical literature and knowledge was due to the ongoing efforts of a large group of naturalists and observers who, always receptive to new discoveries, continually sought to unlock the secrets of nature. Although they held their classic, the Han *Shen-nung pen-ts'ao ching*, in great respect, its insights represented only a starting point for their own concerns and not, as was the case for followers of the *Huang-ti nei-ching/Nan-ching* tradition, the ultimate and complete stage in a particular field of knowledge. It was the new intellectual climate under the Sung that first transformed the medical thinking of those operating within the conceptual framework of systematic correspondence. It was no coincidence that scholars associated with Confucianism provided the impetus for this development, and it is therefore not surprising that the structural changes in Chinese society sketched above, as well as the fundamental tendencies of Neo-Confucianism, were now mirrored in the concepts of medical literature. The history of medicine under the Sung thus underwent a twofold development. First, we can observe the fragmentation into specialized fields, as well as a tendency toward pronounced reductionism in notions about the cause, nature, and treatment of illness; second, there were intensive efforts to verify the universal validity of the medicine of systematic correspondence by extending it to practical drug therapy. Since changes such as these leave their mark in literature only after a certain interval of incubation, these developments occurred between the time that Sung rule had first been restricted to a southern part of China by the establishment of the foreign Chin dynasty in the North (1115–1234) and the period when Sung rule was completely destroyed by the Mongols, who defeated both the Chin and the Sung, founding the Yüan dynasty (1260–1368). Since the most important exponents of the medical thought fostered by the intellectual atmosphere under the Sung did not compile their works until these subsequent dynasties, they are generally referred to in the context of "Chin-Yüan medicine." To illustrate more clearly the connections with Neo-Confucianism, which is also referred to as "Sung doctrine," it is more accurate to speak of "Sung-Chin-Yüan" medicine.

7.2.1. Reductionism and the Narrowing of Categories

The medical thought and writings of the scholars whom we recognize as proponents of Sung-Chin-Yüan medicine were derived primarily from four sources. In addition to the *Huang-ti nei-ching,* which provided the theoretical foundation of systematic correspondence, and the pen-ts'ao literature, which contained detailed information on the properties of individual drugs, it was mainly the work of the Han author Chang Chi (*tzu:* Chung-ching) as well as T'ang cosmobiology (*wu-yün liu-ch'i*) that influenced the authors of Sung-Chin-Yüan medicine.

7.2.1.1. Chang Chi and the Adoption of Restricted Etiology

Chang Chi (142–220?) is known as the author of two prescription works, the *Shang-han lun* (On Cold-Induced Bodily Injuries) and *Chin-kuei yü-han yao-lüeh* (Survey of the Most Important Elements from the Golden Chest and Jade Container). Although both texts survived more or less intact for centuries, there are several indications that these works exerted only marginal influence on medical thought and literature between the Han and Sung dynasties. While the interest generated by Wang Shu-ho (210–285), for example, in pulse diagnosis had been continued in more than seventy titles by the beginning of the Sung period, and while during the same interval more than ninety works had been devoted to acupuncture and more than fifty to physiology, not even ten authors followed the direction taken by Chang Chi. It was only during the Sung and Chin epochs that a larger circle of scholars became interested in the surviving fragments of Chang Chi; during the course of these two dynasties alone, so many revisions or commentaries appeared on the problems of cold-related illnesses that more than eighty titles have survived to the present day. The contrast becomes even more striking when we compare the ten titles devoted specifically to the treatment of such illnesses written before the Sung period with the more than three hundred encyclopedic works containing prescriptions for all kinds of illnesses that appeared during the same time. The Chang Chi renaissance during the Sung-Chin-Yüan era was due primarily to two characteristics in his writings. To scholars of the twelfth, thirteenth, and fourteenth centuries, it was significant that Chang Chi had been the first to combine the use of drug therapy with the theory of systematic correspondence. In addition, Chang Chi, with his interest in the effects of cold on illness, was the first and virtually only author whose work was devoted exclusively to a specific etiology. All authors of Sung-Chin-Yüan medical texts adopted these elements, which had virtually lain dormant for some 1,000 years, as the point of departure for their own, further-reaching deliberations. Consequently, in almost all of their works, drug prescriptions and theoretical considerations are linked on the basis of systematic correspondence. At a later point I will discuss in detail the development of a pharmacology of systematic correspondence, which represents the true achievement of Sung-Chin-Yüan scholars. In addition, each of these authors concentrated on a specific etiology. Here, too, considerable advances beyond Chang Chi's original impulses were made. While Chang's particular interest had been in cold as merely one of many causes of illness, several of the Sung-Chin-Yüan scholars identified highly specific personal or nonpersonal factors—which is why I speak of reductionism—that they regarded as responsible for the vast majority of human illnesses. Each of these theoreticians, who were all practitioners as well, focused on a narrow etiological category, which then served as the basis for diagnosis and treatment of individual suffering. This procedure stands in stark contrast to the contents of the *Huang-ti nei-ching* and, even more so, of the *Nan-ching* where, although we can find the indication that wind, for instance, is responsible for numerous afflictions, the emphasis nonetheless is on initial observation of the victim's condition, followed by an individual course of therapy that was not dependent on the cause of the condition.

7.2.1.2. *The Cosmobiological Concepts* Wu-yün liu-ch'i

The notions of a correspondence between cosmically determined seasonal cycles and phenomena in the existence of individual organisms, which Wang Ping had introduced to the *Su-wen* during the T'ang period, did not raise great interest until the Sung epoch, when such concepts were even adopted as an examination topic. Since such a significant part of the theoretical framework of Sung-Chin-Yüan medicine is unintelligible without an understanding of the five phases of circulation (*wu-yün*) and six climatic influences (*liu-ch'i*), it will be necessary to discuss briefly the basic outline of these concepts.

The five phases of circulation are five different time periods that together constitute a cycle. All are of equal duration, encompassing a total of one year. A distinction was drawn between "primary" phases and "guest" phases. The former are the phases that theoretically correspond exactly to the calendar, while the latter are the actual seasonally related phases, which are subject to certain fluctuations from year to year. Each of the five phases of circulation is associated with one of the Five Phases of change (*wu-hsing*). An older calendrical system was also incorporated, the so-called celestial stems (*t'ien-kan*), a system consisting of ten symbols, in which the odd-numbered symbols are associated with yang, while the even-numbered symbols are each associated with yin. Two symbols from the ten celestial stems, namely one "odd" yang and the following fifth—that is, even—yin, are associated with each of the five phases of circulation. The five phases of circulation ensure the orderly progression of seasons and formation of corresponding climatic conditions. In systematic correspondence the circulatory phase *chia-chi* (symbolized by the first and sixth celestial stems) corresponds to soil and stimulates the formation of moisture. The circulatory phase *i-keng* (symbolized by the second and seventh celestial stems) corresponds to metal and engenders dryness. The phase *ping-hsin* (symbolized by the third and eighth celestial stems) corresponds to water and produces cold. The phase *ting-jen* (symbolized by the fourth and ninth celestial stems) corresponds to wood and gives rise to wind. Finally, the phase *mou-kuei* (symbolized by the fifth and tenth celestial stems) corresponds to fire and brings forth heat. Since the cycle of five phases together encompasses a period of one year, each phase lasts one-fifth of a year, or a total of seventy-three days.

Irregularities can appear within the relationships between phases of circulation and climatic conditions: the influence of a phase, for example, can be only partly developed (*pu-chi*), producing an insufficient supply of the expected seasonal climatic circumstances. Moreover, each phase can also be excessively developed (*t'ai-kuo*), resulting in the exaggerated presence of normal climatic conditions.

In addition to the five phases of circulation, the year was divided into a cycle of six climatic influences (liu-ch'i), which were also associated with the yinyang duality and the Five Phases. In order to achieve correspondence between the groups of six and five, one of the Five Phases or agents had to be further split; in this system, therefore, "fire" is replaced by the two phases "ruler-fire" (*chün-huo*) and "minister-fire" (*hsiang-huo*).

A second calendrical system, the twelve so-called terrestrial branches (*ti-chih*), was used to designate the six climatic influences. Each influence was associated with two symbols—the first and following sixth terrestrial branches.

The six climatic influences encompass the entire range of climatic conditions (ch'i) that affect man during the course of a year. Once again, a distinction was drawn between two constellations: namely, the constellation of "primary influences" (*chu-ch'i*), the unchangeable climatic influences that theoretically should occur during the yearly cycle, and the constellation of "guest influences" (*k'e-ch'i*), the actual weather conditions. Both constellations correspond to the progression of an entire year. Climatic influences of the first half of the year are associated with heaven and thus with yang; those of the second half are associated with earth and therefore with yin. Each half of the year is further separated into three climatic periods of sixty days each. This produces a total of six climatic periods, each of which is itself divided into four sections of fifteen days corresponding to specific weather conditions. Consequently, a year encompasses twenty-four different climatic periods.[20]

The functions of the human organism, it was believed, are to a great extent determined by the influences that affect it during each season. Liu Wen-shu, who in 1099 published one of the best-known works on the theory of the five phases of circulation and six climatic influences, went so far as to claim that each season was dominated by certain climatic influences that inevitably caused certain illnesses, giving rise to the concept of "illness caused by seasonal influence" (*shih-ch'i ping*). Other authors, however, rejected or modified this extreme interpretation of *wu-yün liu-ch'i* theories. They argued that good health was completely possible if man was able, through appropriate conduct, to adapt himself and, should climatic irregularities occur, take appropriate therapeutic measures to rectify a condition of excess or deficiency of influences from the yinyang or Five Phases categories.

7.2.2. Individual Contributions to Contemporary Trends

The Sung-Chin-Yüan epoch provides an instructive illustration of two factors that together determine the nature of cognitive progress. These are, first, the effects of the general intellectual climate as determined by ideological and social structures on the great, overriding tendencies of the development of knowledge and, second, the intellectual achievements of certain individuals who are nonetheless able to shape the direction of science in a highly personal manner within the boundaries of these tendencies. To illustrate the spectrum of alternative approaches within this unifying conceptual framework, I will now turn to the views and works of four theoreticians of the Sung-Chin-Yüan period.

7.2.2.1. Liu Wan-su

Liu Wan-su (1110–1200), whose origins and life remain largely obscure, regarded the theory of the five phases and six climatic influences as the basis for all healing. In the introduction to one of his works, the *Su-wen hsüan-chi yüan-ping-shih* (The Original Forms of Illness in the Obscurity of the *Su-wen*), he wrote:

> If we consider medical practitioners, we find that [in the diagnosis and treatment of illnesses] they take into account only whether [the affliction] belongs to the yin or yang category or whether a symptom of deficiency or excess exists. The [sole correct] procedure, however, for achieving understanding about illnesses [is as follows]. Only when the influences that give rise to illness have been investigated as to the changes in the [normal course] of the five circulatory phases and six climatic influences, can the [nature of illness and its treatment] be perceived clearly.[21]

Liu Wan-su subscribed to the view that a normal progression of circulatory phases and climatic influences is possible without pathogenic consequences for man, criticizing, as he called it, the "mechanistic" approach of Liu Wen-chu. Liu Wan-su taught that only cosmic deviations from the normal progression of events or the failure of man to adjust to this progression cause illness. In this context he also observed that of the five phases of circulation, four were one-dimensional, while the fifth—associated with fire—was subdivided into ruler and minister, and thus constitutes a point of special emphasis. In addition, he determined that among the six climatic influences—wind, dryness, dampness, cold, summer heat, and fire—the first four each possessed independent and unmistakable attributes, while summer heat and fire ultimately formed an integral entity. These observations led Liu to the conclusion that fire and heat must have an extraordinary significance in the origin of illness. Analyzing the diseases in the *Su-wen* in this light, he discovered that in fact the overwhelming majority could be traced to these causes. Liu Wan-su therefore concentrated on afflictions due to the climatic influences and phases of fire and heat, thereby founding the "school of cooling" (*han-liang p'ai*) in Chinese medicine. His treatises frequently combined the use of drugs and acupuncture. A few of his prescriptions, as in the seventh chapter of his *Huang-ti su-wen hsüan-ming lun fang* (Prescriptions Compiled and Analyzed on the Basis of the *Huang-ti su-wen*), also advocate the use of Buddhist demonological incantations. The principles underlying his therapies were by no means limited to the relatively simple conceptualization of the hot-cold antithesis, which even today marks the medical thought and practice of numerous cultures, particularly those of Latin America. For Liu Wan-su, an excess of fire influence meant the simultaneous deficiency of water in the body and thus a pathological profusion of yang influences, which in turn corresponded to a lack of vital yin influences. It consequently was necessary to dissipate the former and replenish the latter, utilizing the appropriate therapeutic procedures for the affected palaces and depots as outlined in the *Huang-ti nei-ching*. Liu Wan-su achieved the replenishment of deficiencies primarily through the administration of drugs; in this connection he frequently cited the instructions of Chang Chi in the *Shang-han lun*. For the treatment of heat-related diarrhea, for example, Liu advised the taking of "cold" and bitter medicinal preparations, so as to reduce the excessive heat (by means of the "cold" influences of the drugs), alleviating the obvious lack of fluid in the kidney depot (through the corresponding bitter flavor).[22] This type of approach necessitated an integration of medicinal drugs into the theoretical framework of systematic correspondence as it existed in the *Nei-ching*, a requirement first given a consistent expression in the work of Chang Yüan-su (ca. 1180).

7.2.2.2. Chang Ts'ung-cheng

Chang Ts'ung-cheng (1156–1228) is the second significant medical theoretician of the Sung-Chin-Yüan epoch. As with Liu Wan-su, the circumstances surrounding his life are largely unknown. Although the title of his principal work *Ju-men shih-ch'in* (How a Confucian Scholar Serves his Parents) indicates an intellectual link with Confucianism, it must be remembered that this book was written and published by a disciple and companion of Chang Ts'ung-cheng, possibly even after the latter's death, rendering Chang's influence on the choice of title doubtful. It appears certain that Chang Ts'ung-cheng was an itinerant doctor, for a number of case histories in the above-mentioned work begin with the phrase "When Tai-jen (i.e., Chang Ts'ung-cheng as narrated by his pupil) was passing through."

Like Liu Wan-su, Chang ascribed a decisive significance to the pathogenic potential of climatic influences, but his own deliberations led to markedly different conclusions. Chang stressed the distinction between those influences normally present in the body and those that must be considered pathogenic, which he therefore designated with the classical term *hsieh* ("evil") or *k'e-ch'i* ("guest") influences. Chang's approach diverged considerably from the belief of Liu Wan-su and other contemporary scholars in the organic homogeneity of influences inside and outside the body, a conception which defined illness solely as an imbalance in the distribution of these influences among the various depots and palaces. Chang Ts'ung-cheng, therefore, directed his therapeutic efforts not to the establishment of a state of equilibrium, but to the decisive expulsion of harmful influences. He identified wind, cold, summer heat, dampness, dryness, and fire as potentially harmful influences of heaven; fog, dew, rain, hail, ice, and mud as potentially malevolent influences of the earth; finally, sour, sweet, bitter, sharply seasoned/spicy, and salty as possible harmful influences in food and drink. If someone has fallen ill, there is no other choice, according to Chang Ts'ung-cheng, but to eliminate the responsible foreign influences from the body immediately. For the appropriate therapy, he returned terminologically to the three techniques cited by Chang Chi in the *Shang-han lun*—emetics, sweating, and purgation, thereby incorporating a broad spectrum of therapeutic measures into a classic pattern. Induced salivation, sneezing, lacrimation, as well as all other techniques that eliminate pathogenic foreign influences through upper body orifices, were defined as "emetics." Moxibustion, vaporization, fumigation, lavation, hot compresses, mud packs, needles,

physical exercise, and massage, as well as all other procedures that
eliminate influences through the skin were designated "sudorifics."
Induced labor, increased lactation, diuretics, the unblocking of obstructions, induced flatulation, and all other techniques that eliminate
harmful influences through lower body orifices were called "purgatives." These three general therapeutic categories were further differentiated according to the location and type of illness. On the basis of
these procedures, Chang Ts'ung-cheng is known as the founder of the
"school of attack and purgation" (*kung hsia p'ai*); like Liu Wan-su,
Chang, too, found disciples, but bitter opponents as well, who warned
of the dangers of such one-sided therapy.[23] The appendix of this volume
contains excerpts from four case histories in the *Ju-men shih-ch'in*
that demonstrate the scope of application of Chang's three techniques
for expelling evil influences from the organism. Whether the illnesses
were those that modern Western medicine would term somatic or
those whose treatment today might be a concern for psychologists,
Chang Ts'ung-cheng's conception of the nature of illness enabled in
each case a successful use of emetics, sudorifics, or purgatives.

7.2.2.3. Ch'en Yen

For Ch'en Yen (fl. 1161–1174), not even the exact dates of his life
are known, although he must have been an important medical practitioner and author. He is known primarily for an often-reprinted
handbook of etiology, which has survived under the title *San-yin chi
i-ping cheng fang lun* (Prescriptions Elucidated on the Premise That
All Pathological Symptoms Have Only Three Primary Causes). The
San-yin fang, as the work is usually titled, contains both theoretical
treatises on the etiology and diagnosis of numerous diseases and detailed instructions for the medicinal treatment of these conditions.
Although the use of acupuncture is occasionally cited in the *San-yin
fang,* it did not constitute a part of the specific therapeutic process.
Ch'en Yen frequently referred to the *Huang-ti nei-ching* and adopted
the conceptual framework of systematic correspondence in a consistent
fashion for his own deliberations; but he failed to link the use of
individual drugs in prescriptions directly with his theories, an impulse
so characteristic of most other contemporary medical scholars. In the
work of Chang Chi, so highly esteemed by Sung-Chin-Yüan authors,
Ch'en Yen found another aspect he deemed worth reviving. In the
Chin-kuei yao-lüeh (Remarkable Elements from the Golden Chest),
dating from the Han period, Chang Chi had written the following:

Man is provided the five normal elements of all existence (*wu-ch'ang*); the influence of wind brings man life and growth. Thus the influence of wind can bring life and growth to the ten-thousand things, but it can also bring misfortune to all of them. In this way it resembles water, which both carries and sinks ships. When the original and true influences fill the depot, man enjoys peace and harmony. When he is attacked by foreign influences or evil winds, however, death frequently follows. The thousands of possible afflictions caused by heat are nothing more than [symptoms of] only three illnesses. These are: first, the assault through the transportation channels of evil [influences], which from there then penetrate the depots and palaces. This is an internal appearance [of illness]. Second, if the blood channels between the four limbs and nine body openings are restricted or completely obstructed, the skin is affected externally [by an evil influence]. Third, there are injuries caused by sexual intercourse, weapons, insects, and animals. If all illnesses are investigated in light of this [categorization], all causes are included.[24]

The attempt by Chang Chi to subsume the great number of possible afflictions into only three categories remained as neglected in subsequent centuries as his initial efforts for a theoretically grounded application of drugs and his adoption of a specific etiology. When Ch'ao Yüan-fang (fl. 610), in the seventh century, compiled the first known Chinese work devoted especially to the etiology of illness, the *Chu-ping yüan hou lun* (On the Cause and Course of All Illnesses), he divided the nearly 2,000 syndromes that are described in detail and whose causes are investigated into groups, but there was no underlying, integral scheme. The fifty chapters devoted to illnesses are arranged in part according to principal cause (wind, cold, insects), in part according to where the illness first manifested itself (in the various depots or palaces, etc.), in part according to age and sex of the victim (children, women), but also in part according to known disorders (numerous forms of diarrhea, for instance). Ch'ao Yüan-fang ultimately assigned each individual ailment to a specific etiology, thus ignoring the example set by Chang Chi. The work of Ch'ao Yüan-fang has survived in its entirety; the Appendix 3 contains several translations from his commentaries.

Ch'en Yen was the first to pick up the suggestions of Chang Chi, distancing himself cautiously but explicitly from the methodology of Ch'ao Yüan-fang. In the process he progressed far beyond the rather simple initiatives of Chang Chi, developing a detailed system of assessing individual ailments in terms of "internal," "external," or "neither internal nor external" origin. As external harmful influences he defined, similar to the familiar climatic influences, the effects of cold, summer heat, dryness, dampness, wind, and humidity. Internally, he claimed, illnesses can be caused by certain emotional states such as joy, anger, grief, and brooding. Finally, in the category "neither/nor" he included overwork, idleness, and various violent assaults, such as those from animals, other men, poisons, or accidents. The value or even advantage, however, that knowledge of the category of the cause of an illness provides for its treatment is not apparent in Ch'en Yen's work. Although the text repeatedly states that each treatment must be preceded by determination of the category of origin, there is no indication of the actual or theoretical connection between the author's concrete suggestions for the treatment of a specific illness, on the one hand, and the recognition that the cause is "internal," "external," or "neither/nor," on the other hand.

7.2.2.4. Li Kao

Li Kao (1180–1251) is one of the few medical practitioners of the Sung-Chin-Yüan epoch whose biography can be found in official histories. The annals of the Yüan dynasty indicate that Li Kao came from a family that had enjoyed prosperity for generations; in accordance with the Confucian ideal, he had not learned medicine to earn money or to treat his fellow men, but rather to assist his ill mother.[25] Since it was not particularly flattering for a Confucian scholar to be called a "physician," outsiders, according to the annals, did not dare refer to him as one or ask for his assistance. Li's offers to help in cases where the therapy of others had proven ineffective were spontaneous and not professionally motivated. The distinction between this attitude toward the practice of healing and the apparently financially motivated medical services of Chang Ts'ung-cheng is clear and explains why Li enjoyed official recognition while Chang did not.[26]

The *Huang-ti nei-ching* and *Shang-han lun* also constituted the basis for Li Kao's deliberations. His contribution was twofold. First, he carried on the efforts of his teacher Chang Yüan-su to establish a concrete pharmacology of systematic correspondence. Li Kao's views on the theorization of drug therapy are contained in two medical texts attributed to him, fragments of which have survived. These are the *Chen-chu nang pu-i yao-hsing fu* (Correction of Deficiencies in the Pearl Purse and Poem of Drug Qualities), whose title is a conscious reference to the *Chen-chu nang* (Pearl Purse) of Chang Yüan-su, and the *Yung-yao fa hsiang* (Regularities and Cosmological Correspondences in the Use of Drugs).[27]

The second contribution of Li Kao to contemporary medical thought was the development of a specific etiology, which made him the founder of his own school. These views are recorded in his best-known work, the *P'i wei lun* (On the Spleen and Stomach). It should be noted that according to contemporary thought, the spleen was ascribed the digestive function in the organism.

Li Kao's interest appears to have been provoked by certain statements in the *Huang-ti nei-ching* that stress the central importance of the stomach and digestion for human physiology. He concluded: "When the digestive system and stomach in the body sustain damage, all kinds of illnesses can occur!" Four postulates were offered as proof of this conclusion.

1. Human life is made possible by the yang influence of heaven absorbed by the body. These yang influences must accumulate in the stomach and digestive region.

2. The development of man is made possible by the yin influences of the earth that flow to the body. These yin influences must undergo a transformation in the stomach and digestive region that renders them useful to the organism.

3. For nourishment the human body absorbs yang influences, which collect in the stomach and digestive region.

4. Through yin finest matter (*ching*) the human body achieves longevity. Yin finest matter has its origin in the stomach and digestive region, where it is formed from influences absorbed from external sources.

Should illness occur in the stomach or digestive area, their ability to assimilate, accumulate, transform, and distribute is impaired, and the preservation of a normal state in the body is threatened. In this regard, Li Kao stressed three factors that can lead to such developments.

1. Irregular consumption of food and drink damages the stomach first. If the stomach is affected, it is unable to supply the digestive system with the requisite substances. Finest influences and finest matter, which arise from water and grain in the organism, no longer flow through the body, resulting in depletions.

2. Excessive exhaustion of the body prevents the yang influences, normally radiated by the digestive region, from reaching the four extremities. The results are drowsiness and the need to sleep.

3. Excessive emotions such as joy, anger, sorrow, and fear cause the fire associated with the heart depot to flare up. In accordance with the doctrine of self-genesis among the Five Phases, fire is succeeded by soil, which is associated with the stomach and digestive region.

Ebullition of the fire phase thus eventually spreads to the soil phase, producing harmful effects here, too.[28]

In line with this approach, Li Kao emphasized the necessity for measures that replenish (*pu*) the stomach and digestive area of the affected organism with influences, enabling both organs to resume their functions. Li Kao's doctrine was therefore designated *pu-t'u p'ai* ("the school of replenishing the soil phase") and also *pu p'i wei p'ai* ("the school of replenishing spleen and stomach").

7.2.3. The Pharmacology of Systematic Correspondence

Pharmacology is defined here as the science of drug properties and reactions in the body. The conceptualization of a pharmacology therefore requires an understanding of the processes that occur in the organism between the administration of a substance and the manifestation of its effects. As long as Chinese medical and pharmaceutical literature contained only very pragmatic descriptions of individual drugs, with no consideration of why such substances exhibit their particular properties, we cannot speak of the existence of a pharmacology.

The *Huang-ti nei-ching* mentions about a dozen drug names; occasionally, the term "drug" (*yao*) is employed in an abstract sense. Needle treatments were the sole form of therapy in the *Huang-ti nei-ching;* their results were interpreted on the basis of theories of systematic correspondence. Future philological studies face the difficult task of ascertaining to what extent the few occurrences of the concept of "drugs" and drug names were added to the work only in the second half of the first millennium. A textual comparison of the *T'ai-su* and *Su-wen* versions of the *Huang-ti nei-ching* suggests that the potential for a development of a pharmacology of systematic correspondence was strengthened in the latter.

The *T'ai-su,* that is, the version closest to the Han nucleus of the *Huang-ti nei-ching* scriptures,[29] presents, in the chapter "T'iao-shih" (Regulating One's Diet),[30] a first categorization of primary substance qualities (i.e., "yellow," "green," "black," "red," and "white" as colors, and "acrid," "sweet," "sour," "bitter," and "salty" as flavors) along the lines of the Five Phases doctrine. From these primary qualities, secondary qualities are derived to describe the properties that natural substances can develop in the body, such as "hardening," "collecting," "dissipating," "calming," and "moistening." Through an association of these primary and secondary substance qualities with the five kinds of grains, fruit, domestic animals, and vegetables on the one hand, and with the five bodily depots on the other hand, a conceptual tool was provided to, first, regulate the daily intake of the respective qualities in accordance with a proper balance of the Five Phases, and, second, to add or decrease any of those qualities in accordance with extraordinary conditions, such as illness. Thus, the *T'ai-su* introduced therapeutic dietetics of systematic correspondence.

These tenets reappear in the *Su-wen*, that is, the version of the *Huang-ti nei-ching* that was thoroughly revised and rearranged by Wang Ping during the T'ang period, and then once more under the Sung. Here, however, the dietetic component is rather insignificant; instead one finds an abstract presentation of extended primary and secondary qualities with an emphasis on their usage in the cure of illnesses (see below, pp. 181–186). To the former were added the thermo-influences (ch'i), including "warm," "hot," "cool," and "cold"; the latter were amended by properties such as "penetrating" and "ascending" or "sinking." Furthermore, all of these qualities were now also linked with the two lines of association of the yinyang doctrine.

Thus at the latest by the seventh century (compiled in the *T'ai-su*) or by the eighth century (in Wang Ping's *Su-wen*), the essential prerequisites for the creation of a pharmacology of systematic correspondence were already present in the two versions of the *textus receptus* of the *Huang-ti nei-ching*. Although concrete drug names were not provided, their primary and secondary qualities were interpreted logically—from the taking of a substance to the manifestation of its effects—within the theoretical framework of systematic correspondence. Therefore, it is possible to speak in this context of an *abstract* pharmacology, at least in the *Su-wen* version of the *Huang-ti nei-ching*. The development of a concrete pharmacology of systematic correspondence was undertaken during the Sung-Chin-Yüan period;[31] it signified the attempt to analyze the primary qualities of each medicinally used drug and, on the basis of this information, to ascertain its secondary qualities, so that all dimensions of healing—from symptom and diagnosis to appropriate remedy and its therapeutic effects—could be incorporated within one inclusive theoretical system. In other words, pharmaceutical (pen-ts'ao) literature, prior to the Sung-Chin-Yüan epoch, contained the information that a certain drug x possessed the primary qualities y (thermo-influence) and z (flavor) and that the same drug could alleviate the symptoms a, b, c. There were no indications, however, of a causal connection between y and z, on the one hand, and the effects on $a, b,$ and $c,$ on the other hand.

But the *Huang-ti nei-ching su-wen* contained the information that the primary qualities y and z developed the specific secondary qualities p and q in the body and, consequently, could influence the symptoms a, b, and c. The concrete pharmacology of the Sung-Chin-Yüan era brought these scattered and incomplete efforts together, permitting the argument that a certain drug x, on the basis of its primary qualities y and z, developed the secondary qualities p and q in the body, and therefore could influence the symptoms a, b, and c.[32]

To erect such a system that integrated medical theory and pharmaceutical practice, it was first necessary to establish the exact primary qualities of each individual drug. In addition to the already indicated variables of thermo-influence, color, and flavor, other such empirically determinable qualities as form, odor, and weight were taken into consideration. Second, in order to incorporate each primary quality into the complex system of yinyang and the Five Phases, detailed information regarding both the manner and the location of its effects had to be provided, as required by the physiological insights and diagnostic possibilities recorded in the *Huang-ti nei-ching* and subsequent theoretical texts.

The second of these conditions was already at least partially fulfilled in the *Huang-ti nei-ching*: Sung-Chin-Yüan authors refined and completed this impulse. The drug work *T'ang-yeh pen-ts'ao* (Materia Medica of Boiled Potions) by Wang Hao-ku (fl. 1246–1248) represents the zenith of these efforts. In his work, Wang Hao-ku combined the central concepts of his teacher Li Kao, and Li Kao's teacher Chang Yüan-su, concerning pharmacology with his own deliberations, citing, in addition, other contemporary scholars, such as Ch'eng Wu-i and K'ou Tsung-shih (fl. 1116), who had studied such problems. The following sections illustrate the scope and complexity of the conceptual edifice created by these theoreticians, to the extent required for understanding both the difficulties raised by a desire to combine theory and practice in drug therapy and the solutions that were eventually achieved.[33]

7.2.3.1. *The Fourfold Categorization of Drug Qualities*

In agreement with the *Huang-ti nei-ching su-wen*, Sung-Chin-Yüan scholars assumed that the primary quality flavor (wei) was associated with yin and the primary quality thermo-influence (ch'i) with yang. Following the cyclical transformational character of the yinyang concept, whereby a continuous transition of mature yin (yin in yin) to immature yang (yang in yin) and then to mature yang (yang in yang) and finally to immature yin (yin in yang) occurs before the cycle begins anew, the primary qualities of drugs were now categorized in a four-part scheme. "Strongly developed" flavors (sour, bitter, salty) were identified by Sung-Chin-Yüan scholars as belonging to the yin-in-yin category. "Weakly developed" flavors (acrid, sweet, neutral) were recognized as belonging to the yang-in-yin category. Similarly, the "strong" thermo-influences (warm, hot, balanced) were assigned to the yang-in-yang category, and "weak" thermo-influences to the yin-in-yang category.

An additional possibility of characterizing qualitative distinctions among primary properties at a theoretical level was created by combining flavors and thermo-influence from the four subcategories of the yinyang order. Thus, for instance, a "strong" flavor could be expressed by the combination cold-sour, since cold and sour were both associated with the yin phase of their subcategory. A "strongly developed" thermo-influence could be indicated by the combination warm-sweet, since both warm and sweet belonged to the yang phases of their subcategories.

The secondary qualities developed by drugs in the body were also brought into harmony with this system: the "purgative" (hsieh) secondary quality was assigned to the yin-in-yin category, the "penetrating" (t'ung) secondary quality, for unblocking obstructions, to the yang-in-yin category, the "heating" (fa-je) secondary quality to the yang-in-yang, and, finally, the "dissipating" (fa-hsieh) secondary quality was assigned to the yin-in-yang category. The integration of the empirical dimensions of primary and secondary qualities with the theoretical concepts of yinyang are summarized in the following table:

7.2.3.2. The Sixfold Categorization of Drug Qualities

With the aid of the fourfold categorization, *how* drugs function in the organism could be explained and predicted. An understanding of these functions was, however, not nearly exhausted by the four secondary qualities outlined above. A much more important function ascribed to drugs was supplying individual palaces and depots, in case of depletion, with the necessary influences or, when repletion was present, to dissipate the influences in question. On the basis of these preliminary concepts, the development of a pharmacology required the demonstration of theoretical connections between drugs, on the one hand, and the location of their effects and the conduits leading to these locations, on the other hand. To accomplish this, Sun-Chin-

TABLE 1.
The Fourfold Categorization of Drug Qualities

Theoretical dimensions	yin		yang	
Empirical dimensions	Flavor (*wei*)		Thermo-influence (*ch'i*)	
Phases of theoretical dimensions	yin-in-yin (mature yin)	yang-in-yin (immat. yin)	yang-in-yang (mature yang)	yin-in-yang (immat. yang)
Phases of empirical dimensions	strongly developed flavor	weakly developed flavor	strongly developed thermo-influence	weakly developed thermo-influence
Primary qualities of drugs (1. Definition)	sour bitter salty	spicy sweet neutral	warm hot balanced	cold cool
Primary qualities of drugs (2. Definition)	cold-sour cold-bitter cold-salty	balanced-sour balanced-bitter balanced-salty	warm-spicy warm-sweet hot-spicy hot-sweet	cold-spicy cold-sweet cold-neutral cool-spicy cool-sweet cool-neutral
Secondary qualities of drugs	purgative (*hsieh*)	penetrating (*t'ung*)	heating (*fa-je*)	dissipating (*fa-hsieh*)

Yüan scholars incorporated the drugs into a six-part categorization of yinyang phases that had already been utilized in the *Huang-ti nei-ching su-wen* to indicate correspondences between the conduits and the depots and palaces. To the older notion that conduits in the body could conduct stimuli triggered by needles, heat, or even pressure, theoreticians of the Sung-Chin-Yüan period added the idea that drug properties could also be transported over the same channels. Thermo-influence and flavor were, in the final analysis, nothing more than yin and yang influences, which could be supplied to the body as needed. In his treatise *Chen-chu nang,* Chang Yüan-su therefore included in the description of each individual drug, following the indication of primary qualities, information he considered essential—namely, which conduits the substance could penetrate. During the Sung-Chin-Yüan period, this concept was refined to include the idea of "guiding drugs," drugs that exhibited a particular affinity for certain channels and could therefore lead other drugs directly to the desired location. In addition, scholars recognized that the affinity of drugs for specific conduits, as determined by the primary qualities, could be modified through pharmaceutical or technological means. It was known, for example, that raw drugs worked primarily in the upper half of the body, while prepared drugs acted in the lower half. The yang influence of a drug, and thus its efficacy in yang-associated body regions, could be controlled by treating the substances with wine, since wine itself was defined as a yang substance. The specific type of wine treatment also permitted subtle distinctions. Wang Hao-ku, for instance, commented:

> If the illness is located in the finger tips, in the forehead, or in the skin, the [drugs] *huang-ch'i, huang-lien, huang-po,* and *chih-mu* must be boiled with wine. In this way, the ability of wine to ascend in the body can be utilized. [If the illness is located] below the throat and above the navel, [one need only] rinse [the drugs] with wine.[34]

Numerous additional pharmaceutical-technological measures enabled a very precise control of the path taken by drugs and the location of the effects. The most important paths were the twelve major conduits; the numerous other network branches and secondary conduits can only be touched upon here. Six of the primary conduits were associated with yin and six with yang. Three of the yin conduits ran from the chest to a hand and three from a foot to the chest, and were therefore termed hand or foot conduits. Similarly, three of the yang conduits ran from one hand to the heart or from the head to a foot, and were also termed hand or foot conduits. Within the yin category, one hand and one foot conduit, respectively, was assigned to one of three qualitative phases—great yin (*t'ai-yin*), minor-yin (*shao-yin*), and ceasing yin (*ch'üeh-yin*), while within the yang category, one hand and one foot conduit, respectively, belonged to one of three phases—great yang (*t'ai-yang*), yang-brilliance (*yang-ming*), and minor yang (*shao-yang*). These relationships are summarized in the following table, which also includes information about associated earth branches—indicating connections with cosmic-seasonal tendencies—and the corresponding times of day, enabling the determination not only of the path to be taken by a drug and the desired location, but the desired time of action as well.

Although Chang Yüan-su had included in individual drug descriptions in the *Chen-chu nang* the conduits in which the substance developed its efficacy, and Wang Hao-ku, in the *T'ang-yeh pen-ts'ao*, had been the first to arrange drugs into a twelve-part table according

TABLE 2.
THE SIXFOLD CATEGORIZATION OF COURSE, LOCATION, AND TIME OF EFFECT

Yin				Yang			
Depot	Conduit	Earth branch	Time of day	Palace	Conduit	Earth branch	Time of day
lung	hand great-yin	yin	3–5	large intestine	hand yang-brilliance	mao	5–7
spleen	foot great-yin	ssu	9–11	stomach	foot yang-brilliance	ch'en	7–9
heart-enclosing network	hand ceasing yin	hsü	19–21	triple burner	hand minor-yang	hai	21–23
liver	foot ceasing yin	ch'ou	1–3	gall	foot minor-yang	tzu	23–1
heart	hand minor-yin	wu	11–13	small intestine	hand great-yang	wei	13–15
kidneys	foot great-yin	yu	17–19	bladder	foot great-yang	shen	15–17

to the conduits, in both cases the authors did not indicate which criteria had been used in their classification. A study of individual substances reveals only that drugs assigned to the yin phase in the fourfold categorization are associated here in the sixfold categorization with a yang conduit and vice versa. The reader does not learn why a certain yin drug, for example, is assigned to a yang-brilliance conduit and not to a major-yang conduit. Unlike the fourfold categorization, there is no direct classification of primary drug qualities in accordance with the six-part division. It seems likely that conclusions about the effects of substances within the organism were derived in reverse from the observed reactions.

7.2.3.3. The Fivefold Categorization of Drug Qualities

A third system for the classification of primary and secondary drug qualities which Sung-Chin-Yüan scholars developed on the basis of the *Huang-ti nei-ching su-wen* consisted of arranging the primary properties first in accordance with the five categories of the Five Phases concept. Since these Five Phases were also correlated with the depots and palaces, as well as through the celestial stems with the five cir-

TABLE 3.
THE FIVEFOLD CATEGORIZATION OF DRUG QUALITIES

Phases	wood	fire	soil	metal	water
Depots	liver	heart	spleen	lung	kidneys
Palaces	gall	sm. intestine triple burner	stomach	large intestine	bladder
Flavor	salty	sour	sweet	bitter	spicy
Thermo-infl.	warm	hot	balanced	cool	cold
Celestial stem	*ting-jen*	*mou-kuei*	*chia-chi*	*i-keng*	*ping-hsin*
Yinyang categories	yang-in-yin	yang-in-yang	——	yin-in-yang	yin-in-yin

culatory phases and six climatic influences, the result was an additional method for differentiating the properties of medicinal substances according to location and time. As the following table indicates, a correlation between the fourfold yinyang division and the Five Phases was established, ultimately producing an intricate, extremely complex system of correspondences.

7.2.3.4. The Determination of Primary Qualities

To provide the pharmacological system as described thus far with a concrete significance, it was necessary to fulfill the first condition cited above, namely, to investigate in detail the primary qualities of each drug, so as to establish the connection between a substance and its actual effects, on the one hand, and the pharmacological-theoretical construct, on the other hand. The primary qualities of drugs, it must be stressed, constituted the critical connecting link.

Sung-Chin-Yüan scholars already had access to information on the flavor, thermo-influence, color, and so forth of individual drugs in the older pharmaceutical literature. Such information was, however, incomplete and undifferentiated, and researchers sought to verify their own deliberations by comparing the ideal results, that is, the effects to be expected on the basis of a drug's primary qualities within the theoretical system, with the actual results reported by earlier authors. In addition, they contributed missing information on the primary qualities and had to decide how the flavor and thermo-influence of substances could be determined. Both tasks presented the scholars with difficult problems. There were no objective criteria by which primary qualities, so essential for the pharmacological determination of drugs, could be rendered demonstrable for everyone. Since only a few of the drugs possessed a distinct flavor, to say nothing of the even more formidable task of defining thermo-influence, scholars naturally disagreed. Chang Yüan-su, for example, concluded that the thermo-influence of croton seeds was weak-hot and the flavor weak-bitter. Since the drug was also heavy and descended in the body, he assigned it to the yin category. His pupil Li Kao, in contrast, classified croton seeds as a yang substance, since he determined that it possessed a hot thermo-influence and acrid flavor and, moreover, remained suspended in the body rather than descending. Such a variance in classification, of course, led the authors to different conclusions concerning location, course, and time of a drug's action.

In some cases, it could be shown that the theoretically expected results did not agree with the empirically observed effects of drugs. If so, it was possible to eliminate the contradiction through the notion that each yin phase already contained a nascent yang phase (yang-in-yin) and vice versa. Such an approach, however, simultaneously removed from the system any force of expression and definition. Characteristic of this tendency is a passage from the *T'ang-yeh pen-ts'ao* by Wang Hao-ku:

> [The drug] *fu-ling* has a neutral flavor and corresponds to the *yang* of heaven. [Since it belongs to the] *yang* [category], it should ascend in the body. But why does [the drug] nonetheless function as a diuretic, thus dissipating through the lower part of the body? In the scripture it is written: "That which has a weak flavor belongs to the category *yang* in *yin*." For this reason *fu-ling* is diuretic, dissipating through the lower [parts of the] body.[35]

A second method for eliminating such contradictions was utilized primarily by Chu Chen-heng (1281–1358), the last original thinker of this era, and involved the recognition that each individual drug had at the same time several primary qualities. By arguing that a single substance was simultaneously acrid, sweet, and sour, each effect could be easily explained by means of the theoretical associations of those qualities. It appears that in all these uncertain cases, the theoretical primary qualities were deduced in reverse from the observed actions of the drugs.

The Sung-Chin-Yüan authors appear to have recognized fully the difficulties inherent in their efforts. Their works are marked by detailed annotations that attempt to answer all questions and remove all contradictions. Nonetheless, it must be concluded that they were unable to create a concrete pharmacology that represented anything more than an interpretation of known drug effects derived after the fact on the basis of a universally accepted conceptual framework. It was impossible to take an unknown substance, objectively determine its primary qualities, and, based on this information, deduce the secondary qualities, that is, the expected effects, the path, and the location with such certainty that the subsequently observed reality corresponded to expectations with no significant contradiction. Although practitioners were thus provided with a means of explaining and possibly understanding the use of drugs and effects with old concepts from the *Huang-ti nei-ching,* a more important requirement for a concrete pharmacology went unfulfilled. The practitioner could not, having diagnosed that a patient suffered from repletion or depletion in a depot or palace, and after having qualitatively differentiated the yinyang character of the ailment, as well as having defined the required location and course of action, now consult drug literature for a substance possessing the appropriate primary qualities and initiate therapy on that basis. It is therefore not surprising that drug works of the Sung-Chin-Yüan era, in addition to numerous theoretical explanations, also contained a section labeled simply "Treatment of Symptoms." Here, without any pharmacological embellishment, the reader was advised to use the drug x for headache and, for some other illness, the drug y.

If this discussion of these efforts and their results has a negative tone—since it appears that Sung-Chin-Yüan scholars ultimately failed to develop a concrete pharmacology—we should nevertheless ask ourselves if such a critical assessment is perhaps not historically incorrect, since it is based on our own criteria for a concrete pharmacology. We do not know whether it was even the intention of Sung-Chin-Yüan researchers to provide practitioners with just such a tool. Perhaps they desired only to integrate existing pragmatic pharmaceutical knowledge into classical theories of systematic correspondence without fulfilling our own notions of the practical implications of a pharmacology. As long as we lack any explicit statements from any of the theoreticians involved, we must restrict ourselves to a presentation of the events themselves and judge their success, if at all, only with great reservation.

8. Medical Thought during the Ming and Ch'ing Epochs: The Individual in Search of Reality

8.1. POLITICAL AND INTELLECTUAL DEVELOPMENTS

8.1.1. The Ming Epoch (1368–1636)

At approximately the end of the first quarter of the fourteenth century, the Mongol rulers of the Yüan dynasty faced the first uprisings of the Chinese people. The inability—or unwillingness—of these horsemen from the steppes to comprehend Chinese intellectual culture and the accompanying lack of understanding for the civil service system of a country highly dependent on agriculture and trade, led to such intolerable conditions that socially motivated revolutionary movements sprang up at several locations, quickly expanding into widespread civil war. The Mongol leaders themselves were fractionalized and paralyzed by brutal internal strife; numerically at a great disadvantage, they were unable to suppress the Chinese rage for very long. Finally, when highly nationalistic elements joined social revolutionary forces in the struggle against foreign domination, thus providing the Chinese aristocracy with a justification for entering the rebellion, the Mongols were driven into the northern steppes, where they remained a political factor for several centuries. In 1368, Chinese troops occupied Peking, and the Ming dynasty was proclaimed in the same year. Chu Yüan-chang (1328–1398), the son of an impoverished peasant family, who had risen from a simple gang leader to be the most important commander of the rebels, was named the first emperor.[1] Some of the governmental and political reforms that he initiated were to shape political, intellectual, and cultural life during the subsequent centuries of the Ming period.

Inseparably linked with Ming rule is the concept of absolutism. Chu Yüan-chang achieved his position through a uniquely balanced constellation of political groups that concentrated institutional power in the imperial office to a degree unmatched by any previous Chinese ruler. Chu Yüan-chang and his advisers did not hesitate to utilize Mongol practices if they served to strengthen their authority.[2] Although the newly achieved peace soon produced renewed prosperity in the empire, the rise of absolutism, it soon became evident, already contained the seeds of the dynasty's decline. The deterioration of the civil service and the encapsulation of imperial control from the rest of society meant in actuality the continuation of the Mongol burden under Chinese rule. Initially, even the eunuchs, who so often had played such a fateful role in conflicts with scholar-officials, were excluded from imperial centers of power. But already by the beginning of the fifteenth century, this situation had changed, and the eunuchs once again occupied decision-making offices. The result was a new outbreak of the old conflict with Confucian officials, although not in the same form as during the Han or T'ang periods, when two largely homogeneous groups opposed each other. Confucianism under the Ming was beset by internal strife, weakened and fragmented into various political and ideological splinter groups, and thus powerless to combat the growing influence of the eunuchs.[3]

It is necessary to examine this development in greater detail since it also had some influence on Ming medical thought. Two aspects of early Ming politics are of particular significance in this regard—the rise of the Neo-Confucianism of the brothers Ch'eng and Chu Hsi to orthodox political and social philosophy, and the "democratization" of the civil service. The emperor and his advisers sought to open a civil service career and its prerequisite, a Confucian education, to broader segments of the population. In this respect, early Ming policies were indeed influenced by the original sociorevolutionary impulses of the earlier rebels. State examinations were standardized and simplified considerably; practical abilities were now judged as more valuable than an extensive literary education.[4] A knowledge of Neo-Confucian ideology was considered an appropriate subject for examination, though the examinations themselves required neither an extensive mental struggle with its concepts nor an internalization of its ethical precepts, but rather simply mechanical memorization of certain passages and orthodox commentaries which were to be recited on cue. Civil service candidates went through the preparation and the examinations as a mere formality, with no expectations that future conduct or political thought had been decisively influenced. The result, as Kuei Yu-kuang (1506–1571) lamented, was that "the status distinctions among scholars, peasants, and merchants have become blurred."[5] Even serfs were now able to receive an education and participate in state examinations.[6] These developments were accompanied by the appearance of numerous writings, in which a popularized Confucianism was presented to a new group of readers previously excluded from a literary education. A general rise in the standard of living, together with an increased demand, produced a flood of printed literature and improved the possibilities for individual writers to publish their works. Thus, not only was the cultural tradition of the upper strata disseminated among the lower segments of the population to a previously unknown extent but, conversely, the views and political objectives of earlier fringe groups found their way to the upper reaches of society.[7]

The ensuing diversity of attitudes during the Ming era is remarkable. It was, moreover, augmented by efforts of many serious Confucian scholars to express concern about the intellectual triviality of official examination requirements through their own ideas of political morality. Since Ch'eng-Chu Neo-Confucianism had been virtually sanctioned by the bureaucracy, numerous thinkers pursued individual solutions, while others, in particular Wang Yang-ming (1472–1529), sought to realize their theories in daily political practice, even if this occasionally produced violent conflicts with the orthodox forces. Several philosophical schools evolved, which operated basically within the bounds of Ch'eng-Chu Neo-Confucianism but which had already reshaped the latter's ideas in a fundamental manner.[8] Other thinkers advocated completely heretical doctrines. The intellectual disorientation of the age was exacerbated by the fact that—although Confucianism had "conquered" the competing philosophies of Taoism and Buddhism since the Sung period—Taoist and Buddhist concepts, under a more or less intended disguise of Confucianism, had influenced Chinese thought to a greater degree than ever before.[9] While an obsolete Neo-Confucianism covered the empire like a hard crust, beneath the surface a vigorous intellectual life developed, increasingly distancing itself from orthodoxy and underlining the growing contrast between the state and its claims, on the one hand, and the expectations and desires of the people and scholarly community, on the other hand. The gap between the divided, strife-ridden civil service and the upper levels of the government, as well as the struggles between individual groups of scholar-officials and their eunuch opponents eventually paralyzed the government, neutralizing its ability to respond effectively to internal and foreign developments. During the late sixteenth and early seventeenth centuries, the widespread mismanagement, which the initial flowering of the Ming era had suppressed, was aggravated by natural catastrophes and failed harvests in several provinces, but there was no reduction in the tax burden of the affected population. During the 1620s, several uprisings occurred which, after scattered initial success, the government was finally unable to contain. In the north, various Tungus tribes had joined together to form a political entity—the Manchu nation. In part with the assistance of the Mongols, they began to invade and conquer outlying territories in 1618, a process that the empire could not permanently withstand. Faced with the disintegration of Ming rule, forced to choose between sociorevolutionary insurgents from within and foreign domination from the north—which could be expected to leave existing privileges intact—the Chinese aristocracy opted for the latter alternative, particularly since it was already known that the Manchus had consciously structured their state after Chinese models before beginning their conquests. The Ch'ing dynasty was proclaimed in the year 1636.[10]

8.1.2. The Ch'ing Epoch (1636–1912)

In stark contrast to the fundamental, far-reaching caesura that accompanied the changeover from Sung to Mongol rule, the transition from the Chinese Ming Dynasty to Manchurian Ch'ing control was marked by a continuity of ideology, structures, and institutions. The new imperial government adopted both absolutism and Sung Neo-Confucianism to reinforce its newly consolidated power. Unlike the Mongols of the Yüan dynasty, the Manchus made a serious effort to understand Confucian values and to become the legitimate heirs of political and intellectual traditions of the subjugated Chinese culture. With three successive, unusually capable and farsighted emperors— K'ang-hsi (reigned 1662–1723), Yung-cheng (reigned 1723–1736), and Ch'ien-lung (reigned 1736–1796)—the Manchu state was in fact able to achieve economic, cultural, and political significance, which, although it did not match the magnificent golden ages of the past, nonetheless represented a new pinnacle of Chinese civilization. But with Ch'ien-lung's voluntary abdication, the cyclical decline in the ceaseless ebb and flow of dynastic history in China began anew; the

Manchu state, in the long run, was also unable to cope with the foreign and internal burdens of China, which perhaps required a totally different philosophical outlook than a Sung Neo-Confucianism reduced to a mere examination topic.

Conservative forces, concerned about the welfare of the Chinese nation, had begun to raise their voices soon after the founding of the Ch'ing dynasty, adding an antitraditionalist component to the already diverse conceptual spectrum of the time. They held the Sung doctrine and its consequences responsible for the decline of the empire that had begun with the collapse of the Northern Sung dynasty. Conservatives cited as proof the fact that, following the humiliation by the Mongols and the relatively brief interlude of the Ming, the establishment of the Ch'ing dynasty signified yet another triumph by northern barbarians over China; thus they believed it was now time to return from the false doctrine of Neo-Confucianism to Confucianism, which had made China strong and whose restoration, it was assumed, was better suited to solving the continuing problems than were all the heresies of a more recent vintage. Opponents of Neo-Confucianism thus steadily retreated through chronologically earlier stages in the development of Confucianism until they had reached Mencius and Confucius himself; then they even began to question the views of these men.

One of the first to attack publicly the "empty philosophizing of Sung doctrine" and proclaim it responsible for China's decline was the scholar Ku Yen-wu (1613–1682). In his view, civil servants trained under this philosophy were incapable of assessing political realities and of guarding the country from internal and external misfortunes. To overcome the "shortsightedness" of Neo-Confucianism, particularly the form of Wang Yang-ming that resembled meditative Buddhism, he proposed the utilization of as many literary sources as possible. Ku Yen-wu believed the Han period commentaries of Confucian classics stood closer to the true insights of antiquity than did the originators of Sung doctrine. He therefore placed particular emphasis on the study of the early texts.[11]

The philosopher Yen Yüan (1635–1704) was also an advocate of the "return to the past." Following initial enthusiasm for Sung teaching, he later rejected all Buddhist and Taoist influences in contemporary Confucian thought, bitterly attacking the "incessant theorizing" of the Neo-Confucians.[12]

Despite all individual attempts to find a conceptual foundation for resolving internal social conflicts and the growing external threat from Western powers, a series of events beginning at the end of the eighteenth century led not only to the demise of the Manchu state but also ultimately to the collapse of imperial rule itself, and with it the conclusion of the Confucian epoch. Contributing to the difficulties of the government were secret societies, particularly the White Lotus, as well as an enormous growth in population, which during the first few decades of the nineteenth century increased in China some 30 percent to 400 million, without food production being able to keep pace. Initially, foreign trade brought significant profits, but the introduction of opium and the subsequent flow of silver out of the country led for the first time to a trade deficit in 1825, an imbalance that quickly became critical. The Opium War of 1839–1842 placed additional severe strains on the Chinese economy; the activities of secret societies continued to grow as a result of internal distress and the humiliation caused by foreign intervention. The conflicts arising out of the T'ai-p'ing rebellion from 1850 to 1866 resulted in destruction of enormous magnitude, claiming many millions of victims. This was soon followed by the Sino-Japanese War and, at the turn of the century, by the so-called Boxer Rebellion, directed against both imperial forces and foreign Manchu domination, which was crushed only by a foreign expeditionary force. All attempts at modernization and reform by the Ch'ing government were doomed to failure under the onslaught of events, as they represented only superficial corrections. When the Manchu leaders announced the abdication of the emperor on February 12, 1912, and proclaimed China a republic, it was not so much a result of an immediate military threat from external or internal sources as an admission of complete perplexity and helplessness.[13]

8.2. MEDICAL THOUGHT

8.2.1. The Intellectual Environment

Medical thought during the Ming and Ch'ing eras adhered closely to general intellectual tendencies of these last two epochs of Imperial China. Certain aspects of Sung-Chin-Yüan medicine—etiological reductionism in particular—were carried on. Another characteristic of Sung-Chin-Yüan medicine, namely, the attempt (resulting from the influence of original Neo-Confucianism) to incorporate medicinal drugs into the framework of systematic correspondence, was not picked up or given fresh inspiration. The reasons behind this last phenomenon are not mentioned explicitly by any author. It might appear that the old theories of the *Huang-ti nei-ching* were regarded as unsuited to resolving the obvious contradictions between the results expected on the basis of specific primary qualities, on the one hand, and the actual observed effects, on the other hand. Such an attempt, however, to explain the end of efforts to establish a theoretical pharmacology of systematic correspondence along this line would rest solely on a Western understanding of science and is therefore useless for an understanding of this phenomenon. It is possible, and perhaps more probable, that the work of Chu Chen-heng provided a satisfactory explanation of drug qualities and usage, even if, from our perspective, it represented only a posteriori theorizing and lacked the prognostic qualities demanded of every science.

Rather than concentrate on a pharmacology of systematic correspondence, important authors of the Ming and Ch'ing eras sought to incorporate demonology—which for centuries had existed independently outside of Confucian doctrine—into systematic correspondence. It will be necessary at a later point to devote a separate section to this development since, along with other phenomena, it constitutes significant evidence of the ongoing synthesis of previously heterogeneous conceptual systems into orthodox medicine.

One way to distinguish between the Ming and Ch'ing approach to medical thought is to recognize that under the Ming, the individual search for reality, begun during the Sung-Chin-Yüan period, was continued, blossoming for the first time in a multiplicity of individual approaches and new interpretations of the ancient classics that far surpassed those of previous centuries. This trend continued during the Ch'ing period, but the widespread belief in the inadequacy of traditional healing influenced some authors to reject vehemently all post-Sung innovations in medical thought and to seek instead a "true" understanding of the ancient sources. The broad influx of Western therapeutic practices beginning in the mid-nineteenth century, in particular anatomical knowledge and the minor surgical skills of Western physicians, as well as the introduction of Western scientific methods, caused a number of Chinese practitioners to lose all faith in their own system.

During the Sung period, when intellectual developments, with the motto "investigate things and affairs and extend knowledge to the utmost" (*ko-wu-chih-chih*), had provided the individual with the legitimate opportunity to establish his own view of the surrounding world and, with the appropriate caution and under the guise of the "correct" interpretation of the classics, criticize past views, Chinese medical thought began a course that ended only with the demise of the empire. Although the precept ko-wu-chih-chih was given a certain new interpretation and significance during the Ming period, the incentive for the individual to develop his own thoughts was even strengthened. The initially intellectual interest in the expansion of knowledge about man's environment, which had marked Sung philosophy, was supplanted during the Ming period by the moral resolve to bring to fruition—through an understanding of things—the knowledge existing a priori in man (liang-chih) that leads us to morally correct action in the real world.[14]

Wang Yang-ming, who had introduced the concept liang-chih to Chinese philosophy, stressed to a much greater degree than did Chu Hsi the oneness of man with the objects of his sensual perception. Chu Hsi had argued that a single organizing principle (li) informed and controlled all things, but he accorded each individual phenomenon a certain separate materialization of this principle that was independent of man's spirit. At this point, Wang Yang-ming and other Ming thinkers diverged by perceiving the reality of environmental phenomena as being preexisting in our mind. They therefore considered the organic unity of the human spirit and the universe to be much closer and all-pervading than did Sung philosophers. The realization of each person's innate knowledge is therefore of enormous significance. Morally faultless conduct that arises from this knowledge produces complete physical and mental well-being, not only in the individual but within all things as well. Personal health and the harmony of the environment are thus partly dependent upon virtuous conduct, which is dictated by the truth of innate wisdom that must be uncovered from beneath many layers of ignorance.[15] To achieve this true wisdom, various thinkers advocated a number of techniques, including introspective meditation which—borrowed from or at least resembling Ch'an Buddhism—assumed a major role. Yet scarcely a single Ming philosopher denied the necessity of supplementing self-investigation with observation of the external world or a concern for the matters of daily life. Representative of this synthesis of self-reflection and active concern with the surrounding world, which sought first to uncover innate knowledge and then to adopt it as a basis for personal conduct, is the work of Ch'en Hsien-chang (1428–1500). In his view, the inner organizing principle of the objects in man's environment could only be recognized through personal experience, that is, direct observation (tzu-te), followed by contemplation. Ch'en Hsien-chang accorded to personal experience an expressly higher value in the formation of knowledge than did the surviving views of the ancient sages, exhorting his readers to:

Have doubts and then undertake investigations! Through investigations man can achieve knowledge! Achieve true wisdom first and then build your faith! Doubt is the starting point of the way that leads to the [recognition] of Tao; Faith is [the true knowledge] that man possesses within himself from the very beginning![16]

The climate fostered by such a philosophy persisted through the Ming to the conclusion of the Ch'ing era, stimulating an extremely fruitful period in medical thought that lasted more than four centuries. But it was a fruitfulness that led to an even greater divergence of opinion; decade after decade saw new theories proposed and older views criticized, with no single approach being able to achieve sufficient authority to displace the others. It is a characteristic feature of this period that its insights remained tied to individual scholars, and that no single approach was sufficiently plausible to convince the majority of medical practitioners and achieve, even temporarily, the position of a generally recognized doctrine.

If the first half of the history of the medicine of systematic correspondence, from the Han to the Sung, is characterized by a naive application of the theories of the *Huang-ti nei-ching* and *Nan-ching* by the few authors who used them, the second millennium following the Sung period reveals a steadily growing unrest, reflected in various reductionistic etiologies, in debates about anatomical and physiological details, and in attempts to expand the theoretical system. The diversity of schools and their conflicting views during the Ming and Ch'ing periods convey the impression that the conceptual framework of systematic correspondence at this time was nothing more than a complex labyrinth, in which those thinkers seeking solutions to medical questions wandered aimlessly in all directions, lacking any orientation, and unable to find a feasible way out. Such a solution came only with the collapse of the Confucian social order and the subsequent weakening of the world view that had prevailed for centuries.

8.2.2. The Spectrum of Conceptual Approaches

8.2.2.1. *Searching the Interior*

Of the countless individual attempts of Ming and Ch'ing authors to sift traditional forms of medical thought and therapeutic procedures and, where necessary, adapt them to contemporary circumstances, several approaches will be sketched in some detail below. One must first keep in mind that all of the Sung-Chin-Yüan authors found adherents during the Ming and Ch'ing periods who adopted the various doctrines and, in more or less modified form, proclaimed them to be eternal truths. Some of these disciples adhered closely to the views of a single Sung-Chin-Yüan scholar, such as Tai Ssu-kung (1322–1405), who had carried on the tradition of his own teacher, Chu Chen-heng. This particular school subsequently became known as *yang yin,* as it was based on the notion that a deficiency of yin influences was the primary cause of human illness. The correct therapy, according to proponents of this school, thus necessitated correcting this imbalance by supplying yin influences with the appropriate substances.

The theories of Li Kao also formed the basis of a long tradition. Known as the *wen pu* course, it gained wide acceptance during the Ming period; its main objective was to supply the body with substances that radiated warmth, in order to replenish the fire in the organism, which was constantly threatened by premature extinguishment.

Around 1550, Hsüeh Chi completed several works in which he sought to synthesize the views of Chu Chen-heng and Li Kao. Hsüeh Chi thus accorded a special physiological significance not only to the spleen and stomach but to the kidneys as well. In the system of the Five Phases, the spleen and stomach are associated with soil. Just as the soil, in order to nourish all living creatures, must retain its fertility during all four seasons, the spleen and stomach must continually radiate fortifying and nourishing influences, so as to strengthen the four extremities and supply the body's depots and palaces with blood. The spleen and stomach perform this central function only so long as they are able to remove vital influences from the basic substances that enter the body from outside. When man falls ill, according to Hsüeh Chi's interpretation of Li Kao's teachings, this processing ability is disrupted and must be restored by the administration of warming substances. To a certain extent, Hsüeh Chi also recognized the necessity of cooling therapy, as the fire present in the kidneys can easily burn out of control, triggering a deficiency of yin influences and producing the corresponding symptoms. It was therefore not unusual for him to prescribe first drugs intended to restore the efficiency of the spleen and stomach gradually, followed by other drugs that supplied the kidneys directly with the required yin influences, all within the course of a single day. Despite these priorities, it appears that Hsüeh Chi was fully aware of the fact that human illness could not be reduced to one or two patterns; indeed, he held open the possibility that his treatment would have to be modified according to the needs of individual patients.[17]

Chang Chieh-pin, an author known through various medical works, was active around the year 1624. Initially Chang Chieh-pin pursued a career in the military, but when this ended in failure, he turned to medicine. From that time on, he viewed illness as his enemy, adopting military terms for the eight different forms of therapy that he developed, such as "battle plans" or "strategic formations" (*pa-chen*); he compared the use of drugs with the employment of troops. Up to the age of forty, Chang Chieh-pin followed the teachings of Liu Wan-su and Chu Chen-heng. But then, as a result of his own experiences, he began to have doubts, and the precepts of Chu Chen-heng in particular—namely, that a pathological surplus of yang influences is frequently present in the body—now seemed to him completely untenable. In accordance with the conclusions of Hsüeh Chi and Li Kao, he too now considered the yang component in the organism to be of primary importance and therefore advocated constant replenishment of the body with yang influences to treat and prevent illness. Chang Chieh-pin's arguments were formulated as follows: The influences that flow through the body form the yang component, while the structure of the body itself constitutes the yin component. Yinyang dualism requires that the yin component cannot exist without a yang component and vice versa. Applied to man, this signifies that bodily structure requires influences to come into existence and that the influences, in turn, require this structure as their supporting medium. All living beings are therefore brought into existence by yang influences and given a physical structure by yin influences. This process of genesis proceeds indefinitely, ensuring the continuation of existence. An imbalance of yin and yang influences leads eventually to death. In this connection, Chang Chieh-pin cited the following two statements in the *Huang-ti nei-ching*:

> When yin and yang influences work together, it is of great importance that the yang influences remain tightly sealed. In this way, strength can be maintained.
> Yang influences possess [for man] the same significance as does the sun for the heavens.[18]

Chang himself remarked:

> This red globe of the sun is of utmost significance for heaven. The original yang influences alone represent the supreme value for man![19]

He then contrasted the precepts of Chu Chen-heng with his own doctrine that the yang component could not form a pathological surplus, further supporting his views as follows:

The only possibility one need fear in regard to the yang component is that it might be insufficiently developed and, in the case of the yin component, that it might be overly developed. The yin component is, however, by itself incapable of reaching a state of excess; for this it requires a deficiency of yang [influences]. The animation of all things is dependent upon yang [influences]; similarly the death of all living beings is dependent upon yang influences. But the yang [influences] themselves do not kill, for life itself arises where yang influences are present. Death occurs where yang [influences] fail to appear![20]

In this view, therefore, it is impossible to assimilate an excess of yang influences.

The function of the kidneys played a significant role in sixteenth- and seventeeth-century discussions about the physiological priorities of individual body depots and palaces. At the center of debate was the so-called Gate of Life (*ming-men*), a concept that found contradictory interpretations in classical literature. In the *Huang-ti nei-ching,* the term *ming-men* is employed repeatedly to designate the eyes.[21] For many subsequent centuries the authoritative statement stemmed from the *Nan-ching,* whereby man had two kidneys, the left of which was the actual kidney, while the right constituted the Gate of Life. In men, according to the *Nan-ching,* the Gate of Life served as a sperm depot; in women, as the womb.[22] Hsüeh Chi and Chang Chieh-pin had supported this view. Chao Hsien-k'o, however, a contemporary of Hsüeh Chi, deemed it necessary to introduce a new idea, which called into question the traditional hierarchy of bodily storage facilities. His convictions rested on two passages in the *Su-wen,* which had apparently remained unnoticed up to that time. The chapter "Ling-lan mi-tien" contains the following passages: "The heart is the ruling official" and, somewhat later, "If the ruler is not enlightened, this denotes danger for the twelve officials." Since "twelve officials" refers to the six body depots (including the heart-enclosing network) and the six palaces, the heart—generally considered to be the ranking official in the depots—can thus not be the foremost ruler in the body, whose "enlightenment" (*ming*) is required to ensure the activities of the twelve officials. From this Chao Hsien-k'o concluded that the true ruler had to be the Gate of Life, finding support for this contention in the *Su-wen.* The chapter "Tz'u-chin lun" contains the following statement:

Adjacent to the seventh vertebra, in the center [of the body], lies the minor-heart (*hsiao-hsin*).

Chao Hsien-k'o interpreted the term "minor-heart" as merely an obsolete designation for the Gate of Life, pointing out that the kidneys were also located next to the seventh vertebra. He concluded:

> When Yüeh-jen [i.e., Pien Ch'io, the purported author of the *Nan-ching*] maintains that the left [kidney] is the true kidney, while the right is the Gate of Life, this claim is false. The Gate of Life is located between the two kidneys, one *ts'un* and five *fen* distant from each, exactly at the midpoint of the body. Here is the real master, the true ruler.[23]

Despite the detailed measurements, it is not totally clear whether Chao Hsien-k'o considered the Gate of Life to be a concrete anatomical structure. He argued that the two kidneys should be understood as water, separated by an amorphous fire, the Gate of Life. While physical fire is extinguished by water, he continued, formless fire is created by water, a fact that explains the position of the Gate of Life between the two kidneys. But this dependency is mutual, for the Gate of Life is the point of origin for all essential influences. If a deficiency of influences occurs in one of the depots or palaces, illness will result. Insufficient radiation by the Gate of Life to the kidneys results in a diminished sexual drive. If the Gate of Life does not supply the bladder with sufficient influences, the water passages become obstructed. If the spleen and stomach lack influences from the Gate of Life, they lose their ability to digest substances and to direct the five flavors that are assimilated from foodstuffs to the appropriate regions of the body. If the liver and gall bladder are insufficiently supplied, the victim's decision-making and planning abilities are affected. The small and large intestines require influences from the Gate of Life in order to convert foodstuffs; a deficiency in this area produces a blockage of the urinary and anal openings. Finally, an insufficient supply of influences to the heart causes a disorientation of the mind and abnormal reactions to external impressions. According to Chao Hsien-k'o, these results confirmed the claim in the *Su-wen:* "If the ruler is not enlightened, this denotes danger for the twelve officials!"[24]

Chao Hsien-k'o's fundamental therapeutic principles were derived from the implications in the above-mentioned considerations that the continuation of human life is dependent on the intensity of the internal fire. A weakness, as well as an excessive intensity, of this fire, results in illness and, possibly, death. Treatment of such pathological conditions, however, can only be accomplished by means of the kidneys, which—associated with water—control the fire of the Gate of Life.

In this connection, Chao Hsien-k'o returned to the relationship between physical water and physical fire, advocating, if the fire were too
intense, augmenting the water of the kidneys and, if the fire threatened
to go out, the drawing off of water.[25]

At the end of the sixteenth century, Sun I-k'uei dealt with the concept of the Gate of Life. He agreed with Chao Hsien-k'o that it was
located between the kidneys, arguing that the kidneys and Gate of
Life together constituted the first morphological element of the future
human body, which comes into existence after the coalescence of male
yang and female yin influences but before the future being has been
differentiated sexually. During the entirety of human existence, he
continued, the Gate of Life contains the original influences (*yüan-ch'i*),
which he also designated—redefining a term used in another sense in
classical literature—*tung-ch'i* ("driving influence").[26]

Some fifty years later another author, Li Chung-tse (died 1655),
forged the concepts of Hsüeh Chi, Chao Hsien-k'o, and Sun I-k'uei,
on the one hand, and Chang Yüan-su and Li Kao, on the other hand,
into a synthesis. Like Hsüeh Chi, Li Chung-tse also regarded the spleen
and stomach as well as the kidneys as the most important organs of
human physiology, but he justified his conclusions with a new argument. In his view, the basis of human existence can be compared to
the roots of a tree or the source of a stream. For man, however, this
foundation is two dimensional, for it consists of both the "roots of
early days" and the "roots of late days." Li Chung-tse saw in the
kidneys the roots of early days and in the spleen the roots of late days,
arguing as follows:

> Why are the kidneys the roots of early days? Even before the fetus
> assumes any form, the two kidneys are already in existence. They there-
> fore constitute the roots of the depots and palaces, of the twelve blood
> channels, the roots of inhalation and exhalation and the source of the
> triple burner. The very beginning of human existence depends on the
> kidneys. Therefore it is said that the source of early days lies in
> the kidneys. Why is the spleen called the source of late days? When
> the fetus has assumed its form and does not eat for a day, it becomes
> hungry. When it has received no nourishment for seven days, the in-
> testines and stomach dry up and the fetus dies. In the classic it is written:
> "Wherever sufficient nourishment is present, existence flourishes; where
> the supply of food is interrupted, life is doomed!" If the influences of
> the stomach have finally been destroyed, all medicines are of absolutely
> no use. As soon as the body assumes its physical form, it requires the
> influences contained in foods. Foods first enter the stomach and are
> then freshly stored in the six palaces. The foods then release their in-

fluences, which are blended in the five depots, bringing about the formation of blood. For the entire course of his life, man depends on these influences; thus we speak of the roots of late days.[27]

Li Chung-tse did not regard the numerous diverging doctrines advocated by previous authors, which were based on various specific etiologies, as mutually exclusive positions and even defended the originators against the criticism of one-sidedness. According to Li Chung-tse, these men were concerned above all with correcting certain flaws in the writings of their predecessors and thus contributed to an increasingly complete whole. Those practitioners, however, who specialized in one or another of these doctrines, obviously had only a superficial knowledge of the literature, since they followed only the corrections and not the original works that had been revised.[28]

The words of Li Chung-tse serve as a bridge to a short discussion of an eclectic tradition known as the School of Compromise (che-chung p'ai). Its followers did not propose any of their own theories, selecting instead those insights and instructions from the extensive medical literature that they found useful. It appears that the School of Compromise shared the concern of numerous Confucians that medical knowledge could become so highly specialized that only experts would be able to master the field. Such experts, however, were viewed with great suspicion, for Confucians were highly conscious of the fact that with specialization comes the formation of groups within society, which in turn has consequences for the distribution of decision-making powers. To prevent such developments, orthodox Confucians required of each individual sufficient medical proficiency to provide assistance to relatives in case of emergencies.[29] Ni Wei-te (fl. 1370), one of the earliest eclectics, wrote the following passage on the problem of specialized knowledge:

The art of healing is one of the matters of concern for every Confucian; when the two paths went their separate ways, I do not know. Father and mother are man's closest relatives. If they should fall ill, and one entrusts their treatment to a stranger, life and death of the parents are in the hands of a man not even close to them. A single mistake is all it takes, and their life is over. If, however, a person during his entire life has treated his fellow man with human kindness, why should he not demonstrate this same concern for his parents! . . . This is why the art of healing belongs to the concerns of every Confucian. Whether it be suffering caused by cold, internal injuries, feminine disorders, or children's illnesses, a practitioner must be equally adept in all of these areas. I do not know when all of these fields split into specialized branches.

Today, when someone is knowledgeable in a certain area, it is said of him, he has devoted himself to some specialty. If, in addition, he can demonstrate some further knowledge, it is said he is equally competent in two specialties. And if he can even point to a third field, it is said that he is not competent in any specialty. It apparently has been forgotten that Pien Ch'io lived in antiquity. At some point in his life he recognized the problems of older people to be especially acute, and therefore treated the elderly. Later, he considered the problems of women and young girls to be urgent and therefore treated them. Or he found the problems of small children to be of primary concern and consequently treated small children. What end would it have served to divide these procedures [into different specialties]?[30]

8.2.2.2. Searching the Exterior

The preceding section introduced a small selection of Ming and Ch'ing authors concerned primarily with clarification of physiological questions. But other authors of therapeutic literature exhibited little or no interest in such problems. Kung T'ing-hsien (fl. 1615) is one of those who carried on the naive application of theories and practices of the classics in the style of the first millennium. He avoided contemporary debates almost completely and, on the evidence of his handbooks and pharmaceutical works, appears to have been more interested in practice than in theory. The concise theoretical accounts that introduce his books or individual chapters seem more like obligatory gestures. This also explains his relatively uncritical attitude toward demonology, which is reminiscent of such accounts as the eighth-century *Wai-t'ai pi-yao* of Wang T'ao. I will return to this matter in more detail in section 8.3.

Kung T'ing-hsien carried on one phase in the development of healing during which an understanding of the cause of illness was far more important than knowledge of the processes at work in the affected organism. In his works, reprinted to the present day, Kung T'ing-hsien was therefore able to draw upon an important element in the *Huang-ti nei-ching,* even though he did not follow the advice of the classic in other questions, such as demonic medicine. For Kung T'ing-hsien, wind was the most important source of illness. Wind had been mentioned in this context as early as the Shang oracle bones; in the *Huang-ti nei-ching,* the concept was elevated to a primary etiological principle recognized by numerous authors during all subsequent centuries. Kung T'ing-hsien distinguished among various areas in the body that can be affected by wind. Symptoms vary, depending on whether the wind has affected the depots, palaces, blood vessels, or transportation conduits; Kung T'ing-hsien's recommended therapy generally involved the use of medications; he devoted little attention to physiological connections between cause and symptom.

Kung defined cold, heat, dampness, fire, incorrect foods, and also overexertion in sexual activity as wind-related sources of illness. During the Sung period, these etiological categories had been incorporated by Ch'en Yen into the system of external, internal, and neither-external-nor-internal causes of illness. But Kung T'ing-hsien had no interest in Ch'en Yen's system and did not develop his own.

Wu Yu-hsing (fl. 1644) is another well-known author of the sixteenth century whose system of healing was based on etiological principles. Contemporaries regarded him as belonging to the School of Attack or Purgation (kung-hsia p'ai) of Chang Ts'ung-cheng, since he, too, felt the primary therapeutic objective to be the suppression or elimination of evil influences that had penetrated the body. Wu Yu-hsing's reputation rested largely on his Wen-i lun ("On Warmth Epidemics"), in which he recorded experiences gathered during an epidemic that struck the provinces of Shantung, Honan, and Chekiang in the years 1641–1644. The victims' symptoms included head, back, hip, and eye pains, deafness, vomiting, alternating hot and cold fits, urine retention, constipation, abdominal pain, and sensations of repletion, and thus resembled cold-induced maladies (shang-han), known for centuries from both practical experience and medical literature. To the astonishment of all medical practitioners, the instructions of Li Kao's wen-pu school proved completely ineffectual, although suffering induced by cold, that is, a surplus of yin and a deficiency of yang influences, was considered the fundamental provenance of this field. Wu Yu-hsing, however, recognized the true origin of the epidemic, and through the use of saltpeter and other drugs, was able to achieve convincing success. In the Wen-i lun he revealed the secret of his highly effective therapy. He had noticed that the presence of seasonally inappropriate influences was insufficient to explain the mass epidemic. Such an imbalance, he concluded, could only result in isolated cases of illness. He thus decided that the victims had been struck by an unusually virulent evil influence (li-ch'i):[31]

This illness resembles injuries caused by the influence of cold, and yet it is the result of something totally different. Cold-related afflictions enter the body through the ends of the hair, and from there reach the blood channels. They continue to penetrate farther into the body, eventually entering the conduits. From the yang region they invade the yin region and drive deeper and deeper into the body. Epidemics due to warmth enter the body through the mouth and nose, finally settling on the diaphragm. The affliction is thus located between inner and outer regions and can subsequently manifest itself in nine-fold form.[32]

Since this particularly hideous evil influence did not initially affect either the depots or the palaces, seeking out instead an area between outer and inner regions of the body, it remained unnoticed at first and, consequently, was not preventable with drugs. Only after a period of incubation, according to Wu Yu-hsing, does the illness become acute and require treatment.[33]

In the second half of the seventeenth century, Ch'en Shih-to (ca. 1687) compiled a therapeutic work entitled *Shih-shih mi-lu* ("Secret Records from the Mountain Cave"). This rather small text was written in the form of sayings by the legendary Ch'i Po, with a commentary by the Han author Chang Chi. The *Shih-shih mi-lu* differs from other works of the time through the inclusion of a highly detailed system of 136 different therapeutic techniques. The logic of these procedures rests primarily on the concepts of the Five Phases doctrine, although occasionally a social metaphor serves to illuminate the physiological relationships among individual body depots and palaces. The 136 techniques are arranged according to various dimensions of illness and therapy. For a certain number of methods, the social status of the patient was decisive; different forms of therapy were advised for poor and rich, old and young, residents of the northwest and those living in the southeast, men and women, cataleptics and the unconscious. A second group of techniques was directed at the specific type of suffering; in this connection, it was necessary to distinguish among illnesses of the depots, palaces, or blood, determine whether the afflictions were warmth epidemics, prior to or subsequent to birth, chronic or acute afflictions, colds, or conditions of excess or deficiency, or whether a period of convalescence was necessary. A third large group of the 136 techniques was arranged according to the required therapeutic procedures. The practitioner had to decide, for example, whether treatment should be carried out quickly or over a longer period of time, whether a mild or vigorous therapy was called for, whether the patient should stand or lie down, whether one or more conduits were to be used simultaneously, and whether inhalation, exercise, or rest was indicated.

To illustrate Ch'en Shih-to's argumentation, two of the procedures will be sketched here. Under the heading "direct healing" (*cheng i-fa*), Ch'en described the treatment of lung ailments. Possibly influenced by such anatomical data from the *Ling-shu* version of the *Huang-ti nei-ching*, he pointed out that the respiratory passages and the esophagus were separated by a tonguelike structure (*wei-yen*). This flap sealed the air passages tightly during eating, so that food can enter the stomach. But when someone talks too much while eating, the flap may open, causing choking and coughing. On the basis of this knowledge, Ch'en argued that lung ailments cannot be treated directly with drugs, since only air can enter the lungs. Consequently, treatment must be indirect, and the theory of the Five Phases provided the necessary basis. Since soil brings forth metal, the spleen, associated with soil, can be strengthened with drugs, producing a fortifying influence on the lungs, which are associated with metal. Another possibility was to use drugs to bring the liver into harmony. This removes from the metal of the lungs the continuous obligation of cutting the wood of the liver, thereby providing it with a period for recuperation. A final alternative recommended by Ch'en Shih-to included the medicinal strengthening of the heart; the effect was based on the notion that the fire of the heart, which requires nourishment from the outside, does not then need to consume the metal of the lungs, thus providing it with the opportunity to regenerate itself. In each case, Ch'en Shih-to indicates the appropriate drugs for achieving the desired effects; information on pharmacological connections between individual substances and their effects, however, was not provided (see appendix 10.1).

Under the heading "Reversing Treatment" (*ni i-fa*), the author, again on the basis of the Five Phases, describes a different approach to the treatment of lung ailments. To make his argument plausible he utilized the logic of the relationships among the symbols water, soil, fire, wood, and metal, as well as the logic of social relationships, in this case, that between a mother and her son. The kidneys are the child of the lungs, since metal engenders water. At night when man sleeps, Ch'en Shih-to argued, the influences of the lungs return to the kidneys, just as a mother finds shelter with her son. In a family, a son can undergo financial ruin and receive help from his mother's savings. If this support continues, not only the son but the mother, too, becomes penniless. Both are now at the mercy of creditors; the mother seeks refuge with her son, and death may provide the only way to end the disgrace. To help both, the son must be given a loan. Not only will this help the mother, but the creditors will also withdraw. Accordingly, some lung ailments are in reality caused by the exhaustion of the kidneys, due, for instance, to excessive sexual activity. A depletion of influences in the kidneys forces the lungs to supply their own influences to the kidneys. When, as a result of the continuing stress on the kidneys, deficiencies arise in both depots, evil influences from outside the body are able to take over the storage facilities, perhaps even causing death. When such a situation arises, it is necessary to strengthen the kidneys with the aid of drugs (see appendix 10.2).

Ch'en Shih-to adopted a medical axiom here that runs through virtually the entire literature of systematic correspondence. The attack of malevolent influences from outside is frequently a result of deficiencies of vital influences within the body, a situation brought on by the victim himself. A healthy life, without extravagance, and the medicinal correction of, for example, seasonably induced imbalances in the supply of "correct" external influences, are the most effective means for preventing illness.

In several passages following the extensive presentation of 136 therapeutic techniques, Ch'en Shih-to addresses purely theoretical questions. But Ch'en Shih-to by no means limited himself to traditional concepts and was able to offer his readers new information. In the section "On the Depots and Palaces," he argued that in the future it would be necessary to speak of six depots and seven palaces. As the sixth depot, equal in importance to the heart, lung, kidneys, liver, and spleen, he named a channel connecting the heart with the kidneys. In women, the upper part of the passage is narrow and widens further down, while in men, it is narrow for its entire length. In the channel are generated those influences that—when joined in the relationship between man and woman—produce conception. The seventh palace, according to Ch'en Shih-to, was the organ *tan-chung,* already mentioned in the *Su-wen.* The prevailing view, however, had always been that this term designated the heart-enclosing network (*hsin pao-lo*) and thus constituted the sixth depot, since the yinyang duality required a division of storage facilities into three groups of two. Ch'en Shih-to's views remained his own; neither his anatomical findings nor his therapeutic system found any significant proponents.

8.2.2.3. Searching the Past

When influential scholars in the seventeenth and eighteenth centuries, in particular Ku Yen-wu (1616–1682) and Yen Yüan (1635–1704), began to question the merits of Sung Neo-Confucianism as a binding political and moral doctrine, the necessity arose for those conservative forces supporting this view to determine the nature of the true and genuine Confucian teachings. Tai Chen (1724–1777) is generally regarded as one of the originators of ensuing efforts, utilizing careful philological study to identify the authors of the most important surviving Confucian writings and to distinguish genuine concepts of antiquity from later interpretations and corruptions. In this way, it was hoped, the original doctrine that had made China strong could be recovered, in contrast to Sung Neo-Confucianism, which within just a few centuries had twice been helpless to prevent the loss of the entire empire to northern invaders. Even the period of Chinese rule that separated these two foreign dynasties was too reminiscent of Mongol political structures to serve as a model for Confucian scholar-officials. The resulting so-called *Han-hsüeh* movement, a return to the teachings of the Han, was also reflected in medical literature. Indeed, efforts to reveal the innovations of Sung-Chin-Yüan authors as falsifications are evident in this area even earlier than in the realm of political philosophy. It is possible that the nonpolitical subject of healing revealed tendencies of conservative Confucianism at a time when it was not yet opportune to express corresponding political concepts.[34]

Medical literature of the *Han-hsüeh* tradition, which continued to appear until late in the Ch'ing period, is marked by the efforts to restore the original forms of the classics of healing. Apparently, the surviving version of the *Huang-ti nei-ching* itself was regarded as a pre-Sung text, since the interest in reconstructions was directed mainly to the *Pen-ts'ao ching* of Shen-nung, the classic of pharmaceutics, and to the *Shang-han lun* of Chang Chi, the first known prescription manual.

Fang Yu-chih (born 1522, fl. 1593) was one of the earliest proponents of the medical *Han-hsüeh* tradition. The wisdom recorded by the ancients in their writings was no longer understood by later centuries or had been passed down only in a distorted form. He therefore devoted twenty years of his life to establishing the true substance of the works of Chang Chi and Wang Shu-ho, compiling a book entitled *Shang-han lun t'iao-pien* ("Analysis of Individual Sections of the Shang-han lun").[35]

At the beginning of the seventeenth century, Lu Fu (fl. 1616) initiated a series of philological studies concerning the reconstruction of the *Shen-nung pen-ts'ao ching;* by the end of the nineteenth century, more than a dozen, in part quite well-known scholars had carried on his work, including Miu Hsi-yung (ca. 1625), Hsü Ta-ch'un (1693–1771), and Sun Hsing-yen (1753–1818).[36]

Hsü Ta-ch'un, in particular, stands out as a brilliant thinker. Born into a family with a long medical tradition, he acquired, in addition to a comprehensive medical education, a thorough knowledge of astronomy, music, geography, and philosophy. Not only his numerous medical books but his commentaries on Taoist classics and even a work on the control of rivers found wide acclaim. To a degree virtually unmatched by any contemporary, Hsü Ta-ch'un took into consideration the history and contemporary situation of medicine, publishing his conclusions in frequently critical and ironic words that did not shy away from open attack. Like Li Chung-tse before him, he rejected all traditions that cultivated the teachings of one or another of the Sung-Chin-Yüan authors as a complete system of healing. Hsü Ta-ch'un argued that every medical practitioner must possess an overview of all significant ancient literature and must combine classical theories with the realities of practical experiences.[37] He expressed particular criticism of the maxims of Chang Yüan-su (ca. 1180), who had claimed that the therapeutic instructions of the ancient sages were unsuited to the treatment of contemporary illnesses. In the same way that this statement of Chang Yüan-su had symbolized the philosophical and political view of Neo-Confucianism, Hsü Ta-ch'un's response reflected the belief of contemporary conservative forces that only the political-moral precepts of antiquity could resolve the present internal and external problems. Among others, Hsü Ta-ch'un sought to refute one of the most important innovations of Sung-Chin-Yüan medicine, namely, Chang Yüan-su's doctrine that medicinal drugs reach the intended locations through specific transportation channels.[38] Hsü termed such notions "nonsense" (*ch'uan-tso*).[39] His general assessment of Sung-Chin-Yüan authors is evident in the following passage:

> The darkness enveloping medical teaching has continued now for a long time. During the Ming period, the instructions of the Four Great Masters were followed, and Chang Chung-ching [i.e., Chang Chi], Liu Ho-chien [i.e., Liu Wan-su], Li Tung-yüan [i.e., Li Kao], and Chu Tan-hsi [i.e., Chu Chen-heng] were revered as the founders of medicine itself. This is nothing but ignorant and inane foolishness! Chang Chung-ching was truly a sage whose renown will continue throughout eternity. He is like K'ung-tzu, the ancestor of Confucianism. Liu Ho-chien and Li Tung-yüan, however, left us only ill-considered teachings. Chu Tan-hsi did nothing more than reflect on and rearrange the views of all earlier authors, leaving out something here and borrowing something there. He thus created an easy entrance for beginning students. And these men are generally called renowned physicians![40]

8.2.2.4. Searching Down Below

In my discussion of the approaches to healing taken during the Ming and Ch'ing periods, I have so far only dealt with those that remained within the medicine of systematic correspondence. Chao

Hsüeh-min (ca. 1730–1805) initiated an entirely new perspective. Of the twelve works that he completed, only two have survived—a work on drugs, the *Pen-ts'ao kang mu shih-i*,[41] and a collection of prescriptions entitled *Ch'uan-ya*.[42] Little is known about his life. It is possible that he came from a lower social stratum; in any case, nothing is known about how he gained his comprehensive education. On the basis of information about individual drugs in the *Pen-ts'ao kang mu shih-i*, Chang Tzu-kao concluded that Chao Hsüeh-min had possibly never left his native province of Chekiang. All material in his work pertaining to drugs from outside this region was gathered, according to Chao Hsüeh-min's own words, from travelers, returning officials, or relatives, while he himself attested to information regarding Chekiang.[43]

Chao was apparently interested in alternative approaches. A significant portion of the *Ch'uan-ya* is based on the recollections of an itinerant country doctor, whose personal notes Chao Hsüeh-min was able to consult. The *Ch'uan-ya* (A Series of Outstanding Guidelines) offers a remarkable look at healing procedures expectable from eighteenth-century itinerant practitioners who served that segment of the Chinese population whose access to the medicine practiced by literate, educated, and established physicians was prevented by various geographical, economic, and social factors. What first strikes the reader of the more than 1,000 drug descriptions and guidelines of the *Ch'uan-ya* is the virtually complete absence of yinyang theories and of the Five Phases doctrine. Although in a preface Chao mentions that itinerant doctors were familiar with these concepts, the remark can be viewed as an attempt to reduce somewhat the completely heterodox nature of the practice of these doctors. The *Ch'uan-ya* is the sole Chinese medical work prior to the arrival of modern Western pharmacology that offers an alternative explanation of how drugs function in the body, providing us with an indication of notions prevailing among the lower strata of the population, views that diverged greatly from those found in the scholarly writings of the upper levels of society. The *Ch'uan-ya* distinguished among drugs whose effects ascend in the body, those that descend, and those capable of interrupting an illness or some organic event (such as when a tooth is extracted). The group of "interrupting" medications was further divided into three sections, according to whether the intended interruption was directed at a specific location in the body, was to develop a netlike effect extending over the entire body, or was an effect radiating in various directions from a single point. Whereas drugs that ascended, descended, or interrupted were meant only for illnesses perceived as organic disturbances in the body, a fourth group of medications, the so-called repelling (*chin-yao*) drugs were available to combat pathological agents that attack the body or mind from outside, and thus are capable of penetrating the organism.[44]

The use of medicinal drugs represents the most significant, but not the sole, therapeutic dimension of the *Ch'uan-ya*. Some fifty guidelines pertaining to the use of incantory pictograms and exorcistic techniques were of purely demonological origin. In addition, the author also recommended acupuncture and moxibustion, as well as smoke and steam treatments, lavation, plasters, hot compresses, breathing techniques, and other methods from the practice of itinerant doctors.

The *Ch'uan-ya* was written in 1759 and even reached Japan in manuscript form. But almost a century passed, until 1851, before a publisher expressed willingness to publish this work. The attempt to sift approaches from the lower strata apparently did not reveal concepts attractive to a large number of scholars.

8.2.2.5. Searching Far Ahead

Perhaps it was the general atmosphere of skepticism toward surviving tradition that attracted the interest of Wang Ch'ing-jen (1768–1831), provoking him to compile a work that, at least in part, tore away the conceptual foundation in the classics of the medicine of systematic correspondence. Wang Ch'ing-jen was in Luan-chou in 1797 when an epidemic broke out, claiming the lives of hundreds of children. The bodies of children from poor families were buried in shallow graves in a public cemetery, so that stray dogs could dig up and devour the corpses. This custom, it was thought, protected the next child in the family from premature death. Wang Ch'ing-jen, according to the sources, had to pass by the cemetery every day and, at first, always held his nose in disgust at the stench. But his interest was soon sparked by the numerous dismembered bodies, and he began to study systematically the internal anatomy of the corpses. The dogs ate primarily the heart and lungs, leaving behind the stomach and intestines. The diaphragm was always torn, so that Wang was unable to determine if the heart was located above or below it. Despite such unfavorable conditions, he felt he detected considerable differences between the reality of what he saw here and the statements of medical literature. After his curiosity had been aroused, Wang devoted the rest of his life to this question. Two years after the events in Luan-chou, he had an opportunity to witness the execution of a woman sentenced to dismemberment, but since he was a man, he was not permitted to approach closely, and had to have the executioner show him the heart, liver, and lungs after the sentence had been carried out. Two decades later, in 1820, he was finally able to attend the execution of a man sentenced for matricide, but once again, the diaphragm tore before he was able to examine it closely. Only after forty years did he find an official who had seen numerous executions and consequently was able to describe the structure of the diaphragm. At the age of sixty-three, shortly before his death, Wang Ch'ing-jen published the results of his investigations under the title *I-lin kai-ts'o* (Correction of Errors from Medical Literature).[45] The following passage from this work, which also included illustrations by the author, demonstrates some of the many contradictions that Wang Ch'ing-jen believed could be resolved through anatomical study:

In ancient times the people used to say: "If I can't be a good minister of state, I wish to be a good physician!" They thought it was easy to be a good physician and difficult to be a good minister. I say, this is not so! Through the ages there have always been good ministers to govern the state; but there was not one single perfect man who has written books as a good physician. And what is the reason that there has never been one single perfect man? The reason is that the people in former times in compiling medical books were mistaken when they wrote about the depots and the palaces, and later people then respectfully followed [these ancient statements] and built their theories on them. They missed the basis of the illnesses. Now, if the basis of the illnesses is missed, one may have a pen to embroider tigers or to engrave a dragon, one may have the abilities to cut the clouds or to fill the moon, but he will definitely not be able to reconcile the circumstances of an illness with the [actual condition of the] depots and palaces. This is the reason why there is not a single perfect man in medicine. Anybody who practices medicine, in diagnosing an illness he must first of all understand the body's depots and palaces. I have examined what the people in ancient times had to say on the depots and palaces, and [I have also investigated their] illustrations. In their teachings they contradicted one another again and again. For instance, when the ancients spoke of the spleen, they remarked it corresponds to the soil. The soil is the master of tranquility and should not move. If the spleen moves it is not at peace. Now, if it is said [in one place] that the spleen is not at peace if it moves, how can it be said later on that the spleen moves when it hears a sound and that, because of this moving, it rubs the stomach which [as a result] digests the food. If the spleen does not move, the food is not digested. These, then, are their misconceptions concerning moving and nonmoving of the spleen. When they spoke of the lung, [they said] it is empty like a beehive and has no opening at its lower side. Inhaling fills it, exhaling empties it. Now, if it is said [in one place that the lung] has no opening below, how can it be said elsewhere that the lung has twenty-four holes pointing into all directions as passageways for the influences of all the body's depots? These, then, are their misconceptions concerning the openings of the lung. When they spoke of the kidneys, [they said] that the two kidneys together constitute the kidneys, and that in between the kidneys there are moving influences which constitute the gate of life. Now, if it is said [in one place] that the moving influences in between the [kidneys] constitute the gate of life, how can it be said elsewhere that the left kidney is the kidney while the right kidney is the gate of life? If the two kidneys are one body, why were two names established and what was the concrete basis for this? And if indeed in between [the two kidneys] the moving influences constitute the gate of life, what kind of a thing is there to store these moving influences? These, then, are their misconceptions concerning the kidneys. When they spoke of the liver, [they said] that there is one channel on its left and right side, respectively, and that these are blood vessels originating from the two flanks, moving upward to join with the eyes in the head. [These blood vessels are also supposed] to move downward from the lower abdomen and to reach their destination in the large toes of the feet after having circumvented the sexual organ. Now, if it is said [in one place] that there are channels on the left and right side of the liver, how can it be said elsewhere that the liver is situated on the left, and that the left flanks are associated with the liver? These, then, are their misconceptions concerning the situation of the liver on the left or right. When they spoke of the heart, they held that the heart is the ruler among the officials and that it is the source of spirit-brilliance. Reflection is stored in the heart, reflection is the function of the heart. Reflection is responsible for the mind, and the moving of the mind is called thinking. If plans are made for the future through thinking, this is called consideration, and to place thoughts through consideration is called wisdom. All these five are stored by the heart. [Now, if it is said in one place] that they are stored by the heart, how can it be said elsewhere that the spleen stores reflection and wisdom, that the kidneys are responsible for skills, that the liver masters the planning, and that the gall controls the decision making? According to such statements spiritual mechanisms are distributed over many places, but, in the final analysis, it is never explained clearly which thing creates the spiritual mechanism and which place stores the spiritual mechanism; or what kind of spirit or condition influences the spiritual mechanism from outside! Such is the ambiguity of their statements on the heart. When they spoke of the stomach, [they said that it] was responsible for the digestion of liquid and solid foods. Elsewhere it is said that the spleen rubs the stomach through its moving, [ensuring] the digestion of food. The upper opening of the stomach is called *pen*-gate. [This is where] drinks and food enter the stomach; finest matter and finest influences move upward through the *pen*-gate to be transported to the spleen and to the lung [from where they are distributed] through all the arteries. Such arguments are false; they lack both a real background and a theoretical basis. The lower opening of the stomach is called the *yu*-gate; this is the upper opening of the small intestine. When they spoke of the small intestine, [they said that] it is the receiver among the officials and that the transformation of [all] things starts from here. They said that drinks and food enter the small intestine to undergo transformation. Feces move downward toward the *lan*-gate which is the lower opening of the small intestine. There the clear and the turbid [portions] are separated and the feces are forwarded to the large intestine, where they leave [the body] through the *kang*-gate. The water, however, is forwarded to the bladder and becomes urine. In other words, they said that the urine leaks out from the feces. [If this were true,] its smell should be foul. I have already made use of boys' urine and, in addition, I have asked others who have themselves consumed urine. They told me only that it tastes salty and that it does not have a foul smell. And furthermore, if solid foods and liquids were transformed jointly into feces, the feces should be moist and should flow out. This may be so as far as chicken and ducks are concerned who have no urine, but it is impossible for cows and horses who have urine. How could this be true for men! Look, when they said that the small intestine transforms the food and that the water leaves specifically from the point of the lan-gate, this is so funny that one may laugh about it forever![46]

His understanding of these inconsistencies led Wang Ch'ing-jen to term those practitioners with no conception of the true internal structure of the body blind men, who wander dark streets; to this group he numbered all his colleagues and predecessors. He therefore called his own work just a beginning. He made no claims of omniscience and predicted future progress only when others carried on his work.[47] He could not have suspected that only a few years after his death, the discoveries of medical researchers and practitioners from a foreign civilization, who had already pursued his call for centuries, would raise healing in China to a completely new plane.

8.2.3. Demonology, "Psychiatry," and "Psychoanalysis"

The treatment of emotional problems within its own scientific-theoretical guidelines posed no problems from the very beginning for the medicine of systematic correspondence. The question, for example, which in the twentieth century separated Freud and Jaspers, whether so-called psychic disturbances should be treated on a basis provided by the natural sciences or the humanities (or with a combination of both approaches) simply never arose in traditional Chinese medical thought. The concept of correspondence, of the affiliation of all tangible and abstract phenomena to certain lines of association, enabled a seamless linking of the psychic with the somatic. The biological and psychological dimension of illness constituted here a complete unity; to see in this question two separate dimensions of existence was completely alien to the medicine of systematic correspondence. It was known that the various emotions that had been defined were directly anchored in the biological organism and could also influence it. Excessive anger, it was recognized, eventually led to liver damage; fear strained the kidneys. Conversely, this biological integration of emotions also meant that what initially is a purely somatic effect, such as that produced by the influence of cold or excessive physical exertion, can also cause psychic disorders. Since psychic and somatic disturbances were thus explicable in terms of influences in the body, treatment was directed to correcting deficiencies or excesses in the depots or palaces as indicated by the affected emotions through the lines of association. Acupuncture and, since the Sung-Chin-Yüan period, drugs as well, suited these objectives. From the passage in the *Ju-men shih-ch'in* of Chang Ts'ung-cheng (1156–1228), we have already seen how this system of healing reduced behavioral disturbances to an imbalance of yin and yang influences in the organism that could, in this case, be treated by drugs directed at the biological processes.

The medicine of systematic correspondence was not the only Chinese system of healing concerned with psychological problems. Until modern times the much older demonic medicine, among other approaches, remained a conceptual and, as far as practitioners are concerned, a largely personal alternative. Although precise estimates are impossible, there are numerous indications that, in terms of numbers of patients, demonological healing was the more influential system. In China, as in the West, belief in the existence of evil spirits was by no means limited to the lower or uneducated segments of the population. For this reason, many serious works of Chinese medical literature written by renowned and perceptive scientists contain sections with suggestions for the demonological treatment of certain ailments. Virtually all of the best-known authors of the Ming and Ch'ing periods, including Yü Po (fl. 1515), Li Shih-chen (1518–1593), Li T'ing (fl. 1570), Hsü Ch'un-fu (fl. 1570), Kung T'ing-hsien (fl. 1615), Hsü Ta-ch'un (1693–1771), and Sun Te-jun (fl. 1826), and numerous others, acknowledged the pathogenic influence of demons as a self-evident fact, resembling, in this regard, the *wu* shamans, Taoist priests, or even the itinerant practitioners like Chao Hsüeh-min's informant, for whom the practice of demonic medicine represented all or at least a significant portion of their efforts. Up to the end of the Ming dynasty, the art of spells (chu-yu) constituted one of the official medical specialties at the imperial court and in the academies; the Ch'ing dynasty was the first that deemed it possible to forsake specialists in this field.

The medical literature of the authors cited above integrated demonic medicine in various ways. Li T'ing, for example, author of an "Introduction to Medicine" (*I-hsüeh ju-men*), adopted classical demonological concepts in etiology and therapy. Without regard here to the biological notions within the framework of yinyang and the Five Phases that otherwise dominate his book, he depicted the causes and symptoms of the illness *tsu-chung o-wu* ("sudden attack by evil or hostile agents"). The treatment sought to expel the demons through such means as noise making, burning, and fumigation. The drugs to be employed included peach branches and peach leaves, which symbolized archery weapons constructed in antiquity and which penetrated into the body:

The symptoms resulting from attack by evil or hostile demonic influences (*kuei-ch'i*) appear in the evening or at night when one visits the latrine, goes out into the woods, wanders through empty, cold houses, or stops in places where no man has previously trod. Suddenly, demonlike beings are seen. Their evil influences enter through the nose and mouth, and the victim falls unexpectedly to the ground. The four extremities grow cold; both hands tighten into fists. Clear blood flows from the nose and mouth. Consciousness fades. After a short time, any help is hopeless. The symptoms resemble death; but no sounds can be heard in the abdomen, and the abdomen and sides remain warm.

Whenever someone is unexpectedly unable to move, all his relatives are summoned, and they stand around the victim, beating drums and lighting fires. Or musk, *an-hsi*, *Su* wood, *Chang* wood, or a similar substance is burned. When [the patient] arises again, [the aromatic substances] can be removed and the practitioner can himself withdraw. In certain acute cases, five *ch'ien* pulverized rhinoceros horn, and one *fen* each of cinnabar and musk, both also pulverized, should be taken. Each dose consists of two *ch'ien;* it is given [to the patient] mixed with freshly drawn water. Anyone of a weak constitution should take the [powder] with a boiled potion of peach branches and leaves.[48]

Similar therapeutic principles determined the treatment of the illness *kuei-chi ch'en-t'ung* ("piercing pain caused by the attack of a demon"), also included in Li T'ing's "Introduction to Medicine":

When someone is suddenly attacked by a demon, the [resulting sensation] resembles that of being struck by an arrow. An unbearable pain occurs unexpectedly at a certain spot.

Take a section of peach skin and, after it has been moistened inside, attach it to [the location] of the pain. Then take a spoon and press it on the peach skin. A solid ball, about the size of a walnut, should then be rolled from mugwort leaves and burned on the bowl of the spoon. After a short time, the pain will subside.[49]

A number of therapeutic instructions based on classical demonology are also found repeatedly in the works of Kung T'ing-hsien (fl. 1615), who wrote that such ailments are contracted in old temples, vacant houses, hostels, and inns. He also advocated pungent odors (vinegar, for example), fumigation, and the beating of drums. In addition, he recommended the taking of certain "weapon drugs," such as the plant drug "demon arrow" (*kuei-chien*), as well as swallowing ink, which apparently symbolized the characters found on antidemonic talismans.

Although it appears thus far that demonology was reflected in etiology and therapy in its purely classical form, one difference is nonetheless significant. In the *Shou-shih pao-yüan,*[50] Kung T'ing-hsien argued that the penetration of demonic influences generally, although not always, was first made possible by an already existing organic imbalance. His remark, "in general, misfortune cannot overcome that which is correct," reflects the Confucian ethos of the medicine of systematic correspondence, according to which man, if he conducts his life in the correct manner, provides no target for any kind of "evil." It should be underscored once again, however, that the term *hsieh,* which I have generally translated here as "evil," represents a complex involving such connotations as "heterodox" and "abnormal." The notion that only the incorrect conduct of one's life initiates the somatic and psychic prerequisites for the assault of evil is an ancient one, and can be traced back as far as the classic *Huang-ti nei-ching.* Since the meaning of the term *hsieh,* which in the *Huang-ti nei-ching* was restricted to the excessive influence of cold, heat, dampness, and similar phenomena, had been expanded once again during the Ming and Ch'ing period to include the concept of demons, the way was now clear to integrate demonology into the medicine of systematic correspondence. This process signifies—after the conceptual association of the system of correspondence with practical drug therapy during the Sung-Chin-Yüan period—the second adoption of heterodoxy into quasi-official healing. Even during the Ming and Ch'ing periods, no mandatory standardization of medical knowledge existed, so that attempts at integration by different authors assumed various forms. Several examples will illustrate this process.

In 1515, Yü Po published the *I-hsüeh cheng-ch'uan* (The Correct Tradition of Medicine). Yü Po acknowledged the existence of demons but considered the activities of shamans or sorcerers to be merely materialistically motivated fraud. Although he accorded spells and incantations a mild therapeutic efficacy, he nonetheless rejected their use as heterodox.[51] Using the example of a pregnancy purportedly caused by demons, Yü Po demonstrated that such occurrences can also be viewed from another perspective:

> The question is put sometimes what demoniacal pregnancy is. The answer is as follows: Things thought of in the daytime become visions in the night, and so it is a rule that, if men and women be of lewd disposition, idle, and unoccupied, the fire in their liver and their kidneys flames up at any moment, with the result that, if they are timorous, they dream frequently of intercourse with spectres. So demoniacal pregnancy is unreal pregnancy, by no means a pregnancy produced by actual fecundation by spectres. An ancient recipe says: Where lewd thoughts are boundless, wishes (for children) remain unfulfilled. It is white fluid of lewdness and white foul liquid which, flowing in the uterus, curdle therein and make such pregnancy; it is the blood of the woman herself and her semen which curdle and form a lump that puffs up her breast and her abdomen, and filling these, makes her look as if she were in the family way.
>
> But if it proves to be no unreal pregnancy, what then have we to think of it? Well, in Hwah Poh-jen's work, entitled The Efficacy of Medicines, I have found the following lines: In the temple of Benevolence and Filial Respect the only daughter of the Invoker attached to the building, named Yang T'ien-ch'ing, strolled through the side-gallery in the dim shadows of evening, and saw a spirit in yellow dress. She experienced an agitation of feeling, and that same night she dreamed that she had sexual commerce with that spirit. Her abdomen distended, and she had all the symptoms of being in the family way, when Poh-jen was asked to treat her. He examined her, and said: "this is a case of demoniacal pregnancy," and her mother having related to him all about the cause of it, he cured her by causing her to evacuate by means of blood-breaking and abortive drugs more than two pints of tadpoles, porwiggles, and fish-eyes. Had she not had any real sexual commerce with that spirit? Such commerce may have taken place indeed, but there are no reasons to admit that it actually did, for how would it be possible for an image made of wood and clay to indulge in coition with a human person, and to possess semen which may produce fecundation? Ah, no ghost seduced by a woman was in question here, but a woman bewildered by a ghost. My opinion is, that the girl, advanced in years and yet without a mate, was one of those of whom we might say: where lewd thoughts have no

bounds, wishes (for children) remain unfulfilled. Scholars imbued with correct principles, beware of believing in the errors of such heterodox stories![52]

Just a few years later Hsü Ch'un-fu compiled his "Complete System of Medicine of All Times" (*Ku-chin i-t'ung ta-ch'üan*). The integration of demonology in this work is evident on several levels. Hsü Ch'un-fu made no attempt to conceal his personal view that all demons and similar apparitions were figments of the human imagination. Nevertheless, he cited earlier authors who were of a different mind. Thus we can find, for instance, a classic exorcism, utilizing gesticulative rites and incantations for the treatment of possible asphyxiation due to choking.[53] In another passage, Hsü Ch'un-fu quotes an earlier author who argued that the sudden assault of demons was only occasionally responsible for illness, while in the most cases, a previous weakness on the part of the victim had first made the attack possible. Accordingly, exorcistic incantations were deemed appropriate in some cases to expel demons, while in others, drugs to eliminate the underlying somatic problem and thus drive out the demons, were indicated (see appendix 8.4). Hsü Ch'un-fu placed special emphasis on the purely psychological benefit of incantations, since some illnesses, although caused by fears and doubts, required somatic treatment. In such cases, he advised therapy combining drugs and incantations:

If these two methods of treatment are combined, inner and outer are forged into a whole, producing a prompt cure of the illness. Anyone who engages an exorcist and avoids the application of drugs will be unable to eliminate his illness, for a principle is lacking that could bring about a cure. He who takes only drugs, and does not call upon an exorcist to drive out existing doubts, will be cured, but relief will be achieved relatively slowly. Consequently, the inner and outer must be treated together; only in this way is rapid success possible. This is the reason for the introduction of the "exorcism of the cause" (*chu-yu*).[54]

In his *Lei-ching* (Classic Arranged According to Topics), published some fifty years later in 1624, Chang Chieh-pin also advocated exorcistic healing as the thirteenth specialty. Of the authors known to us, Chang Chieh-pin carried out the most consistent integration of demonology into the conceptual framework of systematic correspondence. He also considered demons to be creations of the human mind and therefore not phenomena of the real world. He thus regarded the appearance of demons as merely subjective symptoms of specific disturbances in the psychosomatic organism of the victim. Emotional states, for instance, that bring on such hallucinations are caused primarily by continued one-sided attraction or aversion toward an object of the phenomenal world. Excessive attraction or aversion can lead to an imbalance of certain influences in the organism, since these emotions stimulate an increased production in certain body depots. This situation, in turn, can produce mental disorientation associated with the respective depots. Such mental illusions or other similarly caused weaknesses of the body's own spirit, which is located in one of the five depots, enable a foreign "evil" to establish itself. While for some authors this evil consisted of demons that entered from outside the body and had to be expelled through one method or another, Chang Chieh-pin viewed such apparitions as hallucinations brought on by the victim's own senses. These illusions can also be generated by seasonally related imbalances in the climatic influences assimilated by man from the macrocosm. Each of the five body depots is, of course, associated with a specific color. When illness affects a depot, the victim may perceive demons, whose color can enable the practitioner to determine the affected depot or depots.[55]

From a Taoist text, the *Kuan yin tzu,* Chang Chieh-pin cited a passage claiming that the heart was controlled by various emotions and thus can be seized by specific demons.[56] In all those cases in which a specific emotion was the primary source of illness, Chang advised first an analysis of the inclinations or aversions of the patient; therapy could then take a number of courses. One can simply remove the object of aversion; this procedure was used by Chang Chieh-pin in the case of a woman who suspected her husband of having a mistress. He advised her that the lover had died (see appendix 9.1). Another possible technique involved the use of the mutual relationships among the Five Phases, with which all emotions are associated. If the pathogenic emotion to be eliminated has been identified, one need only stimulate mildly the emotion which, according to the relationship of mutual destruction, destroys the former, and the cure is effected. Chang Chieh-pin illustrated this approach with the example of a woman who fell ill following constant brooding upon the death of her mother. Since, according to the *Huang-ti nei-ching,* the emotion anger overcomes brooding, it was necessary to arouse anger in the woman (see appendix 9.1). In a third case, a man had been afflicted by the influence of cold. Chang recognized the affected depot by means of the color of the demons seen by the victim and recommended normal drug therapy (see appendix 9.1).

With regard to the treatment of behavioral disorders, Ch'en Shih-to (fl. 1687), author of the *Shih-shi mi-lu,* represents the opposite pole of the position taken by Chang Chieh-pin. The emotional source that drove a patient to madness, for instance, was of no interest to him. Madness, he argued, was the result of too much mucus being produced in the heart. (The character for "mucus" consists of the two elements "burning flame" and "sickbed.") Since it is too dangerous to dissipate directly the flame responsible for this overproduction, it is necessary to strengthen the soil region of the body (spleen and stomach). According to the Five Phases, fire engenders soil, so that this therapy removes from fire its function, enabling it to reduce itself. A restriction of fire, that is, of the function of the heart, results in a decrease in mucus production and, consequently, the desired cure of the behavioral disturbance, in this case madness.[57]

In the eighteenth century Hsü Ta-ch'un cited "irrefutable evidence" of the influence of ancestors, demons, and victims of unjust and un-avenged deeds on the well-being of man. He was convinced, in addition to the direct actions of demons, that illnesses were primarily a result of situations in which a weakening or even loss of the body's spirit first permitted an attack by external demons. For Hsü Ta-ch'un, de-mons constituted only one category of many in the spectrum of natural forces, and he compared evil spirits to wind, cold, summer heat, and similar phenomena. Just as a deficiency of yang influences enables cold and a deficiency of yin influences permits heat to penetrate the body, emotional fatigue allows demons to gain entrance. Since a weakness of the spirit originates in fears and doubts, it is necessary, in mild cases, to identify and eliminate them. For more serious cases, however, Hsü Ta-ch'un advocated medicinal treatments, using both classic "weapon drugs" as well as physiologically efficacious drugs (see appendix 11.1–11.3).

Sun Te-jun (fl. 1826) is the best example of a well-known author who as late as the nineteenth century included purely classical de-monological guidelines and concepts in serious medical literature. For the illness "curse of evil" (*hsieh-sui*) the author, following a depiction of the physiological symptoms of the affliction, cited an unnamed source that claimed the taking of drugs was counterindicated for this illness; only amulets and incantations were of any use. According to the author's definition, hsieh-sui is the "curse of malevolent demons and pathogenic agents" (*hsieh mo kuei sui*). Additional definitions and illustrations cited from earlier works also imply the actual existence of demons. Various medicative measures were advised for treatment, such as a pill from the *Wan-ping hui-ch'un* by Kung T'ing-hsien against demon attacks, made up of tiger skull bones, cinnabar, realgar, rhizomes of the demon-vessel plant (*kuei-chiu*), feathers of the demon-arrow plant, black hellebore, orpiment, and elm fruit. According to the directions, the pill is to be carried in a small pouch, on the left arm by men and on the right arm by women: "This prevents spirits from approaching, heals women from sexual intercourse with demons, and protects against epidemics of warmth."[58]

8.3. THE HETEROGENEITY OF CHINESE MEDICINE DURING THE DECLINE OF THE EMPIRE

In the present and preceding chapters I have dealt almost exclusively with developments within the confines of the medicine of systematic correspondence. It is therefore appropriate to recall once more the total spectrum of healing systems operating at the time when China was confronted with Western civilization and, consequently, Western medicine.

Until the beginning of the twentieth century, the concepts of systematic correspondence dominated Chinese medical literature and undoubtedly the approaches of educated practitioners and self-healing private citizens as well, at least among the upper strata of society. The common underlying conceptual basis of all these practitioners, however, was exceedingly narrow, being limited to the acknowledgement of certain surviving works as classic texts and a belief in the fundamental truth of the central theories of the Five Phases and the all-encompassing dualism of yinyang. But even the interpretation of the universally revered classics, as well as the application of these theories to the concrete realities of daily life, gave rise to numerous contradictions, fragmenting the large community of private scholars and professional medical practitioners seeking solutions to health-related problems into countless individuals, groups, and traditions. In the preceding sections I have surveyed some examples of the various directions taken during the last centuries of Imperial China in the search for solutions to disturbing circumstances. When current Western publications devoted generally to the history of medicine in China attempt to present the concepts of systematic correspondence as "*the* Chinese medicine," the result is doubly misleading. Such an attempt gives the erroneous impression of a philosophically well-defined system with standardized notions about the morphology of the body and physiological laws governing the organism. In addition, a concentration on concepts of systematic correspondence as synonymous with "Chinese medicine" conceals the fact that alternative therapeutic approaches were cultivated in all segments of society until this century and even dominated medical care among the Chinese masses. Actions based solely on experience, along with religious, demonological, and magical practices for the prevention and treatment of illness shaped the daily life of the majority of Chinese people. In his 1891 history, *I-ku*, Cheng Wen-cho's comments are thus by no means to be understood as disparaging:

> The specialty "exorcism of causes" (*chu-yu*) is today used to designate a procedure that enjoys widespread acceptance among the people of Hupeh. There are printed talismans and spells for the treatment of the most unusual conditions. The rate of success is quite high. A parallel exists here to the incantations practiced by the *wu*-shamans in antiquity. Those who pursue this art today visit the victims and determine the cause of the illness. They then write down the name of the victim, recite incantations to the spirits or give [the patient] certain influences to swallow or talismans to be consumed with spectre-water. This technique resembles the art of interdictions (*chin-shu*), as both utilize no [medicinal] prescriptions.[59]

Henry Doré has extensively documented such practices arising from Buddhist, Taoist, or religious-syncretic conceptions.[60]

In comparison with the extensive corpus of writings on the medicine of systematic correspondence and pragmatic drug therapy, the amount of literature devoted solely to the various alternative concepts and techniques of exorcistic and incantory therapy, despite numerous medical titles in the Taoist and Buddhist canon, is smaller; apparently, under the pressure of political circumstances, such traditions were frequently passed down orally or in the manuscripts of esoteric circles. One exception was the *Mi-ts'ang i-shu shih-san k'o* (Secretly Preserved Thirteenth Specialty of Medical Literature). The work consists of a description of numerous calligraphic amulets purportedly discovered on stone tablets as early as 1118 during dike construction on the Yellow River and identified by a Taoist named Chang I-ch'a. Subsequently in the fifteenth century, a preface explains, a man named Hsü Chin-hui had expanded the documents to their present form.

The current edition of this work was printed in red in 1895 in Shanghai. Two prefaces are followed by six exorcistic incantations that are to be recited over the water, ink, paper, and brush required for the written amulets, as well as over the appropriate characters themselves and during the writing process. A following general spell recommended for the healing of illness is structurally similar to formulas in the "Classic of Interdictions" of Sun Ssu-miao; significantly, however, the contents have been influenced by Confucian and Buddhist values:

> When heaven and earth were separated, the five thunders rolled independently for the first time, the three original principles [of finest matter, of finest influences, and of the spirit] were created; the eight trigrams were given their form and man was afflicted by illness and suffering. All this was due to the effects of the Five Phases. Earlier, during the time of Huang-ti and Shen-nung, the arrangement of illness and regulations for the use of drugs were subject to a definite order. Within the body, they regulated the five depots; outside the body, they brought about harmony among the seven emotions. Since man possessed an upright mind, his feelings always achieved their objectives. The mountain has five peaks, the Great Wagon seven stars. May the laws of Emperor Hsüan Yüan achieve their complete effects on the symptoms that I describe to you here. No matter how much they strive to conceal themselves from your legions, they shall nonetheless be quickly destroyed and healing will soon occur. Let the magic power unfold immediately! Quickly, quickly, this has the force of a command of the supreme and original One who is both compassionate and merciful![61]

This passage is followed by two chapters containing simple and compound calligraphic amulets and spells to be used against a broad spectrum of diverse illnesses. The simple amulets, in particular, are frequently to be charred and then taken in combination with other equally intricately described boiled potions, containing incense, ginger, realgar, orange peel, plaster, cinnamon, and many other drugs. The complex amulets, in contrast, are to be carried out in conjunction with sword motions in the air or drawn at some other indicated location. Frequently, the sense of these written amulets is virtually impossible to decipher; some, however, bear a clear relationship to the indications in question. The compound characters generally comprise an upper element *shang*, meaning "responsible" and a lower-left element *shih*, meaning "food; to consume." The lower-right element varies according to the specific indications. Some easily understood examples are presented below; my description focuses on the variable, indication-related element:

Cures afflictions caused by wind[62]

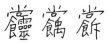

Yü, use magic power to drive out!

Cures swellings[63]

Penetrate through the shell; level all!

Cures those who have fallen victim to wine and drink themselves to intoxication[64]

Indication of the character for "wine"

Cures those exhausted by excessive contemplation[65]

to rest

Cures burning eyes and eye pains[66]

wind

In 1894, a widespread outbreak of bubonic plague was reported in southern China. Several representatives of modern Western medicine traveled to Hong Kong in order to track down the cause of the illness using modern scientific methods. In the same year, the French physician and microbiologist A. Yersin (1863–1943) announced his discovery of the plague virus. In 1896 the colonial government of Hong Kong published a medical report on the 1894 epidemic and included in the document a "Chinese View of the Plague," which the British editor introduced as follows:

> The following translation from a Chinese publication gives the latest theories and treatment of the plague, and as it is a peculiar document I give it in full. The translation has been kindly supplied by Mr. J. Dyer Ball. It should be noticed that the author lays great stress on what one might term the "disinfection of the family well." I am convinced with a considerable amount of reason. Although the various wells through the City of Victoria are much better built than some of those I have seen in other Chinese places, and in the foregoing report I have given a guarded opinion as to the question of their pollution in Hongkong, still I feel pretty certain that in Canton these wells had a good deal to do with the propagation of the Epidemic. The treatment recommended closely resembles what I saw in the Chinese Hospitals here and represents the most advanced views of Chinese medicine.[67]

The Chinese document that provoked such keen interest on the part of British colonial officials is, in fact, a significant historical source in several ways. Evidently, it is a publication of a "Society for the Performance of Good Deeds" influenced by both Buddhist and Confucian values, in which the public learned the views of the God of War on the causes of the plague as well as on effective countermeasures, made known through planchette revelations. The opening lines of the Society's introduction are as follows:

> Whereas we have heard that calamities are caused by atmospheric influences and destiny:—Good deeds can cause an avoidance of them. The terrific plague has recently been prevalent; it depresses the hearts and is painful to the sight. Although already people of the whole place distribute prescriptions and medicines free, and offer up all manner of prayers to avert the calamity, which means are the best that men can devise as preventives, yet the noxious influences have not been kept away. The reason of this failure is because the people have not done all the good deeds that they should to move Heaven and gain its approval.[68]

The subsequent planchette revelations show the ultimate cause to be the depravity of the victims. The decline of morality was perceived to be widespread and already visible in the behavior of small children. Honorable ideas were scarce, animals were slaughtered for sacrificial purposes, money was wasted on sacrificial paper, incense, and candles; man deceived his fellow man. In addition, a coal mine near the city had radiated poisonous substances. Nevertheless, according to the God of War, effective prevention is completely possible. Plague demons do not afflict those who practice filial piety and remain true to friends. For those who previously have exhibited a poor attitude, atonement for past conduct is still possible. The rich must demonstrate their virtue through regular generous gifts to charitable institutions. The poor can provide the same proof by reciting a certain liturgy. But the liturgy may be read only by one who has already demonstrated loyalty, honesty, virtue, and filial piety. In addition, in order to achieve protection, at least 5,000 families in each city must fulfill these requirements. As a sign that they are truly complying with the demands of the God of War, these families should draw his halberd, and beneath it add the characters for "assisting superintendent in the Office of Epidemics. Seal of the Official. . . ." If this sign has been attached to the entrance of the house, the plague demons will stay away. Anyone who has fraudulently drawn the halberd, however, will himself be destroyed by this weapon.

As the next step, the God of War advised the burning of water-purifying amulets in the family well and throwing garlic as well as the drug *kuan-chung* (Rhizome Cyrtomii), whose insecticidal properties were known, into the water. This measure was necessary because the wells were poisoned during the plague primarily by decaying rats, which found their way in from sewer drains. If despite such preventive measures, fever and boils should appear, the God of War advised the taking of a boiled potion containing seventeen drugs, as well as lancing the boils and applying external treatment.

The religious import of the planchette revelations is thus characterized primarily through linking adherence to socioethical norms with the origin of illness. In addition, medicinal measures were recommended, coupled with the call for the "disinfection" of water. Moreover, the role played by rats in the spread of the disease was indicated. Although the document contains the usual identification of "evil influences" as pathogenic agents, there is otherwise absolutely no mention of classical theories of orthodox Chinese medical thought. It would certainly be misleading, on the basis of this one document, to draw far-reaching conclusions about the significance of the Five Phases and yinyang theories of Chinese healing at the beginning of this century. But the fact that the revelations cited above could be designated the most recent insights of Chinese medicine is a sign of both the diversity of healing concepts in China at the end of the empire and of the lack of a dominant theoretical system that could have confronted Western influence.

9. Medicine in Twentieth-Century China

9.1. A SURVEY OF INTELLECTUAL CURRENTS IN THE TWENTIETH CENTURY

The establishment of the Republic of China in late 1911 and the formal abdication of the last Chinese emperor several weeks later; the "iconoclastic" movement of May 4, 1919, for a radical renewal of China along Western lines, which grew out of a protest against provisions of the Versailles treaties that ceded former German colonial possessions in China to Japan; the establishment of the Chinese Communist Party in 1921; the slow rise of communism and its struggle with the Kuomintang nationalists, which culminated in the civil war of the 1940s; the founding of the People's Republic of China in 1949; the "Great Leap Forward" of 1958 and the "Great Proletarian Cultural Revolution" of 1966, as well as more recently the seizure of power and "Smashing of the Gang of Four"; these events in the recent history of Chinese civilization represent only the most obvious politically and historically significant indications of a long-term metamorphosis, encompassing much more than the transition of a particular state from one political order to another. It is pointless to speculate on how politics and philosophy in China might have developed without the powerful military, technological, and ideological influence of Western culture beginning in the mid-nineteenth century. It should be remembered, however, that at the time of its momentous encounter with the West, China had become so impotent internally that it was completely unable—politically, economically, or intellectually—to cope with an external threat totally unlike any of the earlier "barbarian invasions." The encounter with Western civilization, unlike previous contacts with foreign peoples, expanded the Chinese world view, leading some thinkers to revise the belief prevailing for many centuries "in the uniqueness of indigenous culture and in the universality of its underlying principles."[1]

The impulse behind this highly painful and still ongoing process of adaptation to the new situation arose in China at a point in history when the search by individuals and groups for a new ideological orientation had already produced a multiplicity of diverse and competing approaches and beliefs. Western civilization—completely unexpected and uninvited as well—stepped as a mediator into internal debates, opening a number of possible solutions to the Chinese. Christian missionaries were the first to arrive, but they achieved no lasting success. A magic word, however, soon appeared in China and promised, in the eyes of numerous influential thinkers, a better future; this word was *science*. Within a few decades this initially alien concept of the dynamics of knowledge, of the methodical search for objectively reproducible truth, exerted such a fascination in China among those seeking both a renewal of Chinese culture and an adaptation to the changed realities of internal and international political circumstances, that Hu Shih, in a subsequently oft-cited remark, could declare in 1923:

> Ever since the beginning of reformist tendencies in China, there is not a single person who calls himself a modern man and yet dares openly to belittle science.[2]

The concept of "science" thus proved to be the first influential contribution of Western civilization to Chinese intellectual development. An ideological gulf subsequently opened between proponents of a Western and adherents to a Chinese course for the future. But the persuasive force generated by conservatives, who sought guidelines and values for the solution of modern social, economic, and technological problems in China's past, was apparently so weak that yet another Western philosophical system, Marxism, found acceptance and, in its Chinese form, was able to shape recent history decisively. If the older Chinese world view continued to play a certain role, it was evident, as Bauer has shown, in various epistemological concepts with which Mao Tse-tung modified Marxism, as well as in political consequences that he derived from them, primarily the notion of a permanent revolution.[3]

The concepts of Chinese medicine and pharmacology faithfully followed the historical developments sketched here. The polarizations and tensions generated by the clash of Chinese tradition, modern science, and Marxism were also reflected in medical thought, particularly in discussions concerning the fate of traditional "Chinese medicine."

9.2. THE APPEARANCE AND SPREAD OF WESTERN MEDICINE IN CHINA

9.2.1. Concepts of Modern Western Medicine

The history of Chinese ideas about the nature of illness and the optimal treatment of physical and mental suffering is only comprehensible when perceived as an integral component of the larger context of sociopolitical objectives and developments. The reflective character of therapeutic conceptual systems also clearly reveals modern Western medicine to be the product of social and economic factors in the history of Western civilization. Despite its sometimes extremely close ties to "neutral" discoveries of modern natural science, Western medicine, especially etiology and therapy, is shaped by the prevailing values of modern European society. It is important to bear this fact in mind as we seek to understand the reactions of social groups in China to what may be the most potent healing system of all time and the difficulties that stood in the way of its general acceptance from the very beginning.

An important feature of modern Western medicine is its true freedom to seek solutions to medicotherapeutic problems without obvious ideological restraints. This freedom, which we regard as both a necessary prerequisite and the point of departure for the development of a diagnostic and therapeutic system whose effectiveness, despite numerous inadequacies, is unique, grew out of a historical compromise that ended centuries of conflict between seemingly ideologically irreconcilable opponents.

On one side stood natural scientists requiring only their own empirical observations, who since the time of Hippocrates had increasingly recognized the connections between the organism and its natural environment as a primary source of illness. They had noted the significance of diet, physical exertion, and climatic factors for the maintenance of well-being and began to systematize this knowledge as a basis for therapeutic efforts. At approximately the same time that the concept of "wind" in China found acceptance as the primary cause of all illnesses, the Hippocratic author of the work *Peri physon* attributed all suffering to this same natural element.[4] The overriding theory that developed out of this was the so-called humoral pathology, that is, the doctrine of body humors, which permitted the inclusion of an empirically validated materia medica from older times as well as more recent drug discoveries.

This development of a purely natural healing—free of any metaphysics—was significantly impeded during the first half of the European Middle Ages by the rise of Christianity to a dominant political force. Christian dogmatists recognized in natural conceptions about the origin and cure of illness a threat to the success of their teachings. In the Bible itself, only three causes of illness are identified—transgressions by the victims themselves (or their ancestors), acts of God that reveal His omnipotence, without the victim having committed any offense, and demonic possession.[5] The sole procedure to prevent illness, according to biblical etiology, was a life free from sin, that is, a life in accordance with Christian morality; similarly, the only course of therapy was the plea for God's infinite mercy, a remedy to which even demons must yield. Belief in the natural origin of illness and the medicinal efficacy of natural substances, as well as the emphasis on a dietetically regulated life for the avoidance of illness, liberated man from the fear of any consequences of "sin," removing any obligation to preserve well-being by pursuing a life based on Christian doctrine. This antagonism explains the hostility with which influential proponents of the Christian Church viewed natural healing. Tatian (120–173), for example, perceived in the apparent efficacy of medicinal drugs nothing more than the deceitful machinations of demons to take from man his fear of God and replace it with a faith in herbs and roots.[6] In a similar vein, Justin (100?–165) compared drugs to thieves, who demand from their victims not ransom, but rather their belief in God.[7] The use of plants and other medicaments was tolerated (and even supported) by the Church only when an ideologically satisfactory procedure had been developed to raise, by means of blessings, inherently worthless substances to agents of divine healing power.[8] Christian notions of the efficacy of drugs thus by no means required actually taking them; it was fully sufficient to carry on one's person consecrated substances as phylacteries or amulets, to keep them in the house or stall, or bury them in the fields.

Only with the gradual weakening of ecclesiastic power and the increased influence exerted by secular groups on daily life and the developing structure of knowledge was natural medicine slowly able to regain its position. At the same time, from approximately the twelfth

century on, those within Christianity who regarded the conflict between natural science and religious belief as reconcilable and thus
strove for a "compromise" that we have termed "conceptual diversity,"[9] gained in persuasive power. Natural explanations of the mutual
interaction of phenomena were accorded a fundamental reality while,
at the same time, the hand of God, or even the actions of demons,
were recognized in all things. This prepared the foundation for the
harmonious coexistence of natural investigation and Christian doctrine, for it removed the almost paralyzing effect of two irreconcilable
ideological alternatives on the free cultivation of knowledge. For the
first time, it was now possible for Christian, Jew, or atheist, either
collectively or individually, to deal with the same scientific or, in this
case, medical problem and to exchange results without the fear that
their views might conflict with those of certain ideologically fixed and
politically influential groups. It is true, for instance, that in 1772 several
priests in England initiated a movement against Boyer's smallpox in-
noculation as a "dangerous and sinful practice," and "the work of
the devil,"[10] and that shortly after Jenner's discovery of the smallpox
vaccine, a group of physicians and priests in the United States formed
an Anti-Vaccination Society in 1782, claiming that God's Law prohibited such practices.[11] As late as the mid-nineteenth century, English
and Scottish clerics rejected as sacrilegious Simpson's discovery that
chloroform facilitated birth, since such assistance alleviated the consequences of the original curse on women.[12] But these occurrences are
only isolated examples of a waning conflict that illuminate the expansion of medicine into unknown and previously unthinkable areas
of knowledge and therapy.

It is no coincidence that the evolution of a harmonious plurality of
Christian and non-Christian beliefs fostered in the nineteenth century—first in England and France and, after 1850, in Germany as
well—a historically unique period of medical progress. In the space
of a century, until the 1950s, intensive and broad-based fundamental
scientific research produced all the achievements that have brought
Western medicine to its unchallenged preeminence in world health
care. The compromise produced by conceptual diversity permitted the
fruitful exchange of ideas between all those in Western societies seeking
solutions to acute health problems and those interested in expanding
the boundaries of scientific knowledge. The medical system that evolved
out of these conditions incorporated certain experiences, concepts,
remedies, and vocabularies from the past, but its recent innovations
derived solely from the application of the four fundamental principles

of scientific method. These are: (1) the empirical principle, in which observation precedes hypothesis, hypothesis precedes experiment, and experiment, in turn, is followed by renewed observation; (2) the quantitative principle, based on a belief in the measurability of real processes and, consequently, on the need for precise measurements; (3) the mechanical principle, expressed in the search for regularity among causal relationships and the formal abstraction of these relationships; (4) the principle of progress, which rests on an understanding of the incompleteness of present knowledge and the accompanying belief in the need for research.[13] Yet despite such seemingly objective methods, the newly developed etiological concepts and therapeutic concerns incorporated values and structures that appear to mirror the industrial society of the nineteenth and early twentieth centuries. The free economic system, with an emphasis by all significant groups on the individual and on individual achievement, and the concept of free competition, in which the industrious individual thrives while the less capable must assume a socially inferior position, not only rendered Darwin's ideas of the "survival of the fittest" plausible but also made germ theory, which regarded the physical condition of the individual and hygienic efforts as decisive for illness and well-being, the most popular explanation of individual suffering. Just as it was necessary in daily life to defend oneself constantly against the efforts of competitors in order to ensure economic survival, the individual faced a constant struggle with the ever-present germs in order to preserve physical well-being. The decline of holistic thought, evident in so many areas of modern civilization, led medical thinkers step by step from the theory of humors, with its notion of the unity of somatic and emotional processes (which was accepted in some circles until the beginning of the nineteenth century), to the primarily isolated and individual observation of organs and processes in the body.

Before I turn to the arrival and spread of this system of healing in China, it should be noted that what I term here "Western" medicine has undoubtedly been preeminent in the West for a century, but nonetheless has been unable to dislodge all competing systems. Just as can be documented for many centuries in China, there existed (and still exists) in modern industrial nations of Europe and the United States a diverse plurality of therapeutic approaches. Orthodox Jews and Christian fundamentalists still follow faithfully the precepts of their holy scriptures; for the Catholic church, the demonic origin of suffering—now as then—remains an unshakable element of its faith; tens of thousands of healers practice folk medicine outside of any official control, utilizing in part concepts of magic. In addition, new systems have evolved, which appear to correspond to the personal and social objectives of more or less large segments of the population, such as Christian Science, or in Central Europe, the healing art of anthroposophy. Yet none of these alternative systems appears sufficiently adapted to the modern industrial age, in terms of values and structures, to provide any serious competition to biochemical/biophysical medicine and the corresponding chemical, physical, and surgical treatment of illnesses. It therefore becomes understandable why it was biochemical/biophysical medicine that became identified as "Western" medicine and began its impressive march throughout the entire world. This phenomenon is undoubtedly in part due to the system's unparalleled ability to influence the processes of the organism in a desired and predictable manner. In addition, however, the rise of "Western" medicine to world medicine is an indication that the universal efforts of virtually all states to industrialize and match living standards in the West, including mortality and morbidity statistics, require a universal healing system as well. When to the present day in China, groups have repeatedly rejected Western medicine, or at the very least, sought to relativize its significance, this reaction must also be understood as resistance to Western economic models and their accompanying social structures.

9.2.2. The Medical Missionaries: Objectives and Methods

It is not completely without irony that it was Christian missionaries who brought Western medicine to China, utilizing it to demonstrate the superiority of their beliefs and the uniqueness of their God. Following unsuccessful efforts by Jesuits in the seventeenth century to disseminate European anatomical and physiological concepts, it remained for Protestant physicians and missionaries in the nineteenth century to introduce Western healing to all provinces of the Chinese Empire.

At first, Western medicine had precious little to offer. Robert Morrison, the first Protestant missionary in China, and J. Livingston, a physician of the East India Company, opened an apothecary shop together in Macao in 1820, in which they treated patients for one or two hours daily. Morrison had attended medical lectures in addition to his theological studies in London and had received brief clinical training in Saint Bartholomew's Hospital so that he could treat himself and colleagues in case of illness. Average life expectancy among missionaries in East Asia was still approximately five years in 1835,[14] a situation that underscored the necessity of equipping some of them with the rudiments of healing skills. When Morrison and Livingston opened their practice, the primary objective, according to their own words, had been to establish friendlier relations between the Chinese and foreigners. Since therapeutic knowledge available to Western physicians at the time was still not yet sufficient to occasion an attitude of superiority, Morrison and Livingston immediately sought the assistance of a respected Chinese practitioner, as well as a native apothecary, whose entire stock of drugs they purchased. In addition, the two compiled a library containing some 800 works of Chinese medicine, demonstrating their special interest in learning native healing techniques.[15]

Only a few years later the situation had changed markedly. The dynamics of the expansion of Western medical knowledge characterizing the entire century from the 1840s through the 1940s showed an immediate influence on the attitude of Western medical men toward Chinese health care theories and practices. Between 1851 and 1858, Benjamin Hobson, an English physician, together with his Chinese collaborator Kuan Mao-ts'ai, published in Shanghai in Chinese language a series of four titles on anatomy (1851), internal medicine (two volumes, including materia medica) (1858), gynecology/pediatrics (1858), as well as on Western medicine in general (1857). A fifth book (1855) was devoted to the sciences; its subjects included physics, optics, astronomy, and zoology. The demand for such materials, all of which were skillfully illustrated, is demonstrated by Chinese reprints. Dr. Hobson's books were introduced to Japan as well; a first facsimile edition appeared there as early as 1858.

A translation of two paragraphs from the first chapter of Hobson's "Summary of Western Medicine" (*Hsi-i lüeh-lun*) of 1857 should be of interest here. Hobson's assessment of the standards of health care in his host country may be seen as an early indication of an antagonism which has marked the relationship between Western and Chinese medicine ever since.

On Chinese and Western Medicine:
    The sciences of today, as for instance the writings on astronomy, mathematics, and geography, are more sophisticated than in former times; why should medicine be an exception? Two centuries ago the principles of vascular blood circulation were not yet fully understood

by Western medicine. Nowadays one understands this clearly. And there
are further [areas], including cerebral nerves and pancreas duct, about
which men of former times had nothing to say. When I asked my Chinese
friends [I was told that] Chinese medicine is worse today than in ancient
times. Two reasons account for this. In the West, medical scholars must
pass a series of examinations. Those who take a degree will have a title
and may then go out to practice. The value [of such a degree] is similar
to the Chinese titles of *chü-jen* or *chin-shih;* and its regulations resemble
the example of Chinese literary scholars who earn it through an examination. This is why those who practice [medicine in the West or
literary scholarship in China] ever seek refinement in what they do.
Medical scholars in China are men who train themselves. They do not
pass any official examination and they do not add any tokens of distinction [to their names]. This is the first reason of their being unsophisticated. The human body, the organs and the entire organism are
like a clockwork. If one does not open it and take it apart, there is no
way of knowing how it functions and what are the reasons for its failure.
This is why Western countries permit the dissection of corpses. If in
any home for the aged, for the insane, or for the deaf and mute there
is someone who dies without any [person] to whom he could be returned, the Bureau of Medicine is authorized to dissect [the corpse] for
the purpose of teaching students. Once an examination has been completed, someone is ordered to dress and bury [the corpse] in accordance
with the regulations. As a result, all Western physicians comprehend
the mysteries of the organs and of the blood vessels. Chinese who study
medicine do not even have one single such [experience]. Old physicians
who have [practiced for] decades still do not know the shape of the
organs. If they are confronted with a strange and incurable symptom,
they will never know where the origin of the illness was. This is the
second reason of their being unsophisticated. I wish China would establish a Bureau of Medicine authorizing medical scholars to dissect
and examine criminals who were sentenced to death. As a result, medicine in China would inevitably become more sophisticated than [the
medicine] of the men in the past.[16]

On Drugs:

   I have heard in China Shen-nung's *materia medica* included 360 drugs.
Through the ages these were amended until, at the time of the Ming,
Li Shih-chen wrote the *Pen-ts'ao kang mu*, listing almost two thousand
samples. This represents, indeed, a highly complete *materia medica*. But
when I take a close look at it, it includes some items of great use, such
as ginseng and rhubarb, and some of no use at all, like dragon or tiger
bones. The commentaries and explanations of all authors, in general,
take the association of the colors and tastes with the Five Phases to
differentiate their correspondences with the organs. How could they
know that drugs must first enter the stomach where anything colored
is transformed into something without color, and where anything with
taste is transformed into something without taste. There is no reason
[for drugs] to enter different organs each according to their color and

taste. There are those who say that a consumption of pork-loin strengthens the inner kidney, that a consumption of brain strengthens the head, and that a consumption of legs strengthens the feet. These are definitely prejudices. Food must first of all enter the stomach where it is digested. From the stomach it proceeds toward the small intestine where it meets with bile and pancreas secretions. Its essential liquids are squeezed out and absorbed by small ducts which move them to the *hui-kuan* [?]. They reach the heart and become blood. If the items eaten have any beneficial contents, their effects are distributed throughout the entire body; there is no reason why they should benefit only one particular place. As to statements to the effect that tortoise urine nourishes the kidneys, that the placenta nourishes the water, that metals and minerals reduce deficiencies and that hares' droppings warm the blood, I do still less know what might be a concrete basis of such claims.[17]

As a consequence of their increasing self-confidence and of their general inability to gain access to more fundamental concepts and theories underlying Chinese health care, Western physicians saw little attraction in a cooperation with their Chinese colleagues. Furthermore, those who, in the coming decades, practiced Western medicine in China as medical missionaries, either honestly considered or pragmatically utilized Western medical knowledge as a direct manifestation of a superior civilization based on Christian faith. It could not be in their missionary interest to support any doubts about that superiority by seriously investigating traditional Chinese medicine as a possibly preferable alternative.

The actual age of the so-called medical missionaries began in 1835 when Peter Parker, the first Protestant missionary with complete medical training, opened a clinic in Canton and, in a space of a few years, treated thousands of patients solely utilizing techniques of Western medicine. At the time, the development of chemotherapy still lay decades in the future. Although European pharmacology was already familiar with some reliable, efficacious natural substances, such as digitalis and, since the isolation of morphine in 1804, various pure alkaloids, it is doubtful whether this represented any fundamental advance over Chinese healing. At the beginning of his activity, Parker was also unfamiliar with antisepsis and anesthesia, so that it was primarily minor surgical procedures, such as the removal of external tumors and the treatment of superficial ailments, as well as spectacular cataract operations, that quickly made him famous and brought an incessant stream of patients from near and far.

As welcome as such successes were for Parker as a practitioner, they hampered his effectiveness as a missionary, an objective he regarded as primary.[18] The directives of the American Board of Commissioners for Foreign Missions, Parker's sponsoring organization in the United States, expressly permitted medical activity only to the extent required for the dissemination of religion.[19] The medical missionary was not to concentrate on the Chinese body, but rather on the Chinese mind;[20] it was not the number of patients cured that mattered, but the number of Chinese converted.[21] When it eventually became known in America that Parker had devoted too little time to his real task, the missionary society withdrew its financial support.[22] Nevertheless, observers saw in Parker's work a clear indication of the possibilities inherent in a combination of medical and missionary efforts, if both elements were kept in the proper proportions. After a visit to Parker in 1847, a representative of the Missionary Society of the Church of England reported enthusiastically:

> at the present time the Missionary Hospital is the most hopeful agency for effecting good on an extensive scale by disposing the minds of rulers and people most favorably towards foreign teachers.[23]

This conclusion did not go unheard. In 1850, 10 missionary hospitals had already opened; by 1889 the number had risen to 61,[24] and shortly after the turn of the century, medical missionaries were active in 362 hospitals with fixed treatment facilities and in an additional 244 devoted solely to ambulatory care.[25]

So as not to neglect their spiritual obligations and the desire for conversions because of the heavy medical burdens, some missionaries devised detailed procedures for the integration of both objectives. The following plan was deemed highly promising and had already proved its practical worth in at least one hospital when the author published and recommended it to his colleagues:

> As the out-patients begin to gather, the evangelist and his helpers, instead of keeping up a continuous preaching performance as is so often the case, mingle with the patients, and get into general conversation with them one by one. They find out where they have each come from, and what it is that has brought them to the hospital, at the same time explaining to them, in a simple way, the procedure that is to follow— how long it will be before the doctor comes; in what order they will be seen; where they will get their medicines; what they will have to do if they need to be admitted to the wards, etc. In these and similar ways they gain the confidence of the patients, and make them feel that they have their interests at heart.

About twenty minutes before the clinic is to open a bell is rung, and an announcement is then made that a short service will be held, at which all are asked to sit quietly, special stewards being appointed to show into their seats any fresh patients who may arrive during this time. The service opens with a brief introduction, in which the evangelist, or better still the doctor himself, explains simply why such a gathering is held. He tells them of the great Gift which the hospital tries to represent, and points them in simple language to the Father who cares for them all.

Having made this introduction, and shown them how that Father may be approached by all who care to do so through the use of prayer, he asks them all to stand reverently in their places while he offers up an intercession on their behalf. Prayer concluded, an earnest address is given, usually on some incident in the life and teaching of Jesus Christ, and a strong appeal is made to all to study for themselves the truths of the gospel.

As the hour for the opening of medical work strikes, a second bell is rung, and at this signal the evangelist and his helpers leave the platform and mingle once more with the people. The earlycomers, whose registration number will entitle them to be seen first, are directed to the proper door, while the evangelist sits with those who have some time to wait, explaining in more detail what has been said during the service, offering portions of the Scriptures or other books for sale, and attempting to draw them into conversation. In this way he soon learns to recognize those who are coming regularly for treatment, and in some cases is able to obtain an invitation to visit them in their own homes, there to follow up the impression that has been formed.[26]

It may appear that the difficulties of combining missionary objectives and medical activity were solved here in a harmonious fashion, but a fundamental conflict between theologians and medical practitioners nonetheless marked the efforts of medical missionaries in China during the entire nineteenth century and well into the second decade of the twentieth. The missionary societies and Christian congregations in Europe and the United States who provided the financial support for the establishment of hospitals were not particularly interested in providing exemplary models of Western healing to China. The attitude of these groups was expressed by the medical missionary J. L. Maxwell in 1905 in the following words to his colleagues:

It does not matter very much in what kind of building your medical and surgical work is performed, provided it gives you an opportunity of preaching the gospel to your patients; and, further, that seeing that the spiritual results are the chief thing, there is no special call to lay yourself out for and to be ready to deal with difficult cases. Such cases will take up a lot of time, and will give the medical missionary a good deal of anxiety and trouble; therefore, it would be well to cultivate only those cases that can be easily and quickly managed.[27]

But the majority of medical missionaries active in China, as well as the medical societies in Europe and the United States, to the extent they were able to observe the activities of their colleagues in East Asia, were of a different mind. They saw in the practice of the medical missionaries first and foremost a chance to demonstrate the benefits and effectiveness of modern medicine, whose almost daily advances in these decades must have inspired every physician. A widespread enthusiasm about the future role of healing in politics and society, coupled with the related possibility, for the first time in history, of the medical profession to achieve social prominence on the basis of actual achievement and not solely because of purported motivations, caused representatives of the medical profession to view with suspicion any development that resembled a renewed subordination of medicine to theology. Thus as early as 1855, the editor of the British medical journal *Lancet* entitled an editorial in which he criticized the linking of missionary and medical activities "Medicine Independent of Theology."[28] But China was located far away, and European and American professional organizations were much too occupied with overcoming the shadows of the past in their own lands, solidifying their new status, reforming the system of medical training, and controlling structurally the rapid advancement in specialized fields, for Chinese problems to play a significant role. Until about 1920, financial support by missionary societies determined the image of Western medicine in China, an image that only rarely corresponded to medical standards in Europe and the United States. The results of a 1920 study by the China Medical Missionary Association, which encompassed some 80 percent of all missionary hospitals in rural and urban areas, revealed some startling deficiencies:

92% of the hospitals have no pure water supply and only 6% have running water in all suitable rooms.
73% of the hospitals have no means of sterilizing bedding or mattresses.
50% of the hospitals seldom or never bathe their patients.
43% of the hospitals have no laundries or only inadequate facilities for dealing with hospital linen.
34% of the hospitals have no pressure sterilizer for their dressings.
31% of the hospitals have no laboratory of any kind.
82% of the hospitals have no bacteriological incubator.
87% of the hospitals have no x-ray machine.[29]

The fact that the China Medical Missionary Association was forced to call public attention to this unfortunate situation, in order to bring pressure on European and American missionary societies to reconsider their policies, was owing primarily to two developments. First, mission hospitals are now no longer the only hospitals known to the educated classes in China. Hundreds of students and merchants who have travelled in Europe, in America, or in Japan, have had personal experience of modern hospital treatment in those countries, and are increasingly conscious of how far away many mission hospitals fall short in scientific equipment and modern nursing methods.[30]

Second, hospitals that met the highest contemporary standards were now also being built in China by both national and foreign secular agencies, in particular the Rockefeller Foundation, making the contrast to the majority of mission hospitals obvious to all. Some mission hospitals were therefore closed in 1920, and when Yale University, at about the same time, decided to establish a modern medical school to "train [Chinese students] in science, humanities, and medicine, and bring them closer to God," because it was still generally felt that "medical work . . . is in general the surest and strongest way of introducing missionary operations in any part of China," Dr. Hume, in charge of planning for the undertaking, warned the trustees in New Haven: ". . . it would be a great mistake for medical work to be done on any but the most scientific lines; for us that means the standards of Johns Hopkins!"[31]

At this point, the history of Western medicine in China finally entered a new phase. The anachronistic attempt to combine a primitive variety of modern healing with Christian dogma and thereby render it useful for the missions was replaced by the progressive alliance of the newest medical achievements with modern science, which for an untold number of Chinese signaled the philosophy of the future.

9.2.3. Science and Scientific Medicine in Twentieth-Century China

Decades of humiliation by Western powers and, ultimately, by Japan— which despite the numerical inferiority of its forces, easily emerged victorious from the war of 1895—as well as the increasingly obvious fact that China's own intellectual and material resources were inadequate to resist the threat from without and ensure the national existence, led a steadily growing number of Chinese politicians and intellectuals, beginning in the final third of the nineteenth century, to focus their attention beyond the borders of their own civilization. More and more, the view prevailed that it was not enough to imitate Western techniques of arms production, but rather that a serious confrontation with the intellectual, social, and political principles un-

derlying this technology was unavoidable.[32] Christianity had been able
to secure only a small number of Chinese followers; it was, however,
another "religion" of the West—that is, the promise of scientism—to
which the vast majority of those skeptical about the intellectual traditions of China would turn. The force of these tidings of modern
civilization could not remain hidden to anyone who turned his eye to
Europe. The fervor of Western scholars to search for ultimate truths
with the aid of scientific methods had, by the mid-nineteenth century,
crossed beyond the bounds of natural science, culminating in the conviction that it must be possible to uncover these same truths in every
other field of endeavor, including, of course, the harmonious coexistence of men. Virchow, possibly the most prominent advocate of scientism in Germany, ascribed to the scientific method in law, economics,
health care, education, morality, and conscience, the role that "in
earlier times had fallen to the transcendental strivings of the various
churches."[33] At last, happiness and freedom no longer appeared to be
concepts of a distant utopia. The power of this gospel reached China
undiminished and remained influential during the first two or three
decades of the twentieth century, at a time when a more sober assessment of the potential and limits of science for human existence
had long since regained the upper hand in Europe.

But how can one explain the unparalleled attraction and persuasive
force that the concept of modern science, which was so foreign to the
Chinese, exerted on reformers of all possible political beliefs at the
beginning of this century, such that for a period of time the term
science was synonymous with "modern civilization"?[34] Certainly the
desires of many to adopt Western values and even the entire Western
culture, in order to restore to China the international greatness that
had marked its foreign relations during past periods of glory, was just
as decisive as the model of Japan, which in a short time had been able
to assimilate significant elements of Western civilization. Yet the speed
with which scientific salvation became the philosophy of so many and
gained influential adherents among those in public life can be understood only in light of the centuries-long uncertainty among Chinese
thinkers regarding the limitless diversity of interpretations of Confucian doctrine and fragmentation of the Chinese world view in general. At a time of highly threatening national humiliation, searchers
encountered the fascinating illusion of a new doctrine, whose comprehensive validity encompassed all natural and social dimensions of
existence and whose apparent universality fulfilled the same requirements as the old Chinese doctrine of the correspondence of all phe-

nomena, but in an incomparably more promising fashion. The motto on the frontispiece of the first issue of the journal *Young China,* which appeared in 1919, was programmatic of the hopes of both reformers and revolutionaries: "In service to society, under the guidance of the scientific spirit, for the realization of our ideal of the creation of a New China."[35]

At the same time, however, the outbreak of World War I raised the first doubts about the suitability of "science" as a social theory. Critics of a total Westernization pointed to the catastrophe of the war as evidence of the bankruptcy of Western culture, calling for a return to the intellectual values of China. Subjectivity instead of cold objectivity, a synthetic world view in place of the analytic dissection of the universe, intuition instead of logical methods, as well as freedom of the will and belief in the uniqueness of each individual instead of in the uniformity of all of nature and its processes—these were the values that conservative circles called for the Chinese youth to restore.[36] Opponents of this philosophy of life and proponents of a fundamental break with the past found it not difficult, on the basis of the past 2,000 years, to demonstrate the failure of these values to ensure China an honorable existence. The conservative argument that China possessed a humanistic tradition while Western civilization was purely materialistic caused Ting Wen-chiang, the best-known spokesman of adherents of scientism in the 1920s, to recall the facts from his perspective for his contemporaries:

> From Confucius to Mencius to the thinkers of the *Li* schools of Sung and Ming times, the accent was on the cultivation of inner life with the result being a kind of "spiritual civilization." Let us now see the result of this kind of spiritual civilization in history.
>
> The Sung had more than just one of these *Li* scholars who advocated the art of inner control; the most obvious was the school of Lu Hsiang-shan. The scholars of the time, fortunately, still emphasized learning and had not yet become entirely addicted to empty talk. During the Southern Sung, though, it was alarming how the scholar-literati lacked ability and common sense. The result was that we were for a hundred years controlled by the barbarian Mongols, and the southern people were butchered by the millions, and the Han culture all but died. . . . Toward the end of the Ming, the schools of Lu [Hsiang-shan] and Wang [Yang-ming] were popular everywhere. They were even more backward than the people of the Southern Sung. In their eyes, to study was a frivolous affair and a wasting away of the ambition, to attend to affairs was injurious to the dilettante ideal. . . . The scholar-literati did not

know the present or the past . . . like insane people they became completely ineffective in time of need. The two bandits of Shensi became the vanguards for the Manchus. The slaughtering in Szechuan by Chang Hsien-chung alone amounted to more than the total deaths in the first World War, not to speak of the atrocities of the Manchus in a few of the southern provinces. Let us ask ourselves fairly what price this spiritual civilization![37]

But the price appeared to be too high, and by the end of the 1920s, the few remaining voices that continued to call for a philosophy based on humanistic civilization once again lost the attention they had enjoyed for a brief period. The desire for a fundamental revolution and for an alternative completely removed from the values of the past only increased, shaping the intellectual situation until the 1940s. Increasingly, the debate focused on the concept of dialectical materialism, whose attraction was by no means restricted to members of the Chinese Communist party, which had been founded in Shanghai in 1921.[38] Not only avowed communists, but central theoreticians of the nationalist party of the Kuomintang, as well as other groups of the nonaligned intelligentsia, had finally found the doctrine that provided a kind of final building block for erecting a complete antithesis to the past. It constituted a comprehensive conceptual structure, which in all of its individual aspects stood in radical contrast to tradition, but which perhaps found such rapid and persuasive acceptance in Chinese thought because it paralleled so faithfully the familiar superstructure of the Confucian era. Modern science assumed the role of the doctrine of systematic correspondence, whose magic-derived concepts of yin-yang and the Five Phases were now spurned as fully inadequate for the solution of new technological problems. Marxism, which appeared in China claiming to be a scientific social theory, replaced Confucianism, whose sociotheoretical concepts and view of history had been closely associated with the old "natural science" of systematic correspondence. Imperial rule, which had been legitimized in the notion of the "Son of Heaven" and the desirable harmony of man with universal nature by both Confucianism and systematic correspondence, was now inevitably replaced by democracy, whose ideals of man's control over his own destiny and his environment appeared to offer the hope of turning the concepts of Marxism and modern science into political reality. Science, Marxism, and democracy—these were the key elements of the formula to which one wished to entrust the shape of the future. Mao Tse-tung expressed this in 1940:

New-democratic culture is scientific. Opposed as it is to all feudal and superstitious ideas, it stands for seeking truth from facts, for objective truth and for the unity of theory and practice. On this point, the possibility exists of a united front against imperialism, feudalism and superstition between the scientific thought of the Chinese proletariat and those Chinese bourgeois materialists and natural scientists who are progressive, but in no case is there a possibility of a united front with any reactionary idealism.[39]

The primacy of the sciences in the superstructure of the "New Democracy" initially meant an unrestricted esteem for the scientific medicine of the West as well. The early reformers K'ang Yu-wei and Liang Ch'i-ch'ao were already aware of the significance of a modernized medicine for the renewal of society that they sought. Their writings laid the foundation before the turn of the century for a radical reassessment of professional medical activity, castigating the traditional disinterest of the Chinese state in institutionalized healing. Viewed from our own perspective, Western medicine at the turn of the century was still far removed from the diagnostic and therapeutic achievements of today; it appears that reform-minded Chinese found two aspects of scientific healing in particular to be superior to their own medical traditions. The first of these was health-care policy and public hygiene. Liang Ch'i-ch'ao, haunted by the vision of a possible annihilation of the Chinese race in a struggle for survival among nations, regarded governmental support for medical sciences and the establishment of public health programs as a basic prerequisite for the strength of Western nations. Liang therefore called for an improvement in both the mental and physical circumstances in China. K'ang Yu-wei, repeating Virchow's boldest demands, even went so far as to entrust medical officials in the new society with the supervision of all spheres of human life.[40]

The second aspect that made Western medicine so attractive during those decades at the turn of the century was actually grounded more in expectations than in actual medical reality. As with the natural sciences themselves, medicine was also buoyed by a certain conviction in the fantastic potential that a consistent application of scientific methods held for the future. Traditional medicine, in contrast, whose progress was evident only in centuries of debate among an ever-growing number of authors concerning the correct interpretation of the ancient classics, offered no such optimistic perspective.

This contrast became readily apparent when, at the end of the epoch of medical missionaries, the actual capabilities of Western medicine were impressively demonstrated in China itself in highly modern training facilities and hospitals. Ch'en Tu-hsiu, one of the most prolific advocates of scientific modernization in China (and later the first secretary-general of the Communist party), unmistakably summarized his faith in the new and contempt for the old in 1919 in his famous "Appeal to the Youth":

> Our men of learning do not understand science; thus they make use of *yin-yang* signs and beliefs in the five elements to confuse the world. . . . Our doctors do not understand science: they not only know nothing of human anatomy, but also know nothing of the analysis of medicines; as for bacterial poisoning and infections, they have not even heard of them. . . . The height of their wondrous illusions is the theory of *ch'i* which really applies to the professional acrobats and Taoist priests. We will never comprehend this *ch'i* even if we were to search everywhere in the universe. All of these fanciful notions and irrational beliefs can be corrected at their roots by science, because to explain truth by science we must prove everything with fact.[41]

The subsequent fate of Western medicine in China has experienced two phases. The unconditional support of scientific-medical practice and research by reformers and radicals continued until the mid-1950s. By 1920, 900 Chinese doctors with modern training were already practicing, including a number of outstanding specialists, in addition to some 600 foreign colleagues.[42] By 1927, the number of Chinese physicians had grown to nearly 3,000; two years later the total reached 9,000 Chinese practitioners of Western medicine.[43] Much of the ideological support for these practitioners came from the early Marxists, such as Lu Hsün, Pa Chin, and Lao She, who expressed in particularly drastic literary form the senselessness and disastrous dangers they associated with traditional medicine.[44] Not until 1954 was there an indication of any revision in the political assessment of Western medicine, when in conjunction with the campaign against bourgeois attitudes, extensive skepticism was directed against the unaltered appropriation of Western medical practice for the formation of a socialist society. As early as 1940, Yang Ch'ao and T'an Chuang had pointed to the "capitalist, imperialist, and colonialist" context of Western medicine and, perceiving traditional Chinese medicine as inseparably linked with the feudalism of the past, called for the creation of a "new democratic medicine."[45] These impulses were picked up again in 1954/55. The fact that Western medicine had aided the missionaries in promoting their own goals of conversion was as clear to the Chinese as the concrete economic motivation underlying the medical activities of the Rockefeller Foundation in China.[46]

As the first difficulties in controlling the political views of Western-educated doctors became evident,[47] suspicion arose regarding the circumstances of initial Chinese contact with modern medicine and about the ideological reliability of its present representatives, a significant percentage of whom had studied at European and American universities. Criticism of Western-trained practitioners was, at least initially, limited to such trivial concerns as the purported insufficient preparation for dealing with health problems of the masses. Not until the beginning of the 1970s, perhaps encouraged by the prevailing political influence of the radical leftist Shanghai faction, did analyses appear in which, as far as can be determined from available sources, the central core of Western medicine, namely its therapeutic concepts, was subjected to an epistemological critique from a Marxist-Maoist perspective. In his well-known essay of 1937, "On Contradiction," Mao Tse-tung, drawing upon corresponding statements of Marx and Engels, had defined the epistemology of dialectical materialism primarily through its contrast to "bourgeois metaphysics," arguing:

> The metaphysical . . . world outlook sees things as isolated, static and one-sided. It regards all things in the universe, their forms and their species, as eternally isolated from one another and immutable. Such change as there is can only be an increase or decrease in quantity or a change of place. . . . Metaphysicians ascribe the causes of social development to factors external to society, such as geography and climate. They search in an oversimplified way outside a thing for the causes of its development, and they deny the theory of materialist dialectics which holds that development arises from the contradictions inside a thing.[48]

In various contributions to the journal *Dialectic of Nature* (*Tzu-jan pien-cheng-fa*), which—significantly—appeared in Shanghai from 1973 to 1976, these sociotheoretical concepts were transferred to the medical sphere. Thus, many aspects of Western medicine had to be condemned as bourgeois and metaphysical, including modern diagnostics, which treats individual organs and organic functions as well as associated illnesses in an isolated manner; modern etiology, which virtually without exception seeks the sources of illness in external pathogenic agents; and the medicamentous, physical, and surgical therapy of Western medicine, which is based less on the principle of the combined efforts of a therapist and an active patient to stimulate the inner defensive forces of the body in the struggle against disease than of using external measures to produce changes in a passive patient, that is, to discover and remove or destroy pathogenic agents that have penetrated from outside. Thus, a quarter-century after the founding of the People's Republic of China, at least a small number of Maoist dogmatists had recognized in contradictions between Western concepts of the origin, nature, and treatment of organic crises, on the one hand, and the views of Mao Tse-tung on the rise, nature, and solution of social crises, on the other hand, the fallaciousness of the unconditional equation of Marxism with science and science with modern medicine that had taken place during the 1920s and 1930s. Both equations are inaccurate. The "scientific" principle of Marxism, dialectical materialism, is not the basis of natural sciences, and although modern medicine utilizes numerous scientific discoveries, its fundamental concepts of etiology, prophylaxis, and therapy are by no means as neutral as may at first appear. It still remains to be seen whether the critical voices in China that demonstrated this have—with the fall of the Shanghai "Gang of Four"—been permanently silenced.

9.3. TRADITIONAL MEDICINE IN THE TWENTIETH CENTURY: CHANGES IN CONCEPTUAL LEGITIMATION

Following the collapse of imperial China, which marked the official end of the Confucian era, traditional Chinese medicine was faced with the problem of establishing a new ideological legitimacy. The strength of a healing system in society rests only partly on objective successes; equally important for its continuing acceptance and support is the anchoring of its medical notions in the world view and, especially, in the sociotheoretical concepts of a population or individual political groups. Such an assertion is supported by the fact that there has not yet been a system of healing that, detached from the values and structures of a specific culture or subculture, would have been objectively able to deal successfully with the entire spectrum of "health" problems as defined by a specific population. Even the success of Western medicine is only partial, and although in this respect it appears superior to all other existing healing systems, there nevertheless remains a considerable void, that is, problem areas in which Western medicine is helpless. Into such voids, whose extent, in turn, is dependent on ideological definitions of illness, step competing systems—in part with the justified claim of better results—thus contributing to the overall plurality of medical approaches in the world. The practical successes of historically documented and existing healing systems may justify claims for support, but not, however, for exclusivity. History teaches us that exclusive attitudes in the support and legal recognition of medical systems by political groups was, and remains in many places today, the rule. The fact that in the United States, for instance, hundreds of thousands of patients continue to seek—and find, according to their own testimony—sympathy and treatment in alternative systems is not reflected in governmental support for medicine. The enormous sums that flow year after year into medical research and practice benefit only orthodox medical doctrine.

A similarly exclusive policy toward Western medicine is evident in China as early as 1914, when the minister of education—responsible for such matters—made the following declaration to a group of traditional practitioners seeking official recognition for their medicine: "I have decided to abolish Chinese medicine and to use no more Chinese remedies as well."[49] This shocking revelation must have convinced the traditionalists of the true dimensions of their present situation, and it did not remain without repercussions. First, it was now necessary to close ranks and face the opponent united; second, it was imperative, following the loss of ties to Confucianism, so frequently invoked in past centuries,[50] to forge a new conceptual alliance. For this, several courses lay open.

Initially, the external threat reduced the internal spectrum of competing Chinese interpretations of the classics. When the first voices were raised in defense of the indigenous medical tradition, the increasingly obvious lack of direction exhibited by Chinese medical practitioners since the Sung-Chin-Yüan period, apparent in the steadily growing number of competing and frequently antagonistic doctrines, seemed suddenly forgotten. The great diversity of individual efforts to reconcile insights from personal experience with the ancient theories of yinyang and the Five Phases, as well as with other older views about the structure of the body, disappeared behind the illusion of a so-called Chinese medicine (chung-i), supposedly well-defined and with theory easily converted into practice. This term thus lumped together the basic principles and therapeutic techniques of the medicine of systematic correspondence, practical drug therapy as recorded in prescription literature and in the purely pharmaceutical pen-ts'ao works, as well as certain other pragmatic techniques, such as the traditional treatment of injuries. This situation, in turn, has given rise to the historically misleading impression that these diverse elements, like the concepts and practices of Western medicine, constituted a unified, coherent system. Demonic medicine, whose influence continued uninterrupted at least until the 1940s[51] and whose concepts corresponded to the attitudes and socioeconomic conditions of broad segments of the Chinese people, particularly among the rural population, was as ignored as "Chinese medicine" as the Buddhist oracle medicine practiced by the faithful in innumerable temples.

Traditional practitioners and conservatives, who opposed the Westernizing tendencies of their culture, were in accord that Chinese medicine should be preserved from destruction, but the question of future legitimation for this healing system was marked by disagreement. Some sought to demonstrate that all Western discoveries had already been anticipated in classical Chinese theories and that the lack of any surgery since the time of Hua T'o could be explained by the fact that medicine had advanced beyond this particular phase of therapy and that such problems could be treated with medication. Other authors stressed that Chinese medicine expressed the "spirit of the nation" (kuo-ts'ui); they condemned Western medicine as "materialistic," viewing Chinese medicine as an integral component of the supposedly humanistic civilization of China that was to be preserved. More moderate conservatives attempted to differentiate the practice of Chinese medicine from the older theories by arguing that the former was empirically grounded while the latter were faulty interpretations of later times.[52] Representatives of such a differentiated approach consequently had no reservations about using scientific methods to analyze the practices of Chinese medicine, so as to retain that which was useful while eliminating harmful or meaningless aspects. Although highly conservative circles protested such attempts, claiming that Chinese medicine was degraded in this manner to a mere component of Western medicine, the "scientization" of Chinese medicine constituted the compromise reached after 1929 by the nationalist party of the Kuomintang and after 1950 by the Chinese Communist party as well.[53]

Despite the clear preference of Marxist thinkers for natural science and scientific therapy during the 1920s, 1930s, and 1940s, the fate of traditional medicine had by no means been determined when the Communists assumed power in China in 1949. Only seventeen years after the Marxist T'an Chuang had termed Chinese medicine the "collected garbage of several thousand years" in 1941,[54] Mao Tse-tung formulated his famous dictum of 1958: "Chinese medicine is a great treasurehouse! We must make all efforts to uncover it and raise its standards!"

Western secondary literature generally suspects the reasons for this rehabilitation of those elements of medical tradition that—unlike demonic medicine and Buddhist temple medicine—were not disqualified from the very beginning as "superstition" and thus remained outside the bounds of discussion, to lie in quantitative considerations by the Chinese leadership. Indeed, until recently, modern medicine—in part because of the still relatively small number of its practitioners—was unable to offer the entire Chinese population one or another form of health care. But to resolve this dilemma, other political solutions would have been conceivable; the intensive ideological support for Chinese medicine since the 1950s cannot be explained solely by the numerical indispensability of its practitioners. Perhaps, in substituting "treasure-house" for "collected garbage" in the internal party debate, Mao Tse-tung had come to the conclusion, inconceivable for early Marxists, that certain essential elements of both theory and practice in Chinese medicine were significantly closer to Marxist notions of epistemology and social practice than was the case for Western medicine. To be sure, Mao Tse-tung was unable to provide Chinese medicine with an unqualified statement of support; the call to "uncover the treasure-house and raise its standards" clearly indicated this while simultaneously containing a program for the future, namely, a combination of the positive elements of Western and Chinese medicine with the establishment, along Marxist lines, of a "new medicine."

9.3.1. The Combination of Western and Chinese Medicine and the Emergence of a New Therapy

At first, the desired synthesis of Western and Chinese medicine appears to have consisted solely of various gradual attempts to integrate traditional drugs and techniques into the theoretical framework of modern natural sciences. Such investigations from the 1950s to the present are directed primarily to an explanation of acupuncture as well as a pharmacological analysis of active ingredients in the traditional materia medica. Only since the beginning of the 1970s, as a result of the rejection of "bourgeois" and Western influences compelled by the Shanghai faction, are there publications that redefine theory and practice of Chinese medicine from a Marxist-Maoist viewpoint, introducing a "new medicine" freed of the bourgeois "metaphysical" values of Western medicine.

Such articles and books apparently first stressed the contribution of Chinese medicine to the new therapy, but already this involved an "uncovered" core, increasingly removed qualitatively from the substance of its earlier basis in systematic correspondence. Accordingly, the doctrines of yinyang and the Five Phases experienced a reassessment:

The [doctrines underlying] the theory of Chinese medicine—yinyang and the Five Phases—represent a kind of original materialism and spontaneous dialectic. They are an expression of opposition to the religious and superstitious doctrine of the existence of spirits; they incorporate the understanding that the world is composed of matter; they include the knowledge that all things are related to one another and that in all things the two forces yin and yang are present in mutual dependence and mutual conflict. By adopting such perspectives to provide information about the prevention and treatment of illnesses, Chinese medicine has—over the course of history—been of enormous benefit for the development of our native medicine. This fact must be acknowledged. Chairman Mao teaches us: "The dialectic of antiquity, however, possesses a spontaneous, primitive character; in accordance with the social and historical conditions of the time, it could not yet assume the form of a complete theory and was unable to provide a comprehensive interpretation of the world." The same is true for the doctrines of yinyang and the Five Phases. They constitute but one comprehensive explanation arising from a general mode of perception of the diverse contradictions within the human body, but not, however, a concrete and exact overview that would result from a scientific analysis of even the most minute details. Thus there exists between the doctrines of yinyang and Five Phases, on the one hand, and the dialectical materialism of present-day science, on the other hand, a distinction that is fraught with contradictions, and we must deal with these doctrines from the perspective of "dividing one into two." This is especially true for the doctrine of the Five Phases. Although it acknowledges the reciprocal relationships existing between all inner elements of the body and the entire external world, the limitations of the historical situation [in which it was conceived] have prevented it from adequately portraying the true character of these relationships. The conclusions and deductions derived from the Five Phases that result in the formation of associative categories, the mechanical conclusions produced [by this doctrine even in] complex situations, as well as the subjective guessing games [associated with this doctrine] inevitably lead [those who utilize it] to sink into idealism and metaphysics.

We must therefore strive to comprehend the original significance of the doctrines of yinyang and the Five Phases and develop it critically from the perspective of dialectical and historical materialism, in order to uncover the medical treasure-house of our homeland even better.[55]

Not only were the primary theories of traditional medicine reevaluated during the rule of the extreme leftist Shanghai faction; the entire development of healing was viewed in the context of what was now propagated as a central aspect of imperial Chinese history, namely, the purported 2,000-year struggle between the (evil) Confucians and the (good) Legalists. The latter, it was now proclaimed, had continually striven for a "progressive and materialist" medicine, while the former, because of their social interests, had always endeavored to suppress such efforts. Such a facile interpretation, which virtually ignores the diversity of conceptual systems in Chinese medical history, was possible in part only through the gross manipulation of available source material, a procedure demonstrated by a document published in 1974 in the Shanghai journal *Dialectic of Nature* (*Tzu-jan pien-cheng-fa*). The complete text is included in the appendix of this volume as a particularly striking example of questionable historical writing.[56]

After such arguments had largely removed from traditional therapy its conceptual basis in systematic correspondence and in the formerly so obvious link to the prevailing world view of imperial China, a changed legitimation manifested itself in the emphasis on those precepts of Chinese medicine that corresponded to Marxist-Maoist values and were foreign to Western medicine. Several examples will illustrate this process.

One of the central features of the "New Medicine" became the activation of the patient and his internal bodily defense mechanisms. Mao Tse-tung had written:

> Dialectical materialism . . . holds that external causes are the condition of change and internal causes are the basis of change, and that external causes become operative through internal causes. In a suitable temperature an egg changes into a chicken, but no temperature can change a stone into a chicken, because each has a different basis.[57]

On the basis of this insight, it was now necessary for practitioners to consider the internal causes of illness and healing as the "basis" of the transformation from well-being to sickness and from sickness to well-being again, and to view external pathogenic agents that penetrate the body as well as therapies applied from outside as the "essential conditions" for this metamorphosis, which produce their specific effects only by means of the "basis." The etiology familiar from classical literature, in which irregularities among the vital "correct" influences (*cheng-ch'i*) enable "evil" influences to penetrate from outside, could be integrated with little difficulty into the dialectical perspective:

The course of illness in the human body is in reality a two-sided struggle between the forces opposing illness, that is, the correct influences, the internal causes, on the one hand, and the elements that bring forth illness, namely, the evil influences, the external causes, on the other hand. The treatment of illnesses is nothing more than a struggle, in which drugs and similar therapeutic measures—as external agents—are employed to assist the organism itself—as internal agent—to overcome disease, resolve the contradiction, and restore well-being. Thus clinical work requires complete concentration on the inner causes, a recognition of the countereffects of this so-called soul, the full activation of the body's own potential energy, and the precise arrangement of the dialectical relationships between correct and evil [influences].[58]

Virtually no other therapeutic technique fulfilled these requirements—namely, the application of a purely external stimulus for transformations that were to occur within the organism—as did acupuncture. This is particularly evident in the so-called acupuncture anesthesia which, unlike the medicinal narcosis of the West, neither rendered the patient passive through sleep nor introduced any foreign substances into the organism that produced the pain-killing effect. This view was expressed by the author of an essay that appeared, in 1974, under the title "Dialectics in Acupuncture Anesthesia":

The most important characteristic of acupuncture anesthesia is that it transforms the functional potentiality of all body regions into actual energy and activity, that it stimulates personal desire in the struggle of the victim with his illness, and that it arouses the body's own defensive elements against disease and pain. . . . Acupuncture anesthesia grew out of the struggle with the metaphysical doctrines of external cause and passivity. The creation of acupuncture anesthesia does not, of course, signify the end of medicamentous anesthesia, which will continue to be refined. Our efforts must be directed against the metaphysical world view and methodology, which hinder the progressive development of anesthesiology; we have no quarrel with medicinal anesthesia as such. Acupuncture anesthesia and medicinal anesthesia should complement and refine each other. But we should also bear in mind that the birth of acupuncture anesthesiology represents a tremendous victory for dialectical materialism over the doctrine of external cause and the doctrine of passivity that will exert a fundamental influence on the further development of anesthesiology.[59]

In addition to the call for the patient's personal responsibility for his own cure and the emphasis on internal causes for illness and healing, the "New Medicine" is to be characterized by a holistic approach as well, which some authors found lacking in Western medicine:

It should be acknowledged that the current state of knowledge concerning anatomy, physiology, and biochemistry, compared with what was known in antiquity about the human body, is much more detailed and complete. We should take full advantage of these discoveries. But the circumstances here are the same as those once described by Engels: "Although in the first half of the eighteenth century the level of scientific knowledge and material production was far superior to that prevailing during Greek antiquity, our theoretical control of these materials and the general comprehension of nature were not equal to the Greeks" (*Nature-Dialectic*). We must therefore also direct our attention to the influence that bourgeois metaphysics has exerted on modern medical thought. As a result of isolated research devoted to individual organs, investigations based on the physiological changes and illnesses in the entire body have all too often been ignored and, instead, a relatively large value has been placed on research into locally restricted pathogenic sources. The cellular-pathological concepts of Virchow are an example of this approach.[60]

To correct these deficiencies of Western medicine, practitioners of the "New Medicine" were to orient themselves on the following saying of Mao Tse-tung: "When a Marxist confronts a problem, he must not view only part of it, but consider it in its entirety."[61] Applied to the diagnosis and therapy of medical problems, the following considerations are involved:

The parts and the whole together form a relationship, in which they oppose one another, but yet at the same time constitute a homogeneous entity. If there are no parts, there is also no whole, if there is no whole, there are also no parts. In therapy it is not permissible to concentrate solely on the partial factor of pathological changes, losing sight of the whole in the process, such as in the case of headache to treat only the head, or in the case of foot pains to treat only the foot. Similarly, one cannot view only the whole and ignore the partial factor of pathological changes, by carrying out a general course of treatment of the entire body while neglecting, at the same time, the individual elements of the nidus. The correct approach is as follows: Proceed from a consideration of the whole; concentrate not only on the parts, but put an even greater emphasis on the entire situation, combining both aspects dialectically. In this manner, a treatment of the parts can be implemented that will also influence the entire body; moreover, a treatment of the entire body can be carried out in such a manner that will, at the same time, affect the parts.[62]

Traditional Chinese conceptions of the mutual relationships and interactions in the body between the "depots" and "palaces," between "outer" and "inner," and between "depots" and "officials" were easily integrated with notions of the dialectical connections between the parts of the body and the whole. Traditional belief in, for example, the mutual bringing forth of the five depots permitted a therapy that not only focused specifically on the affected organ but also took into consideration its position within the nexus of the entire body:

> When one of the depots is afflicted with a condition of deficiency and weakness, one can, in addition to replenishing and strengthening the affected storage facility directly, proceed from the perspective of the entire body, replenishing and nourishing a closely associated depot, namely the mother-depot. Such treatments are known as "For deficiencies, replenish the mother." When, for example, the treatment of a victim of tuberculosis has continued for a long period of time without success, additional therapy can be based [on the fact] that a restoration of the spleen fortifies the lungs. This is the procedure of creating metal by turning over soil; a relatively high rate of success is possible.[63]

An additional Marxist-Maoist value that found its way into "New Medicine" is the importance of experience, "practice," as the source of all knowledge. Mao Tse-tung had expressed this clearly in his well-known 1937 essay "On Practice":

> Knowledge begins with experience—this is the materialism of the theory of knowledge.[64] Knowledge begins with practice, and theoretical knowledge is acquired through practice and must then return to practice.[65]

These are precisely the conditions fulfilled by traditional drug therapy, according to those of its present-day apologists who have largely rejected the doctrines of yinyang and the Five Phases. One of these proponents is Chiao Shu-te, whose book *Yung-yao hsin-te shih-chiang* (Ten Lessons on My Experiences with the Use of Drugs) first appeared in 1977 (second edition 1978). The lessons had originally appeared in the *Journal for Barefoot Physicians* (*Ch'ih-chiao i-sheng tsa-chih*) before the author, "in response to the requests of numerous readers," revised and collected the material in one volume.[66] Chiao Shu-te does not refer to the Five Phases, and yinyang terminology is used only for the traditional designation of certain organic structures in the body; "practice" and "experience" are the sole criteria for the legitimacy of the old drug therapy in modern times. This is also true for prescriptions composed of several drugs, whose collective properties cannot be explained by Western pharmacology:

The men of earlier times went through a long period of medical practice, in which they continually collected experiences in the struggle against illnesses. Gradually, they discovered that when several individual drugs are combined systematically and applied medicinally, the specific virtues of the drug masses are concentrated, the combination of these drugs producing new effective properties that release new forces, improving the rate of success; they also learned that such a systematic combination enables the specific merits of individual drugs to develop even more effectively, and that in this way certain deficiencies or even harmful properties can be corrected, and that [certain ingredients] can be added to or removed from systematically prepared prescriptions, in accordance with the specific symptoms, that is, flexible changes, thereby enormously extending the areas of application. As a result, these men gradually began to use drugs systematically in prescriptions, accumulating in a long-term process a wealth of possible procedures and valuable experiences. It can therefore be stated that the creation of medicinal preparations for the use of drugs was a tremendous achievement and represented a great step forward.[67]

I know of no other source in which an author has so systematically attempted to erase traces of the past from drug therapy and replace them with a Marxist-Maoist orientation.

Of central importance for an understanding of compound prescriptions is the concept of "differential diagnostic therapy" (*pien-cheng lun chih*). This approach necessitates the careful and individual composition of each prescription in daily practice, in order to deal effectively with all differences from patient to patient and in the specific course of each illness. It is no coincidence that the old term *pien-cheng* ("diagnosis") was employed here, for phonetically, substantively, and orthographically it is closely related to the Chinese term for "dialectic" (*pien-cheng fa*). The attempt to modify terminology is characteristic of Chiao Shu-te's efforts. The Chinese term for the concept "drug masses" cited in the passage above—*ch'ün-yao*—is reminiscent of *ch'ün-chung,* a character combination used by the Chinese communists to designate the "folk masses." A similar intention is apparent behind the use of the term *p'ei-wu,* which in the past few years has replaced the previously customary combination *p'ei-ho* to signify the "combination" of drugs in a prescription. The character wu originated in military terminology, symbolizing a combat group of five. Today, the term is closely associated with the concepts "companion" and "comrade." In the theoretical-programmatical context of the passage cited above, Chiao Shu-te used the combination p'ei-wu; at another point in his work, in a more technical context, the term *p'ei-ho* is still found.

Perhaps the most significant terminological modification in Chiao Shu-te's work is to be found in a relabeling of the four classes of drugs in prescriptions as originally defined in the *Nei-ching*. The 2,000-year-old classic had differentiated among chün ("ruler"), ch'en ("minister"), tso ("assistant"), and shih ("emissary") in the drug hierarchy of a prescription; Chiao Shu-te eliminated the first two of these terms, which were too obviously tied to the old society, replacing chün with chu ("leader," as in *chu-hsi*—"chairman") and ch'en with fu ("helper"). Chiao Shu-te illustrated the meaning of "leading drugs" with a topical reference:

> Leading drugs are those [elements] in a prescription that are aimed directly at the illness or the cause of an illness, that are used in treating the primary symptoms, that resolve the main contradictions, and whose medicinal potency plays the greatest role.[68]

Chiao Shu-te's pharmaceutical handbook reads like a manifesto for collectivism and against individualism. The structure that the author desired for the combination of drugs mirrors that of the future socialist society sought by Mao Tse-tung for China. Chiao made no attempt to elucidate theoretically, either through systematic correspondence or modern biochemical concepts, how drugs function in the organism, an explanation that may not have been necessary in a work prepared for the readers of the *Journal for Barefoot Physicians*. The few available sources from the era of the Cultural Revolution (including the period of the "Gang of Four"), however, indicate an attempt, in accordance with the changed political circumstances, to provide traditional drug therapy in China with the third legitimation in its approximately 2,000-year history. Originally based on notions of magic and, then, motivated by the search of certain Taoists for the so-called herb of immortality, the development of Chinese drug therapy from the Han to the Sung continued to rest primarily on Taoist contributions, but it also relied on the completely pragmatic search for remedies by individuals who were not necessarily close to Taoism. During the Sung-Chin-Yüan period, the use of drugs was given additional legitimation by the development of the first Chinese pharmacology, that is, the doctrine of the properties of drugs in the body as explained by systematic correspondence. This process legitimized drug therapy to a certain extent for Confucian circles as well. The opposition of traditional practitioners and conservative groups to an integration of Chinese drug therapy with Western medicine by means of modern scientific analysis, as well as the concomitant inability of modern pharmacologists to explain the collective properties of compound prescriptions have gradually led, in recent years, to a new attempt at legitimation. The emphasis on the practical experience of the population with traditional drug therapy over the course of thousands of years and the adaptation of traditional pharmaceutical values and terminology to the sociostructural circumstances of the present should ensure the traditional pharmacy in socialist society of a chance for survival, as an equal partner with Western pharmacological therapy.

Although it initially appeared as though the traditional elements in "New Medicine" might assume a preeminent position, owing to their Marxist-Maoist reassessment, before scientific medicine, which seemed inseparably linked with its "bourgeois-metaphysical" theories, this advantage was, with the demise of the "Gang of Four" immediately neutralized. At first some publications appeared in which the authors strove for "New Medicine" with a marked emphasis on scientific therapy. An example of this tendency is a pamphlet by Tuan Chen-li, which was published by the People's Publishing House of Honan in 1978, entitled *How to Overcome Chronic Illnesses (Tsen-yang chansheng man-hsing chi-ping)*. In his deliberations, which read like an apologetical eulogy on science, the author cites only discoveries of scientific medicine, which he has elucidated on a dialectical basis. In addition, the author's interpretation of modern knowledge includes concepts taken from traditional medicine. Even in this context, however, the theories of yinyang and the Five Phases, based on concepts of systematic correspondence, were not mentioned. A revealing passage from Tuan Chen-li's pamphlet is included in the appendix to this volume. In the meantime, however, "New Medicine" is no longer a central goal of health care planning in the People's Republic of China.

9.4. THERAPEUTIC PLURALITY IN PRESENT-DAY CHINA

Chinese medicine of today is characterized by a plurality of concepts and practical approaches; thus, it mirrors the multiplicity of ideological tendencies in Chinese society itself. There is evidence indicating that the systems of demonological therapy and of Buddhist temple medicine, still flourishing outside of the People's Republic primarily among the Chinese populations of Hong Kong and Taiwan,[69] survive also on the mainland itself.[70] But even apart from these conceptual systems, the therapeutic spectrum in the People's Republic is diverse and by no means unified in its conceptual orientation. Scientific medicine continues to set the standard, expanding its significance in research, teaching, and practice, particularly since the fall of the "Gang of Four." At the other end of the spectrum is the by-no-means-homogeneous group advocating traditional Chinese medicine. One of its many unresolved issues is the degree of "modernization" that should be attempted in order to compete successfully with Western medicine. The debate concerning this problem is highly reminiscent of its beginnings in the twenties. Current publications reflect the old positions of extreme national conservatism which rejects and deems unnecessary all efforts toward modernization, of cautious reformism which seeks to maintain the unique nature of traditional Chinese medicine while at the same time advocating assimilation of valuable knowledge from modern science, and finally of radical reformism and internationalism which does not believe in the necessity to preserve the old and Chinese if a new idea or technique—wherever it may have originated—proves to be superior.[71]

The efforts of the past decade for a Marxist-Maoist legitimation of certain practices (i.e., acupuncture, application of drugs, and various other techniques) and the flight by some dogmatists forward into the so-called "New Medicine" may, in the long run, have provided more harm to the interests of traditional practitioners than benefit. The elimination of the original theoretical background of systematic correspondence threatened the existence of traditional Chinese medicine as a conceptually independent alternative, thereby contributing to a further, and potentially final, stagnation of this ancient knowledge. This trend, though, has been halted more recently (1980–1981) with the adoption, by the administration, of the policy of the "Three Roads." Under this policy both Western and so-called Chinese medicine are granted the freedom to exist or develop along their respective lines. A third "road" is seen in a conjunction of Western and Chinese medicine wherever this appears feasible. For the time being it seems as if the "New Medicine" demanded by the Marxist-Maoist thinkers of the seventies remains only an ideal which cannot be expanded into a realizable program of practice and research. Two tendencies are discernible in the actual practice of the structured coexistence of Western and traditional Chinese therapy, both of which do not correspond to the requirements of "New Medicine" for a genuine dialectical synthesis of contradictory healing systems. The first of these tendencies consists of the continuation of efforts, begun at the turn of the century, to analyze the effective properties of traditional Chinese therapeutic techniques and drugs with the aid of modern scientific concepts and research. Thus, there have been frequent attempts to explain acupuncture in terms of biochemical and biophysical concepts; modern pharmacological and pharmacobiological investigations of traditional drugs have produced significant results. In addition to this one-sidedly integrative trend of coexistence, there is a second, which can be termed cooperative, meaning that a therapeutic procedure combines Western and traditional techniques or drugs, without any common theoretical basis. Orthopedics and anesthesia are the most well-known areas where Western and traditional insights have been combined successfully in actual practice. The role of acupuncture in the control of pain during surgery, though, is seen more soberly today than in the seventies when so-called acupuncture anesthesia was actively promoted, on purely ideological grounds, in surgical interventions for which it was rather unsuited. The final text in the appendix to the present book reflects this latest tendency; the slogan "Seek truth from facts"[72] indicates a return to a more cautious assessment of the potential of traditional techniques in a modern medical context.

The presently discernible boundaries for the future development of healing in China encompass traditional medicine, which exists on the basis of both a traditional and a modified theoretical legitimation, modern medicine, which is supported on purely scientific grounds by some groups as well as, to a much lesser extent, on a dialectical basis by others, and, finally, the indicated approach of practical coexistence. Which of these perspectives in such a heterogeneous spectrum will eventually prevail, must ultimately depend, as in the past, on factors that lie outside of what are generally termed "purely technical criteria."

Appendix
Primary Texts in Translation

1. *Huang-ti nei-ching t'ai-su*
   (The Most Elementary [Aspects] from the Yellow
   Emperor's Scripture on Internal [Therapy])[1]
COMPILED: Second century B.C.–Seventh century A.D.
AUTHOR: Yang Shang-shan (seventh century) and other
   unknown authors of earlier centuries

1.1. Manifestations of Winds at the Eight Seasonal Turning Points
   (Pa-cheng feng-hou)[2]

The Yellow Emperor: I should now like to hear why it is that in certain
years everyone is struck by a similar illness.
   Shao-shih: This is the result of a manifestation [of the winds] of
the eight seasonal turning points.
   The Yellow Emperor: How is it possible to foresee such occurrences?
   Shao-shih: If one desires to anticipate such occurrences, [it is necessary to consider the following circumstances.] Each year, on the day
of the winter solstice, T'ai-i takes up his position in the chih-chih
palace. In response to his arrival there, the heavens send wind and
rain. If wind and rain blow from the south, it is a depletion-wind that
harms man with great destructive force. If [the wind and rain] arrive
at night, at a time when all of the people lie asleep, no injury shall
occur. In such a year scarcely anyone shall suffer from illness. If,
however, [the depletion-wind] arrives by day, when the populace sits
idle, everyone will be struck by the depletion-wind; great numbers of
people shall fall ill. The depletion-evil invades [the body], settling in
the bones, where it then remains. At the beginning of spring, a great

release of yang influences occurs; the pores open. If, on the first day of spring, the wind blows from the west, the populace is struck once again by depletion-wind. The two evils [namely, that from the winter solstice and the more recent one from the first day of spring] then meet, and the [proper] influences in the transportation channels are interrupted and driven out [by the evil influences].

When one has been exposed to these winds and rain and has been struck by both, this is called "encountering the harvest-time dew."

Whenever the [climate of a] year is harmonious and balanced, and destroyer-winds scarcely make an appearance, only a few people shall fall ill and die. If, however, a year is marked by the frequent evil influences of the destroyer-wind, and warm and cold are not in equilibrium, many people shall fall ill and die.

The Yellow Emperor: To what extent do the depletion-evil-winds cause injuries of a serious or slight nature? And how can this be predicted?

Shao-shih: On the first day of the new year T'ai-i resides in the palace t'ien-liu. If on this day a west wind without rain prevails, many shall die. If at daybreak on the first day of the new year a north wind is blowing, many shall die in the spring. If at daybreak on the first day of the new year a north wind is passing through, 30 percent of the people shall die. If at midday on the first day of the year a north wind prevails, many people will die in the summer. If at evening on the first day of the year a north wind prevails, many people shall die in the fall. If a north wind prevails the entire day, many will be taken ill and of these 60 percent will die.

If the wind on the first day of the year blows from the south, it carries the name "parched land." If it blows from the west it is called the "rattle of bleached bones." [As a result of these winds] misfortune strikes the empire and many people will die. If the wind on the first day of the year comes from the southeast, raises the roofs from houses, and blows pebbles [into the air], catastrophes will plague the entire empire. If on the first day of the new year winds blow through from the southeast, deaths will occur in the spring.

If on the first day of the year the weather is mild and warm and without wind, the grain [later in the year] will be inexpensive and the people shall remain well. If, however, the weather [on new year's day] is cold and windy, the grain will be costly and many will be taken ill.

In this manner it is possible to predict how the depletion-winds will harm man in a [particular] year.

If in the second month [on the day] ch'ou no wind rises, the populace will suffer greatly from illness of the heart and abdomen. If in the third month [on the day] *hsü* the weather is not warm, many people will [suffer] from cold-heat [illnesses]. If in the fourth month [on the day] *szu* the weather is not hot, many will suffer from jaundice. If in the tenth month [on the day] *shen* the weather is not cold, many will die suddenly.

All winds that we have spoken of here [are so powerful that they] can raise the roofs from houses, uproot trees, blow pebbles into the air, blow hair on the head upright, and open the pores.[3]

1.2. The Nine Palaces and the Eight Winds (Chiu-kung pa-feng)[4]

Beginning of autumn	Two	hsüan-wei
Autumn equinox	Seven	ts'ang-kuo
Beginning of winter	Six	hsin-lo
Summer solstice	Nine	shang-t'ien
chao-yao	Five	
Winter solstice	One	chih-chih
Beginning of summer	Four	yin-lo
Spring equinox	Three	ts'ang-men
Beginning of spring	Eight	t'ien-liu

It is customary for T'ai-i to occupy the *chih-chih* palace for 46 days, beginning on the day of the winter solstice. On the day following this he takes up residence for 46 days in the [palace] *t'ien-liu*. On the day following this he takes up residence for 46 days in the [palace] *ts'ang-men*. On the day following this he takes up residence for 45 days in the [palace] *yin-lo*. On the day following this he takes up residence for 46 days in the [palace] *shang-t'ien*. On the day following this he takes up residence for 46 days in the [palace] *hsüan-wei*. On the day following this he takes up residence for 46 days in the [palace] *ts'ang-kuo*. On the day following this he takes up residence for 45 days in the [palace] *hsin-lo*. On the following day he once again occupies the palace *chih-chih* and has thus visited [all] these palaces in turn.

Counting from the palace where he is staying at the time, [T'ai-i also] moves daily in the order one through nine [to the other palaces] and then returns finally to [palace] one. This process is continual and without end. When [a cycle] has reached its conclusion, it begins anew.

On the day T'ai-i advances, the heavens must respond with wind and rain. If on this day wind and rain should arise, it will be a year of good fortune. The people will live in peace and few will fall ill.

If [wind and rain] should precede [the day of advancement] a period of abundant rain [will ensue]. If [wind and rain] should follow [the day of advancement], [the subsequent time] will be marked by wide-spread droughts.

From the changes [in the weather] on the day T'ai-i dwells [in the palace of the] winter solstice, one can foretell [the future] of the ruler. From the changes on the day T'ai-i dwells in the [palace] of the spring equinox, one can foretell [the future] of the ministers. From the changes on the day T'ai-i dwells in the central palace, one can foretell [the future] of the officials. From the changes on the day T'ai-i dwells [in the palace of the] autumn equinox, one can foretell [the future] of the generals. From the changes on the day T'ai-i dwells [in the palace of the] summer solstice, one can foretell [the future] of the people. When we speak here of "changes" [this is what is meant:] If, on the days T'ai-i dwells in one of these five palaces, a strong wind blows over trees and raises pebbles into the air, the extent [of future destruction] can be predicted in accordance with the direction from which the [wind] is blowing in each case. Observe the direction from which the wind is coming, and use these [observations] as the basis for the prediction.

If [the wind] should be blowing from the region where [T'ai-i] is currently dwelling, it is a wind of abundance; it is responsible for the genesis, growth, and nourishment of all things. If the wind should blow from the opposite [direction] and from a great distance, this is a depletion-wind. This wind is harmful to men; it is responsible for killing and injury. The depletion-wind should be watched for with great alertness and avoided. The sages in ancient times avoided this evil and it could not harm them. That is the meaning.

When T'ai-i arrives in the central palace, be alert in the morning for the Eight Winds, so as to be able to foretell prosperity or misfortune.

The wind that blows from the south is called the "wind of great infirmity." It causes injury to man by settling inside in the heart and outside in the transportation channels. Its influences are responsible for the formation of heat.

The wind that blows from the southwest is called the "wind of conspiracy." It causes injury to man by settling inside in the spleen and outside in the muscles. Its influences are the source of infirmity.

The wind that blows from the west is called the "wind of harshness." It causes injury to man by settling inside in the lungs and outside in the skin. Its influences cause the body to dry out.

The wind that blows from the northwest is called the "wind of destruction." It causes injury to man by settling inside in the small intestines and outside in the hand-great-yin transportation channel. If the channel is interrupted, [its contents] are discharged. If the channel is blocked, [its contents] congeal and nothing can flow through. [In such cases] there is a tendency for sudden death.

The wind that blows from the north is called the "wind of great harshness." It causes injury to man by settling inside the kidneys and outside in the bones as well as in the muscles of the shoulder and back. Its influences are responsible for the formation of cold.

The wind that blows from the northeast is called the "wind of misfortune." It causes injury to man by settling inside in the large intestine and outside in the flanks beneath the bones in the armpit, as well as in the joints of the limbs.

The wind that blows from the east is called the "wind of the new-born." It causes injury to man by settling inside in the liver and outside in the joints. Its influences are responsible for the creation of body dampness.

The wind that blows from the southeast is called the "wind of infirmity." It causes injury to man by taking up position inside in the stomach and outside in the flesh. Its influences are responsible for the [formation of] weight on the body.

All eight of these winds come from regions of depletion and therefore are able to cause illnesses in men. When three depletions come together, the result is a violent illness followed by sudden death. If it happens that two abundances and one depletion are present, the victim falls ill with [bladder] dribble and hot and cold [fits]. If, contrary [to all guidelines], one lingers in rainy or damp regions, the result is a loss of strength.

The sages of ancient times avoided the evil wind as one would arrows or stones. If the three depletions are then present and one is [also] partly struck by evil wind, this is a blow from which one falls down, and which results in paralysis on one side.[5]

1.3. The Three Conditions of Depletion and the Three Conditions of Abundance (San-hsü san-shih)[6]

The Yellow Emperor asked Shao-shih: I have heard it said that cold and heat are somehow responsible for whether someone is struck by the eight winds of the four seasons. When it is cold the skin is taut and the pores are closed. When it is hot the skin is relaxed and the pores are open. Could it be that this enables the evil influences of the destroyer-wind to invade [the body]? Or must the depletion-evil of the eight seasonal turning points also be present before man suffers harm?

Shao-shih replied: This is not the case. Whether or not the evil influences of a destroyer-wind strike someone does not depend on the season [of the year]. The necessary conditions are as follows. When [the pores] are open, the [evil-wind-influences] penetrate deep [into the body], quickly reaching the extreme interior and causing a sudden and violent illness. When the [pores] are closed, the [evil-wind-influences] also penetrate [into the body], but they remain at the surface and cause only a gradual illness.

The Yellow Emperor: What if [someone is able to live] in harmony with cold and warmth [and adapt himself to the requirements of the changes in the temperature] so that his pores are not open and yet [this person] nonetheless suddenly falls ill—what is the cause?

Shao-shih: Emperor, are you then ignorant of the ways in which evil [influences invade the human body]? Even if a person conducts his life in an harmonious manner, it nonetheless depends on the time of the year whether or not his pores are open or closed [and his skin] is relaxed or taut.

The Yellow Emperor: Can you tell me more on this subject?

Shao-shih: Man stands in relationship to heaven and earth and responds to [the changes of] the sun and moon. Thus, when the moon is full, the waters of the sea are high in the west. At that time man's blood and his finest influences are pure and his muscles and flesh are present in all their abundance. The skin is clear and the hair firm. The burner-passage is bent[7] and dust and grime cling [to the body].[8] Even if one encounters a destroyer-wind at this time, it will only penetrate the surface and is unable to invade deep into [the body].

During the new moon, however, the waters of the sea are high in the east. At this time man suffers from a depletion of blood and influences; his defense-influences flow away and only the outer form remains. Muscles and flesh decline, the skin hangs loose, the pores are open, the hair loses its deep roots, the burner-passage is released, dust and grime fall [from the body]. If at this time one should encounter a destroyer-wind, it will penetrate deep into the body, causing a sudden and violent illness.

The Yellow Emperor: Which evil, then, is responsible when someone becomes violently ill or dies suddenly?

Shao-shih: When a person is afflicted by the three conditions of depletion [at the same time], he will die quickly and abruptly. When, however, someone is endowed by the three conditions of abundance, no evil can harm him.

The Yellow Emperor: I should very much like to know more of the three conditions of depletion.

Shao-shih: When a person is in the weak phase of the year, when the moon is declining and when [he] loses the harmony with the season and consequently is harmed by a destroyer-wind, this is what is called the three situations of depletion. Thus it is said that a medical man who discusses [illness] without understanding the three situations of depletion is a dilettante.

The Yellow Emperor: I should now like to hear something of the three conditions of abundance.

Shao-shih: When someone is in the flourishing phase of the year, when the moon is full and when [he] is able to exist in harmony with the season, even the evil influences of the destroyer-wind are unable to threaten him.

The Yellow Emperor: That was an enlightening discussion! The principles are bright and clear. I request that [a record of this knowledge] be preserved in the Golden Chests. It shall receive the title "The Three Conditions of Abundance." You, master, are the sole author.[9]

1.4. The Transmission of Evil (Hsieh-ch'uan)[10]

The Yellow Emperor asked Ch'i Po: In their origin all illnesses are called forth by wind and rain, cold and heat, coolness and dampness, as well as joy or anger. Immoderate joy and excessive anger damage the depots. Wind and rain harm the upper [part of the body]. Coolness and dampness harm the lower [region of the body]. . . .

Ch'i Po: Wind, rain, cold and heat are of themselves unable to cause harm to man when they encounter no depletion-evil [in the victim]. When someone is struck by a strong wind or heavy rain and does not fall ill, no depletion-evil was present [in this person]. By themselves, [the strong wind and heavy rain] cannot harm man. For this to occur [a situation must arise in which] a depletion-evil encounters a bodily depletion [and as a result] settles into the [physical] form.[11]

1.5. Longevity, Early Death, Firmness, and Softness
    (Shou yu kang jou)[12]

The Yellow Emperor asked Shao-shih: I have heard it said that the existence of man encompasses firmness and softness, weakness and strength, short and long duration, as well as yin and yang [regions]. I should like to discover in what relationship all this stands to the methods [of therapy].

Ch'i Po: In yin there is yang, in yang there is yin. When one is knowledgeable about yin and yang, he can apply needle treatments methodically. When the origins of illness have been comprehended, the application of needles can be carried out on the basis of the [proper] principles. Carefully assess the causes of the affliction and the correspondences to the four seasons. [The human body] consists of an inner region, comprising the five depots and the six palaces, and an outer region, containing tendons, bones and skin. Thus yin and yang [elements] are present in both inner and outer regions. In the inner region the five palaces belong to the yin and the six depots to the yang [sphere]. In the outer region, the tendons and bones belong to yin and the skin to yang. Therefore it is said that when the illness is located in the yin-in-yin [region], apply needles to the brook transportation [points] of the yin [channels]. If the illness is located in the yang-in-yang [region], apply needles to the confluence [points] of the yang [channels]. If the illness is located in the yin-in-yang [sphere], apply needles to the stream [points] of the yin [channels]. If the illness is located in the yang-in-yin [sphere], apply needles to the network channels. For these reasons it is also said: If the illness is located in the yang [sphere] it is called wind; if it is located in the yin [sphere] it is called rheumatism (*pi*). If yin and yang [regions] have been equally affected by illness, it is referred to as wind rheumatism (*feng-pi*). Illnesses that are manifest but do not cause pain, belong to the yang category. If illnesses are not manifest but cause pain, they belong to the yin category. If they are not manifest but cause pain, the yang [sphere] is healthy while the yin [region] has been damaged. In such cases, the yin [sphere] should be treated as quickly as possible, while the yang [sphere] is left alone. If [illnesses] are manifest and cause no pain, the yin [sphere] is healthy but the yang [sphere] has been damaged. [In such cases] treat the yang [sphere] as quickly as possible and leave the yin [sphere] alone. When the yin and yang [spheres] are agitated, when [an illness] is alternately manifest and not manifest, and when, in addition, heart discomfort occurs, it is said that the yin [sphere] is more severely [afflicted] than the yang [sphere]. This signifies that neither the inner nor outer region alone has been affected by [a single illness]. [Such illnesses] do not remain manifest for long.[13]

1.6. Natural [Phenomena] That Must Be Avoided (T'ien-chi)[14]

The Yellow Emperor asked the following question: The application of needles must be based on the proper guidelines and the appropriate

proportions. I [should now like to learn] which guidelines and proportions [are to be taken into consideration].

Ch'i Po: [Heed] the laws of the heavens and the proportions of the
earth and act only in harmony with the celestial bodies.

The Emperor: This I would like to hear at once!

Ch'i Po: The laws of applying all needles require that one observe
the influences of sun, moon, and stars, as well as the four seasons
and eight seasonal turning points. If [in this manner] one has determined the [condition of] the influences, the needle treatment may be
carried out.

When the heavens are warm and the sun is shining, the blood of
man is pliant and the defense-influences flow easily [through the surface of the body]. Thus the blood flows easily and the influences can
move easily away. If, however, the heavens are cold and the sun is
dark, the blood clots and the defense-influences sink deep [into the
body].

During the new moon the blood and influences are at first pure and
the defense-influences begin their flow. During the full moon, then,
blood and influences are present in abundance; muscles and flesh are
firm. As the moon wanes, muscles and flesh wither; a condition of
depletion seizes the transportation channels, the defense-influences
withdraw and only the outer form remains.

[Needle therapy] should therefore be conducted in accordance with
[the conditions of the] heavens and [the specific characteristics of the]
season.

Thus, when the heavens are cold, needle treatment should not be
carried out; but if the heavens are warm, do not hesitate. During the
new moon [blood and influences] cannot be discharged; during the
full moon [blood and influences] cannot be replenished; during the
waning moon, attempts to regulate are futile.

Let yourself be guided by the orderly progression [of the phenom-
ena] of the heavens, as well as the times of abundance and of depletion,
and determine the point of the needle application in accordance with
the change of light [of sun and moon]. Attend [the specific problem]
in the proper frame of mind.

This is why it is said: when draining during the new moon, depletion
in the depots will ensue. When replenishing during the full moon, this
will cause a violent discharge of blood and influences and total stagnation [of the circulation] in the transportation channels. [This con-
dition] carries the designation "double-abundance." When attempts
to regulate are carried out during the waning moon, confusion in the
transportation channels will occur. The yin and yang [influences] be-

come disordered; proper [influences] and evil [influences] are no longer separated. [The proper defense-influences and the evil-influences] invade deeply [into the body] and settle there. When then a depletion arises in the outer region [of the body] and confusion reigns in the inner [region], evil [influences] are able to reach the surface and rebel.

The Emperor: In what manner, then, is the observation of the stars and eight seasonal turning points carried out?

Ch'i Po: On the basis of the stars one determines the course of sun and moon. On the basis of the eight seasonal turning points one can observe at what time the depletion-evil-[influences] of the eight winds arrive. On the basis of the four seasons it is possible to distinguish whether the influences of spring, autumn, winter, and summer are present.

In order to establish harmony among the influences, the season should serve as the guide. [In this manner] one avoids the depletion-evil-[influences] of the eight seasonal turning points and escapes their assault.

If [during a situation in which] depletion prevails in the body, there is an encounter with a depletion-[influence] of heaven and thus two depletions come into contact, the [evil] influences are able to penetrate to the bones. They invade [the body] and injure the five depots. The medical practitioner observes [the conditions of the heavens and state of the body] and shields [the latter from such situations,] so that no harm can befall the body.

Therefore it is said that it is of utmost necessity to know which [phenomena of nature] must be guarded against.

The Emperor: Very well![15]

1.7. Various Statements on Winds (Chu-feng tsa lun)[16]

The Yellow Emperor: Master, you have said that the evil influences of the destroyer-wind can injure man and in this way cause illness. But there are [people] who do not leave the protection of their homes, who remain well inside and yet quite suddenly are taken ill. Does this not signify that it is incorrect that one must encounter directly the evil influences of the destroyer-wind [in order to become ill]? What, then, is the cause of such [illnesses]?

Ch'i Po: In all these cases an earlier injury caused by the influences of dampness had occurred. These [influences] are stored in the blood channels and in the flesh beneath the skin. They remain there for a long period of time and do not move. [It is also possible, however,] that someone falls down, so that as a result evil blood is present inside the body. The [victim] then tends to display immoderate anger. He no longer eats and drinks in accord with necessity. Whether he wears warm or cool [clothing] no longer corresponds to the seasons. The pores are closed and impenetrable. When they open and encounter wind and cold, the blood and influences are blocked and clump together. The old evils [already in the body] now collide with [these wind- and cold-influences]. The result is cold-rheumatism.

When the [victim, to mention another possibility,] becomes overly warm, he breaks out in a sweat. When sweat breaks out, [the pores open and] permit wind to enter. Therefore, although [such people] do not come into contact with the evil influences of the destroyer-wind, some [earlier] cause must of necessity be present, to which something is added so that [an illness] breaks out.

The Yellow Emperor: What you, master, have brought forth [as causes of illness] are all things of which the victims themselves are aware. But when a person [is certain that he] neither has encountered evil influences nor possesses a fearful or shy disposition, and despite this is quite suddenly taken ill, what is the explanation? [In such a case] is it not solely a matter of demons and spirits?

Ch'i Po: This, too, has its cause. It is due to the fact that an evil remained [long latent in the body], and has not yet manifested itself [as an illness]. When it happens that the senses harbor an aversion to something, or that someone dreams and yearns for something [without such desires being fulfilled], blood and influences within the body become agitated. Both influences [that is, the latent ones of old evil already present and the new ones of unfulfilled emotions] mingle together [and give rise to the illness in question]. The origin of such an [illness] is subtle and can be neither recognized by observation nor perceived by listening. It thus has the appearance of being related to demons and spirits.

The Yellow Emperor: When, in such [cases], exorcism is performed and in this manner a cure is achieved, what is then the explanation?

Ch'i Po: The *wu*-[shamans] of earlier times possessed a knowledge of how one could be overcome by numerous illnesses. Since they knew in advance what the source of an illness was, it was sufficient to perform an exorcism [and in this way know how to achieve the cure].[17]

The Emperor: Very well![18]

1.8. On All Types of Wind (Chu-feng shu-lei)[19]

The Yellow Emperor asked Ch'i Po: When the wind has harmed someone, it causes in some cases cold and heat, or brings about an overheating in the [body's] center, or causes a cold in the center, or causes leprosy, or brings about an unbalanced drying out, or causes destroyer-wind. These illnesses are in each case different and [for this reason] carry different names. In some cases [the wind] penetrates deep into the body, to the five depots or the six palaces. The cause [for this diversity of the effects of wind on men] is unknown to me. I should therefore like to hear your explanations on this subject.

Ch'i Po: When wind-influence is stored in the skin, it is unable to penetrate into the inner region [of the body] or to escape outside. The wind loves movement and makes its appearance in numerous variations. When the pores are open [wind enters and causes sensations] of shivering and cold; [the pores] then close. When the pores are closed, [a feeling of] heat and oppression arises. [This] cold [in the body] causes the muscles and flesh to disintegrate. As a result, the [victim] suffers from mental distress and is no longer able to eat. [This condition] is called "cold and heat."

When the wind-influences enter the stomach by means of the yang [transportation channels], follow the [stomach] channels, and reach up into the inner corners of the eyes, and if the [victim] is well nourished, they are unable to exit the body. Consequently, they produce heat in the center and jaundice of the eyes. But if, in contrast, the [victim] is haggard, [the wind-influences] flow out of the body and [a sensation of] cold arises. This, in turn, gives rise to a cold in the center and causes tears to flow [from the eyes].

When the wind-influences enter through the great-yang-[transportation channels] they travel to all channel-transportation [holes] and are dispersed in the area between the intermediate [-flesh][20] and the pores. The evil of the throughway-influences collides with the defense-influences.[21] Their passage is thus blocked. The resulting [congestion] causes the muscles and flesh to swell and to be damaged. The defense-influences are blocked and remain stationary. Thus the affected flesh grows numb.

Leprosy means that the formative-influences are overheated and decayed. The influences are not pure. Thus, they cause the disintegration of the nasal bone and the destruction of [skin] color. The skin suffers injury and fluid is discharged. Wind-cold establishes itself in the transportation channels and does not move. The name for this condition is leprosy-wind. It is sometimes also called cold and heat.

If someone is injured by wind in spring [on the day] chia-i, the result is a liver-wind. If someone is injured by wind in summer [on the day] ping-ting, this causes a heart-wind. If someone is struck by evil at the end of summer [on the day] wu-i, this causes a spleen-wind.

If someone is struck by evil in autumn [on the day] *keng-hsin*, this causes a lung-wind. If someone is struck by evil in winter [on the day] *jen-kuei*, this causes a kidney-wind.

If wind-influence strikes the transportation [holes] of the five depots and six palaces, this also causes winds of the depots and palaces. [The wind-influence] enters in each case through a specific gate, and thus a one-sided wind arises.

When wind-influence rises into the wind-palace by following the transportation channel, the result is brain-wind.

When wind enters the connection in the head, the result is eye-wind.

When a person is cold while sleeping, if he has drunk and is then struck by wind, draining-wind ensues.

When a person sweats during sexual intercourse and [in this situation] is struck by wind, the result is head-wind.

When wind [remains in the skin] for a long period of time [and then finally] penetrates into the center, intestine-wind ensues and foods are discharged.

When wind remains in the pores, the result is discharge-wind.

Consequently, the wind is responsible for hundreds of different illnesses. Each time it changes, it causes different illnesses. There is no direction from which it blows at all times. Yet [in every case the illness is due] to the presence of wind-influences.[22]

1.9. On the Numerous Manifestations of Wind
   (Chu-feng chuang-lei)[23]

The Yellow Emperor asked Ch'i Po: I should now like to hear how [in all] these [cases] one can diagnose [the cause on the basis of the symptoms] and how each of the illnesses manifests itself.

Ch'i Po: The manifestations of lung-wind [are as follows]: profuse sweating; an aversion to wind; whitish skin color; occasional coughing; shortness of breath; during the day [the illness] is absent; at night [the illness] is acute.[24] The diagnosis is made from the whitish color above the eyebrows.[25]

The manifestations of heart-wind [are as follows]: profuse sweating; an aversion to wind; congestion to warmth; angry temperament; reddish coloring; inability to remain cheerful during great pain. The diagnosis is made from the reddish color of the mouth.

The manifestations of liver-wind [are as follows]: profuse sweating; an aversion to wind; a tendency to grieve; pale-green coloring; dry throat; angry temperament; occasional aversion to women. The diagnosis is made from the greenish coloring below the eyes.

The manifestations of spleen-wind [are as follows]: profuse sweating; an aversion to wind; sluggishness of the body; immobility of the four limbs; light yellowish coloring; lack of desire for food. The diagnosis is made from the yellowish color above the nose.

The manifestations of kidney-wind [are as follows]: profuse sweating; an aversion to wind; puffiness of the face; pain in the back and hips, inability to stand erect; ashen coloring; the hidden sprouts are without discharge.[26] The diagnosis is made from the blackish coloring above the chin.

The manifestations of stomach-wind [are as follows]: profuse sweating on the back of the neck; an aversion to wind; food and drink are unable to reach the lower region [of the body]; the pot[27] is closed and the abdomen exhibits fullness; if the clothing is loosened, [the abdomen] swells up. When cold foods are consumed, [they] are discharged [undigested]. The diagnosis is made from the emaciated condition and swollen abdomen.

The manifestations of head-wind [are as follows]: profuse sweating on the head and in the face; an aversion to wind. One day before the wind appears, the illness is violent; the headache is so severe that the victim desires to be neither outside nor in the house. Then on the day that the wind appears, the illness is minor and [appears] cured.

The manifestations of draining-wind [are as follows]: the victim sweats profusely, yet is unable to [wear] light clothing for any lengthy period of time; after eating he begins to sweat. In violent cases the [entire] body sweats. The victim breathes [heavily] and has an aversion to wind. The clothing is soaked through and the mouth is dry. The victim is thirsty and unable to carry out any strenuous task.

The manifestations of discharge-wind [are as follows]: profuse sweating. The sweat appears [in such profusion] that it flows over the clothing. The mouth is dry; rises.[28] When this wind [is present], one is unable to carry out any strenuous task. There is pain throughout the body and the [body feels] cold.[29]

2. *Huang-ti nei-ching su-wen*
      (Pure Questions from the Yellow Emperor's Scripture
      of Internal [Therapy])
COMPILED: Second century B.C. to Eighth century A.D.
AUTHOR: Wang Ping (eighth century) and other unknown
      authors of earlier centuries

2.1. On the [Preservation of the] True [Influences Endowed by] Heaven in High Antiquity (Shang-ku t'ien chen lun)[30]

In the distant past lived the Yellow Emperor. When he was born his spirit [was already characterized by an] all-pervading magic force. When still an infant he could already speak. In his youth he demonstrated a keen perceptive faculty. When he reached maturity his character was marked by a deep earnestness. When he reached adulthood he ascended to heaven. He put the following questions to the Celestial Master and spoke: "I have heard that the men of our ancient past experienced spring and autumn for one hundred years with no impairment of their ability to move and act. Today, however, it is so that men must limit their movements and actions after only half of a century. Have the times themselves changed or have men, that this [longevity] has been lost?"

To this Ch'i Po replied: "The men of antiquity understood the *tao*. [They therefore strove to adapt their existence to] the rules of the yin and yang [duality] and to live in harmony with numerical calculations. Moderation determined the consumption of food and drink; they arose and slept in accordance with a consistent order. No one depleted his strength through unseemly behavior. The men of antiquity thus preserved both body and mind with their full powers and reached the full extent of life accorded by nature. Death occurred only after one hundred years. The men of today are totally different. They prepare their soup with wine, and unseemly conduct has become the rule. They intoxicate themselves with sexual intercourse, and in [satisfying their] carnal appetite, they deplete the essence [of their existence]. Through careless use they squander man's innate original influences. They are ignorant of how to carry a full [vessel without spilling the contents] and do not provide the spirit with proper care at the appropriate time. They strive mightily to give pleasure to the heart, yet they conduct their lives contrary to the goals of true happiness. When the men of today rise or go to sleep, it is not according to a consistent plan. Because of this they must restrict [their movements and actions] after only half of a century.

"Whenever the ancient sages instructed the people, they repeatedly emphasized that evil [influences, which penetrate the body when a] depletion [arises in the organism], and destroyer-wind can be resisted successfully if met in time. He who is serene and free of immoderate desires shall not lose the original influence; he who keeps watch over [his] essence and spirit, does he not fend off all illness? Wherever emotions are disciplined, desires are held in check; wherever the heart lives in peace, man knows no fears. [The men of antiquity who conducted their lives in accordance with such principles] could place burdens on the body and yet suffer no fatigue. Since the distribution of influences in their body conformed to the laws of nature, they could yield to their desires and still receive that for which they had yearned. For these men, [any] meals provided great pleasure, [any] clothing was a source of happiness, and their customs a cause to rejoice.[31] Those of a high and low station exchanged no empty flattery; of the people themselves it could be said that they lived in a state of original simplicity. There were therefore no excessive desires to exhaust the eyes, no wantonness to confound the heart. No one, whether he was uneducated or a scholar, whether an exemplary man or a good-for-nothing, had cause to fear anything. In this manner they demonstrated their harmony with the tao. That all were able to live for one hundred years, without having to restrict their movements and conduct, was because their potential (te) remained undiminished and was never threatened."

The Emperor spoke: "When people have grown old, they can no longer have children. Is this because their vital forces are exhausted? I ask myself whether it is related to the length of life allotted by nature."

Ch'i Po replied: "When a girl reaches the age of seven, her kidneys are filled with influences. The teeth are transformed and the hair grows longer. With two times seven years, the girl reaches sexual maturity. The controller vessel is now completely open, and the large throughway conduit is now full. The monthly affair commences to descend and [the girl] is now able to bear children. With three times seven years, influences in the kidneys have reached their [ideal] level, so that the wisdom teeth break through and the body grows to its maximum extent. With four times seven years, the muscles and bones have grown firm. The hair has achieved its full length; the body is firm and robust. With five times seven years, the functions of the yang-brilliance conduit start to diminish; the face begins to dry up, the hair to fall out. With six times seven years, the functions of all three yang conduits in the upper [section of the] body start to decline. The face has completely dried out, the hair turns white. With seven times seven years, the controller vessel is empty, and the large throughway vessel reduces its activity. Sexual potency is exhausted and the conduits in the lower body are now obstructed. The body starts to deteriorate and no children are born.

"When a boy reaches eight years of age, his kidneys are filled with influences. The hair grows and teeth are transformed. With two times eight years, the kidneys overflow with influences and he reaches sexual maturity. Essential influences flow out, and when yin and yang [influences] are united, a man can father children. With three times eight years, influences in the kidneys have reached [their ideal] level; muscles and bones are firm and powerful. The wisdom teeth break through and the body grows to its maximum extent. With four times eight years, muscles and bones are in full possession of all their powers; robustness and vigor mark sinew and flesh. With five times eight years, influences in the kidneys begin to decline, hair falls out and the teeth begin to decay. With six times eight years, yang influences in the upper body diminish to the point of complete exhaustion; the face dries out and the temples turn gray. With seven times eight years, influences in the liver decline; muscles can no longer move and sexual potency is exhausted. Essence is present only in minimal amounts, the kidneys' depot is weakened, and the body has reached a turning point. With eight times eight years, teeth and hair fall out. The kidneys regulate water and store essence from all five depots and six palaces. Whenever the five depots are filled to overflowing, [their influences] can be drained [through the kidneys. In old age] all five depots lack [influences]; muscles and bones deteriorate; sexual vitality is exhausted, so that the temples turn gray and the body grows heavy. A man no longer walks fully upright, and he can no longer father children."

The Emperor spoke: "But there are also people who are old in years, yet still have children. How is this possible?"

Ch'i Po replied: "These are the people whom nature has granted a longevity that surpasses the normal lifetime. Their influence vessels remain open and their kidneys contain influences in abundance. Thus, although such [people] are still able to have children, this does not change the fact that in men, at the age of eight times eight, and in women, at the age of seven times seven years, the essence they have received from heaven and earth is completely exhausted."

The Emperor spoke: "But he who lives in full accord with the *tao*, is he not able to have children at the age of one hundred years?"

Ch'i Po replied: "He who lives in accord with the *tao* is able to ward off old age and preserve his body with its complete faculties. Although his body has many years behind it, he nonetheless is still able to have children."

The Yellow Emperor spoke: "I have heard there were true men in antiquity. They controlled heaven and earth; all things associated with yin and yang lay in their hands. In both inhaling and exhaling, as well as in [the utilization of their] essential influences, they pursued only one objective—to protect their spirit [from harm]. Their muscles and flesh appeared never to undergo any changes. The length of their life paralleled the existence of heaven and earth; their time on earth knew no end, for they existed in tao. In the middle ages of antiquity came accomplished men. Their potential was unimpaired; they were completely devoted to tao. They lived in full accord with the yin and yang [components of the universe] and in harmony with the four seasons. They left the world and abandoned all customs. They accumulated essence and preserved their spirit in its entirety. They travelled between heaven and earth, seeing and hearing beyond the boundaries of the eight foreign regions. Through their conduct they increased their life span and achieved strength. Ultimately, they, too, attained the state of true men. Next, there were the sages. They lived in harmony with heaven and earth, following the principles of winds from all eight directions. Their needs and desires conformed to the customs of the times; their heart knew neither anger nor vexation. They had no desire to abandon this world, [unclear] yet when they undertook something, they did not wish to follow custom. Externally, they did not exhaust their bodies with any affairs; within, they were not plagued by any brooding. Quietness and contentness became a guiding principle; for them, success meant self-knowledge. For this reason, their bodies experienced no deterioration; essence and spirit remained undissipated. They, too, reached the age of one hundred years. Finally, there were the exemplary men of antiquity. Their [principles of conduct] stood in harmony with heaven and earth. They strove to resemble sun and moon symbolically. They distinguished [the courses of] the constellations, they followed [in their life-style the pattern of] yin and yang, and they differentiated between the four seasons. They hoped to follow the example of high antiquity and establish harmony with the tao. They, too, improved their destiny and achieved longevity."[32]

2.2. Comprehensive Treatise on the Regulation of the Spirit in Accord with the Four Seasons (Szu-ch'i t'iao-shen ta-lun)[33]

The three months of spring denote genesis and release. Heaven and earth are renewed in every respect; the ten thousand things blossom forth. [He who desires to order his life in accordance with this season] goes to bed at night and rises early. He moves through the house with powerful strides. His hair hangs freely down the back of his neck; he grants his body the serenity of true relaxation. In this manner he is able to cultivate his mind. To create, not kill; to give, not take away; to reward, but not punish; these are [the actions] in accord with the influences that [embrace men] in the spring, signaling the correct way to bring into existence [all things]. He who acts contrary to these [influences] shall harm his liver. Cold will form within him in summer, and very little remains to accompany him into the period of growth.

The three months of summer denote prosperity and abundance. Heaven and earth exchange their influences; the ten thousand things appear in all their splendor and ripeness. Man goes to bed at night and rises early. He does not avoid the sun and guards his mind from vexation. He strives for consummate radiance and causes his own influences to flow away, as if that which he loves lies outside of himself. These are the [actions] in accord with the influences that [embrace men] in the summer, signaling the correct way to stimulate the growth [of things]. He who acts contrary to these [influences] shall damage his heart. In autumn he shall suffer from fever, and little will remain to accompany him into the period of gathering. Severe illnesses will then occur at the winter solstice.

The three months of autumn denote harvesting and weighing [of crops]. The influences of heaven grow violent; influences of the earth turn clear. Man goes to bed early and rises early, together with the fowl. He must be watchful that the mind remains in a state of peace, so as to temper the law of autumn. Man should preserve his spirit and prevent any loss of influence; he must ensure that autumn influences are assimilated in correct proportions. Man no longer directs his mind to phenomena outside of himself, but seeks to clarify influences of the lungs. These are the [actions] in accord with the influences that [embrace men] in the autumn, signaling the correct way to facilitate the gathering [of things]. He who acts contrary to these [influences] shall harm his lungs. Nourishment shall flow away from him in winter, and little will remain to accompany him into the period of storing.

The three months of winter denote securing and storing. Water is frozen and the earth cracks open. Under no circumstances should yang [influences] now be thrown into agitation. Man goes to bed early and does not arise until late; he should wait [before rising] until the sun appears. His mind must remain subdued and imperceptible, as if man had already achieved complete self-knowledge. He avoids cold and seeks out warmth. Influences should not be permitted to flow out through the skin and thus be lost to the extreme. These are the [actions] in accord with the influences that [embrace men] in the winter, signaling the correct way to facilitate the storage [of things]. He who acts contrary to these [influences] shall harm his kidneys and suffer from impaired [virility] in the spring. Little will remain to accompany him into the period of restoration.

The influences of heaven are clear and pure, lustrous and radiant. But [heaven] stores its potential without interruption and does not permit [its light] to reach down. For if the heaven itself were to radiate light, the sun and the moon would be unable to shine. This would allow evil and harmful agents to occupy the gaps [left by the lack of influences from the sun and moon]. If this were to happen, the yang influences would be shut out [from reaching the earth], and the influences of the earth would be turbid [and unable to rise]. Clouds and fog [that is, influences of the earth] would no longer be pure and, consequently, dew [an influence of heaven] would not descend. All this would indicate that the exchange [of influences of heaven and earth] does not take place and that the existence of the ten thousand things would be cut off from the supply [of these influences]. An interruption in the supply [of influences], however, frequently leads to death, even among those plants renowned [for their longevity]. Harmful influences would not disperse, wind and rain would be unpredictable, white dew would not descend. More and more plants would die off and nothing would remain to blossom [in spring]. Destroyer-winds would strike often, frequently accompanied by sudden rainstorms. He who is unable [in such a situation] to maintain [the influences] of heaven and earth as well as the four seasons in a state of mutual accord, and loses his relationship to the *tao*, will perish even before he has concluded half [of the time allotted to him by nature]. Only sages are capable of countering even these [irregularities] with proper conduct. Consequently, they do not suffer from unusual illnesses, they do not lose [control over] anything, and their original influence, upon which their existence rests, does not expend itself.

If one acts contrary to the influences of spring, minor-yang [influences] do not arise, influences already in the liver wither.

If one acts contrary to the influences of summer, great-yang [influences] do not develop fully, and influences already in the heart are eroded.

If one acts contrary to the influences of autumn, great-yin [influences] are not accumulated, and influences already in the lungs burn up completely.

If one acts contrary to the influences of winter, minor-yin [influences] are not stored, and influences already in the kidneys withdraw into the depths.

This means, therefore, that the yin and yang influences [sent out by heaven and earth] during the four seasons constitute the fundament and source [of the existence] of all ten thousand things. The wise man thus will nourish himself in spring and summer with yang influences, but in the autumn and winter with yin influences, in accordance with his foundation. He therefore finds himself in complete harmony with the ebb and flow of all existence on the way of life and growth. He who acts contrary to his basic principles brings harm to his source and destroys his original [influences].

This means, then, that the yin and yang [influences] of the four seasons constitute the beginning and end of the ten thousand things and the source of life and death. If one acts contrary to these principles, catastrophes and harm will ensue. If one conducts his life in accordance with these influences, however, he shall avoid unusual illnesses. This is the significance of the motto: "to achieve the tao."

The sages practice the tao in their daily life, the uneducated turn their back to it. To live in harmony with yin and yang [influences] means life; to act contrary to them means death. To follow signifies order, contrary conduct means chaos. To oppose what is appropriate means contrary action, that is, inner opposition. This is the reason the sages do not treat those who have already fallen ill, but rather those who are not yet ill. They do not put [their state] in order when revolt [is underway], but before an insurrection occurs. This is what is meant. When medicinal therapy is initiated only after someone has fallen ill, when there is an attempt to restore order only after unrest has broken out, it is as though someone has waited to dig a well until he is already weak with thirst, or as if someone begins to forge a spear when the battle is already underway. Is this not too late?[34]

2.3. Comprehensive Treatise on the Phenomena Associated with the Categories of Yin and Yang (Yin yang ying-hsiang ta-lun)[35]

The Yellow Emperor spoke: [The two categories] yin and yang are the underlying principle of heaven and earth; they are the web that holds all ten thousand things secure; they are father and mother to all transformations and alterations; they are the source and beginning of all creating and all killing; they are the palace of spirit-brilliance.

In order to treat illnesses one must penetrate to their source.

Heaven arose out of the accumulation of yang [influences]; the earth arose out of the accumulation of yin [influences]. Yin is tranquility, yang is agitation; yang creates, yin stimulates development; yang kills, yin stores. Yang transforms influences, yin completes form.

When cold reaches its zenith, it creates heat; if heat reaches a zenith, it creates cold. The influences of cold produce turbidity; the influence of heat produces clarity. If clear influences descend in the [body], foods are discharged [undigested]; if turbid influences ascend in the [body], they cause abdominal swelling. Whenever yin and yang [influences] act in such complete contradiction [to their true nature, man] will suffer from this offense against what is proper.

Clear yang [influences] form heaven; turbid yin [influences] constitute earth. The influences of earth ascend and form into clouds; the influences of heaven descend and form rain. Since rain [develops from clouds], its ultimate origin is influences of the earth; since the [formation] of clouds [requires sunlight], their ultimate origin is the influences of heaven.

For this reason, the clear yang [influences] exit the body through the upper openings, while the turbid yin [influences] exit the body through the lower openings. Clear yang [influences] disperse through the skin, while turbid yin [influences] enter the five depots. The clear yang [influences] fill the four extremities, while the turbid yin [influences] enter the six palaces.

Water is yin; fire is yang. Yang [influences] appear as [volatile] influences; yin [influences] appear as [material] flavor. Flavor is dependent upon structure; structure has its origin in [volatile] influence; [volatile] influence arises from essence; essence arises from transformation. [Yet even] essence is nurtured by the transformation of [volatile] influences, and form is nurtured by [material] flavor. Essence arises through transformation; form develops from [volatile] influences. [Material] flavor can harm form; [volatile] influences can harm essence. Essence is transformed into [volatile] influences; thus [volatile] influences] can also be harmed by [material] flavor.

[Material] flavor belongs to the yin [category] and exits the body through the lower openings. [Volatile] influences belong to the yang [category] and exit the body through the upper openings. That which possesses a strongly developed flavor belongs to yin; that which has a weak flavor belongs to yang-in-yin. That which possesses strongly developed [volatile] influences, belongs to yang; that with weak influences, belongs to yin-in-yang. Strongly developed flavor produces discharge; weak flavor produces a drainage. Weak influences produce distribution; strongly developed influences lead to the production of heat.

The influences of a powerful fire weaken themselves; the influences of a small fire increase in strength. A powerful fire feeds on influences;

the influences feed on a small fire. A strong fire dissipates influences; a small fire stimulates the production of influences.

That possessing acrid and sweet [volatile] influences and [material] flavors and producing dissipation, belongs to yang. That which is sour and bitter and produces discharge or drainage belongs to yin. Whenever the yin component predominates [in the assimilation of influences and flavors], the result is a yang illness. Whenever the yang component predominates, the result is a yin illness. When there is an excess of yang, heat arises [in the body]; when there is an excess of yin, cold arises [in the body]. But violent cold develops into heat; a violent heat, in turn, engenders cold. Cold harms form; heat harms [inner] influences. If these [inner] influences have been injured, pain occurs; if form has been affected, swelling takes place. If pain appears first, followed by swelling, the injury to inner influences has affected form. If, however, swelling appears first, followed by pain, the injury to form has affected the inner influences.

Excessive wind causes motion; excessive heat results in swelling. Excessive drought causes aridity; excessive cold allows [yin influences in the body] to ascend; excessive humidity causes discharge.

In nature there are four seasons and five phases. The former bring about genesis, maturity, gathering, and storing. The latter engender cold, heat, drought, moisture, and wind. In man there are five depots, which transform the five influences, producing joy, anger, sadness, sorrow, and fear. Joy and anger can harm influences; cold and heat can damage form. Violent anger injures the yin [components in the organism]; excessive joy impairs the yang [components], causing influences to rise in the body instead of descend; the conduits are filled and their contents leave the body. If joy and anger are not held in moderation, if cold and heat exceed certain limits, life no longer exists on a solid foundation, for strongly developed yin must be transformed into yang; strongly developed yang must be transformed into yin.

Thus it is said: If a person is injured in winter by cold, he will suffer from warmth-illnesses in the spring. If he is injured by wind in the spring, diarrhea will occur in the summer. If he is injured in summer by heat, he will suffer from fever in the autumn. If he is injured in the autumn by humidity, he will cough and gasp in winter.[36]

2.4. Additional Treatise on the Five Depots (Wu-tsang pieh-lun)[37]

The Yellow Emperor asked the following question: "I have heard that some experts of [medical or magic] prescriptions consider the brain and the marrow to be depots and that some regard the intestines and stomach as depots, while still others believe them to be palaces. I should very much like to know how such contradictions could arise. I am not aware of the underlying principle here, and I am keenly interested in what you have to say on this matter."

Ch'i Po replied: "The brain, marrow, vessels, bones, gall, and womb are formed from influences [that man receives] from the earth. They store yin [influences] and correspond to the earth. Thus their function is to store and to prevent discharge. They are called 'extraordinary palaces.' The stomach, large intestine, small intestine, triple burner, and bladder are formed from influences [that man has received] from heaven. Their influences correspond to heaven. Thus their function is to discharge and not to store. They receive the turbid influences discharged by the five depots. They are called 'palaces that transmit and transform.' Similarly, the anus receives liquids and solids from the five depots but is unable to store them for long.

"The so-called five depots collect essential influences and do not permit them to disperse. It is therefore possible for them to be full but never too full. The six palaces transmit and transform things, but do not store them. It is therefore possible for them to have too much [to handle at one point in time] but never to be full. Consequently, liquid and solid foods enter into the stomach through the mouth and can produce a condition of repletion while the intestines are still empty. As the food continues to descend further in the body, repletion occurs in the intestines while the stomach is now empty. Thus it is said: repletion and yet not full; full and yet no repletion."

The Emperor spoke: "Why do the five depots alone determine [what is felt when the pulse is taken at] the [location designated] 'opening [through which the] influences [can be perceived]'?"

Ch'i Po replied: "The stomach is the sea in which liquid and solid foods collect; it is the great source that sustains the six palaces. The five [material] flavors enter through the mouth and are stored in the stomach, from where they then nourish the influences in the five depots. The [location called] 'opening [through which the] influences [can be perceived' also lies on the] great-*yin*-[transportation channel, which carries influences to the depots]. This means that all [volatile] influences and [material] flavors destined for the five depots and six palaces originate in the stomach and—following their transformation there—can be felt at the 'influence-opening.' The five [volatile] influences enter through the nose and are stored in the heart and lungs. When the heart and lungs are affected, the nose cannot function properly.

"In treating illnesses, one must examine all aspects visible to the eye; the vessels must be examined [for a depletion or repletion of influences] and the patient's emotions and attitudes as well as [the severity of] his illness must be taken into account. For someone who believes in demons and spirits it is useless to speak of the virtues of a moral life. For someone who opposes treatment with needles and stones it is futile to speak of utmost skills. Anyone who refuses to allow treatment of his illness must not, under any circumstances, be treated, for such an attempt would be a complete failure."[38]

2.5. Treatise on the Various Methods of Treatment That Correspond to the Four Cardinal Points (I-fa fang i lun)[39]

The Yellow Emperor asked the following question: "How is it possible that one and the same illness can be treated with different techniques, and yet in each case a cure is effected?"

Ch'i Po replied: "This is due to geographic circumstances. The regions in the East were the first to be created by heaven and earth. Here lies the land of fish and salt; ocean sands border the water. The people here eat fish and favor salty foods. They live peacefully in their villages and are content with their meals. Fish generate heat in the human body and salt displaces the blood. Thus these people all have a dark complexion and dried-out skin. Their illnesses can be regarded as sores for which stone treatments are the proper therapy. This means that stone therapy originated in the East.

"The West is the land of metals and precious stones, of sand and minerals. Here heaven and earth have bestowed great abundance. The people live in earthen huts; the winds are frequent; the water and the soil are hard and powerful. The people clothe themselves not in silk, but in fur and bast. Their diet is excellent and thus their nutritional health is good. For this reason, evil [influences] are unable to harm the bodies of these people [from outside]; their illnesses arise from within and require treatment with potent drugs. This means that potent drugs originate in the West.

"The North is the region where heaven and earth secure and store. The land there lies at a great elevation, and the people live in earthen huts. The winds blow cold; the land is occasionally covered by ice and snow. The inhabitants live contentedly in the wilderness, and milk forms the basis of their diet. Their illnesses result from the accumulation of cold in the depots; the appropriate therapy is the burning of moxa [on the skin]. This means that moxabustion originates in the North.

"The South is the region where heaven and earth bestow growth and nourishment, and where yang [influences] are present in abundance. The land lies low; water and soil are soft and weak. Fog and dew are frequent. The people favor sour substances, and their foods give off a strong odor. Thus they all have tightly sealed skin and a reddish complexion. They suffer from deformities and paralyses, for which the appropriate therapy is treatment with fine needles. This means that the nine needles originate in the South.

"The land in the center is flat and damp. Here heaven and earth have engendered all things. Accordingly, the diet of the people is diverse and easily obtained. Illnesses therefore frequently consist of weaknesses as well as cold and hot fits. The appropriate treatments for such afflictions are therapeutic exercises and massages. Thus therapeutic gymnastics and massages originate in the central regions.

"The ancient sages developed different therapeutic [procedures] for the treatment [of illnesses], so that each [region] had its corresponding [technique]. From the fact that disparate techniques are utilized and that all illnesses are cured, it is possible to achieve an understanding of the nature of illnesses and the entire complex of therapy."[40]

2.6.   Treatise on Changes in the [Assimilation of] Essence and on the Transformation of Influences (I ching pien ch'i lun)[41]

The Yellow Emperor asked the following question: "I have heard that in antiquity the treatment of illnesses consisted solely of changing the [assimilation of] essence and of transforming the influences [within the body]; one was capable of exorcising the cause [of suffering] [chu-yu] and in all cases a cure was effected. Today, however, the patient is treated internally with potent drugs and externally with needles and stones, and yet a cure is achieved only in some cases, while in others, treatment is a total failure. What is the reason for this?"

Ch'i Po replied: "The men in antiquity lived among their animals. They pursued a vigorous and active life, avoiding in this manner the effects of cold. They sought out the shade, thereby avoiding the effects of heat. Their inner life knew no exhaustion from emotions, and their external appearance was unaffected by the civil service bureaucracy. In that peaceful and satisfied world, evil [influences] were unable to penetrate deeply into the body. Potent drugs were therefore unsuited for treatment from within, and needles and stones were inappropriate for external therapy. Instead, it was possible to effect a cure through changes in the [assimilation of] finest matter and through an exorcism of the cause [of illness].

"Today, however, the situation has changed completely. Man's life is marked by suffering within and by the misery of his body without. The harmony between [human conduct] and the four seasons has been lost, and man acts contrary to the laws of cold and hot. Destroyer-wind frequently achieves its objective, and in the morning as well as in the evening those evil [influences that utilize] depletions penetrate into the five depots as well as into the bones and marrow, while simultaneously damaging the body openings, muscles, and skin from the outside. It is therefore inevitable that minor ailments develop into severe illnesses, and that severe illnesses eventually lead to death. Thus an exorcism of the cause is today no longer sufficient to cure illness."[42]

2.7. Treatise on the Secrets of Mr. Yü and on the True Depots (Yü-chi chen-tsang lun)[43] (excerpt)

Wind is responsible for many different illnesses. If, for example, wind-cold has penetrated the body, the first symptom is that the fine body hairs of the victim stand erect. The skin seals itself and heat arises. At this stage [wind-cold] can be expelled through sweating. Occasionally, paralysis, loss of feeling, swelling, and pain result. At this point [wind-cold] can still be eliminated with hot compresses, moxabustion, and needles. If no treatment is initiated, the illness penetrates deeper, establishing itself in the lung. It is then called "rheumatism of the lungs" [fei-pi].[44] [The symptoms are] coughing and upward expulsion of influences. If treatment is not begun at this stage, the lung transmits [wind-cold] further, allowing it to enter the liver. The illness is then called "rheumatism of the liver" [kan-pi], or "reversal" [chüeh].[45] Pain occurs in the sides and food cannot be retained. At this stage the appropriate therapy is massage and needles. If no treatment is undertaken, the liver conducts [the wind-cold] to the spleen. The illness is then called "spleen-wind." Jaundice occurs, and heat develops in the abdomen. The heart is distressed and one expels yellow matter. The appropriate treatments at this point are massages, drugs, and lavation. If no treatment is undertaken, the spleen conveys [the wind-cold] to the kidneys. The illness is then called "accumulation-affliction" [shan-chia]. Heat accumulates in the lower abdomen and is accompanied by pain. White matter is discharged. Another name for this illness is ku.[46] At this stage either massages or drugs can be administered. If treatment is not started, the kidneys transmit [the wind-cold] further into the heart. The victim now suffers from violent cramps of the muscles and vessels, and the illness is thus referred to as "twinge-affliction" [ch'e]. At this point moxa should be burned on the skin or drugs administered. If treatment is still not initiated, the victim will succumb after ten days.[47]

2.8. Treatise on Influences in the Depots as Patterned by [the Nor-
      mal Progression of] the Seasons (Tsang-ch'i fa-shih lun)[48]
      (excerpt)

The Yellow Emperor asked the following question: "If, during medical treatment, one desires to establish correspondences between the body of man, on the one hand, and the regular progression of the four seasons and five phases, on the other hand, how is it possible to act in accordance [with these principles] and what would be regarded as contrary conduct? I should very much like to learn what determines success and failure in this regard."

Ch'i Po replied: "The five phases are metal, wood, water, fire, and soil. They alternate in succession between a position of preeminence and one of insignificance. [This transformation] provides us with an understanding of life and death, an insight into creation and decay, as well as helping us to determine the influences in the five depots, the times during which [an illness] is minor or serious, and the ultimate prognosis for life and death."

The Emperor spoke: "I am eager to hear this!"

Ch'i Po replied: "The liver is ruled by spring. Treatment is carried out primarily over the ceasing-yin and minor-yang [conduits] of the feet. The [corresponding] day is *chia-i*. When the liver suffers from strain, something sweet must be consumed at once in order to relieve the tension.

"The heart is ruled by summer. Treatment is carried out primarily over the minor-yin and great-yang [conduits] of the hands. The [corresponding] day is *ping-ting*. When the heart grows sluggish, something sour must be consumed at once in order to restore composure.

"The spleen is ruled by late summer. Treatment is carried out primarily over the great-yin and yang-brilliance [conduits] of the feet. The [corresponding] day is *wu-ssu*. When the spleen suffers from excessive dampness, something bitter must be consumed at once in order to dry it out.

"The lung is ruled by autumn. Treatment is carried out primarily over the great-yin and yang-brilliance [conduits] of the hands. The [corresponding] day is *keng-hsin*. When the lungs suffer from ascending or retreating influences, something bitter must be consumed at once in order to divert these influences.

"The kidneys are ruled by winter. Treatment is carried out primarily over the minor-yin and great-yang [conduits] of the feet. The [corresponding] day is *jen-k'uei*. When the kidneys are dried out, something spicy must be consumed at once in order to restore moisture. In this way the skin is reopened, enabling bodily fluids and influences to flow freely again.

"Illnesses of the liver heal in summer. If a cure is not effected in summer, the condition worsens in autumn. If [the victim] does not succumb in autumn, the illness extends through the winter and recovery occurs in spring. The victim [of such a condition] must not be exposed to wind.

"Victims of a liver ailment recover by *ping-ting*. If the patient is not cured by this date, [the illness] worsens until *keng-hsin*. If [the victim] does not succumb at this time, [the illness] extends through *jen-k'uei* and the patient will rise from the sickbed on *chia-i*. Those suffering from liver ailments grow mentally alert during the day, reaching a high point in the late afternoon; they lie down to rest at midnight. To achieve a dispersing effect in the liver, it is necessary to consume something spicy at once. Spicy foods replenish [influences in the liver], sour foods discharge them.

"Illnesses of the heart heal in late summer. If a cure is not effected in late summer, the condition worsens in winter. If [the victim] does not succumb in winter, the illness extends through spring, and recovery occurs in summer. The victim [of such a condition] may not consume warm meals nor wear excessively warm clothing.

"Victims of a heart ailment recover by *wu-ssu*. If the patient is not cured by this date, the [illness] worsens until *jen-k'uei*. If [the victim] does not succumb at this time, [the illness] extends through *chia-i* and the patient will rise from the sickbed on *ping-ting*. Those suffering from heart ailments grow mentally alert at mid-day, reaching a high point at midnight; they find rest in the early morning. To calm the heart, it is necessary to consume something salty at once. Salty foods replenish [influences in the heart]; sweet foods discharge them.

"Illnesses of the spleen heal in autumn. If a cure is not effected in autumn, the condition worsens in spring. If [the victim] does not succumb in spring, the illness extends through the summer and recovery occurs in late summer. The victim [of such a condition] must not consume warm meals, eat until full, [sit down] on the damp earth, or wear wet clothing.

"Victims of a spleen ailment recover by *keng-hsin*. If the patient is not cured by this date, [the illness] worsens until *chia-i*. If [the victim] does not succumb at this time, [the illness] extends through *ping-ting*, and the patient will rise from the sickbed on *wu-ssu*. Those suffering from spleen ailments grow mentally alert at sunset, reaching a high point at sunrise; they find rest in the late afternoon. To relieve the strain in the spleen, it is necessary to consume something sweet at once. Bitter foods discharge [influences from the spleen]; sweet foods replenish them.

"Illnesses of the lung heal in winter. If a cure is not effected in winter, the condition worsens in summer. If [the victim] does not succumb in summer, the illness extends through late summer and recovery occurs in autumn. The victim of [such a condition] must not consume cold foods or drinks, nor wear cold clothing.

"Victims of a lung ailment recover by *jen-k'uei*. If the patient is not cured by this date, [the illness] worsens until *ping-ting*. If [the victim] does not succumb at this time, [the illness] continues through *wu-ssu*, and the patient will rise from the sickbed on *keng-hsin*. Those suffering from lung ailments grow mentally alert in the late afternoon, reaching a high point at midday; they lie down to rest at midnight. To produce a calming effect in the lungs it is necessary to consume something sour at once. Sour foods replenish [influences in the lungs]; spicy foods discharge them.

"Illnesses of the kidneys heal in spring. If a cure is not effected in spring, the condition worsens in late summer. If [the victim] does not succumb in late summer, the illness continues through autumn and recovery occurs in winter. The victim [of such a condition] must avoid hot, burning foods and warm clothing.

"Victims of a kidney ailment recover by *chia-i*. If the patient is not cured by this date, [the illness] worsens until *wu-ssu*. If [the victim] does not succumb at this time, [the illness] continues through *keng-hsin,* and the patient will rise from the sickbed on *jen-k'uei*. Those suffering from kidney ailments grow mentally alert at midnight, reaching a high point at [unclear]; they lie down to rest in the late afternoon. To fortify the kidneys it is necessary to consume something bitter at once. Bitter foods replenish [influences in the kidneys]; salty foods discharge them.[49]

"The color of the liver is virid; [to counteract the liver's susceptibility to cramps], sweet foods should be consumed. Late maturing rice, beef, dates, and *k'uei* vegetables are all sweet.

"The color of the heart is red; [to counteract the heart's susceptibility to sluggishness], sour foods should be consumed. Small beans, dog meat, plums, and chives are all sour.

"The color of the lung is white; [to counteract the lungs' susceptibility to ascending influences], bitter foods should be consumed. Wheat, lamb, almonds, and shallots are all bitter.

"The color of the spleen is yellow; [to counteract the spleen's susceptibility to indurations], salty food should be consumed. Large beans, pork, chestnuts, and the *huo* vegetable are all salty.

"The color of the kidneys is black; [to counteract the kidneys' susceptibility to drying out], spicy foods should be consumed. Yellow millet, chicken, peaches, and onions are spicy.

"Spicy foods disperse; sour foods concentrate; sweet foods relieve; bitter foods fortify; salty foods weaken. Potent drugs attack evil [influences]. The five kinds of grain provide nourishment. The five kinds of fruits provide support. [The flesh] of the five domesticated animals is necessary for well-being. The five kinds of vegetables constitute the conclusion [of the diet].

"He who harmonizes the assimilation of [volatile] influences and the flavors [of foods] within himself shall replenish his essence and maintain his [inner] influences."[50]

2.9. Blood and Influences, Body and Mind (Hsüeh ch'i hsing chih)[51] (excerpt)

If the body is healthy and the mind suffers, illnesses arise in the vessels. Moxa and needles are the proper treatment.

When both body and mind are healthy, illnesses arise in the flesh. Needles and stones are the proper treatment.

When the body suffers and the mind is healthy, illnesses arise in the muscles. Hot compresses and gymnastic exercises are the proper treatment.

When both the body and the mind suffer, illnesses arise in the throat. Drugs are the proper treatment.

If the body is affected repeatedly by terror and fear, the conduits are obstructed, and illnesses arise in the numbed areas. Massage and medicinal wines are the proper treatment.

These are the five [possible combinations of] body and mind.[52]

2.10. On Yao-Illnesses (Yao lun)[53]

The Yellow Emperor spoke: "All yao-illnesses are caused by wind. In addition, these [illnesses] break out only at certain times. Why is this so?"

Ch'i Po replied: "An outbreak of yao-illness is first visible in the body hair of the victims. If it stands erect, an outbreak will follow immediately. [The victim suffers from] chills so severe that his teeth begin to chatter. At the same time, pain occurs in the hips and back. As soon as the chills diminish, [the victim] feels heat both inside and outside his body. His head begins to ache as though it were about to burst; he is thirsty and yearns for something cold to drink."

The Emperor asked: "Which influence is responsible for these [symptoms]? What is the [underlying] principle here?"

Ch'i Po replied: "Yin and yang influences ascend and descend, falling into mutual conflict. Depletion and repletion also alternate, [reflecting] the mutual displacement of yin and yang [influences]. When yang [influences] enter the yin [conduits], a repletion arises in the yin [conduits], while a depletion occurs in the yang [conduits]. If a depletion strikes the yang-brilliance [conduit] [the patient] will tremble that his teeth chatter; if the great-yang [conduit] is empty pain is felt in the hips, back, head and neck. If all three yang [conduits] are affected simultaneously by a depletion [of influences], an excess arises in the yin [areas]. If, however, there is an excess [of influences] in the yin [conduits], cold develops in the bones, accompanied by pain. Cold is generated in the body and soon fills the body's central area and moves to the outside of the body. If a repletion [of influences] is present in the yang [conduits], the victim feels external heat. If, in addition, the yin [conduits] are affected by a depletion [of influences], inner heat also develops. If the body suffers from heat both within and without, gasping and thirst result, and the victim yearns for cold liquids. All this is the consequence of summer heat, for during this time an abundance of hot influences is present within the skin yet outside of the stomach and intestines. But this is also where the [body's own] constructive influences are located. As a result of this condition, the victim begins to perspire and [his skin] dries out. As soon as the skin opens [to release perspiration], the influence of autumn is able to penetrate. Sweat is thus expelled and combines with the wind. Another way [for the wind, that is, autumn influence, to enter] occurs during washing with water. During this process water-influence settles in the skin, along with the [body's own] defensive influences. These defensive influences flow in the yang [conduits] during the day and in the yin [conduits] at night. The [invading autumn] influence is now able to break out over the yang [conduits], expanding within the body through the yin [system]. This alternating expansion and contraction [of influences] produces the daily outbreaks [of yao-illnesses]."

The Emperor then asked: "How does it come about the outbreaks occur only every other day?"

Ch'i Po replied: "[Autumn] influence has now penetrated deep into the body and expands in the yin [areas]. It can only leave [the body] as an influence of the yang [system]. As an evil [influence] in the yin [conduits], it must remain inside the body. Since yin and yang remain in mutual opposition, no exit is possible. Thus the illness breaks out only every other day."

The Yellow Emperor spoke: "This I understand! But when the outbreaks first occur progressively later each day and then progressively earlier, which influence causes this [symptom]?"

Ch'i Po replied: "The [evil] influence [that has penetrated from outside] remains temporarily in the wind palace [located in the back of the head]. From there it descends along the spine. The [body's] defensive influences also collect in great numbers during the course of one day and night in the wind palace. Beginning on the following day, they descend [along with the evil influence], one vertebra each day. Thus an outbreak occurs progressively later. [The influences] remain at first on the spine. Each time that they reach the wind palace, the skin opens up, and [more of] the evil influence enters. This penetration of evil influence triggers the outbreak of the illness. In this way, [the outbreak is] delayed slightly later each day. When [the influences] have left the wind palace, they descend one vertebra daily. After twenty-five days they reach the lowest vertebra. After twenty-six days they penetrate into the spine and are now located in the spine transportation channel, in which they once again ascend. After nine days they then exit again through the broken vessel [located near the right collarbone]. Day after day the influences rise somewhat higher in the body. Consequently, the outbreaks occur progressively earlier each day. That the outbreaks now take place every second day is due to the fact that the evil influence has expanded in the five depots and permeated the diaphragm membrane. In the process, the distance [to the exit] has grown great, and the influence, which has penetrated deeply, moves only slowly [through the body] and is unable to keep up with the defensive influences. Both can no longer exit together; thus outbreaks occur only every second day."[54]

3. *Chu-ping yüan hou lun*
    (On the Origin and Symptoms of All Illnesses)
    Written at the beginning of the Seventh century
AUTHOR: Ch'ao Yüan-fang (fl. 610)

3.1. Symptomatology of [the Illness] "Hit-by-Wind"
    (Chung-feng hou)

The [illness] "hit-by-wind" means that someone has fallen victim to wind-influence [*feng-ch'i*]. Wind is an influence that is active during all four seasons; it extends throughout all eight directions of heaven. The wind is primarily responsible for bringing growth and sustenance to all things. If the wind originates in the same regions as the people it strikes, the resulting illnesses will only rarely be fatal. If, however, the wind comes from distant areas, people will die in great numbers from the resulting illnesses.

[The influence of wind on the body] can cause [two kinds] of illnesses. In the first, wind-influence collects in the skin, preventing [other influences] from penetrating deeper into the body or from flowing out. In the second, wind-influence invades the conduit vessels, traveling from there to the five depots, where it engenders the illnesses characteristic of the depots and palaces.

When the heart has been struck by wind, the victim desires only to lie down and is unable even to prop himself up. He begins to perspire. If the lips are red and the victim is still perspiring, treatment is possible. One hundred moxa-cauterizations should be performed immediately on the transportation [holes associated with the] heart. If, however, the lips have turned virid, black, white, or yellowish, it means that the heart has been contaminated with water. A fixed countenance and dazed eyes that only occasionally move with sudden fear are the signs that a cure is no longer possible. Death follows after five or six days.

When the liver has been struck by wind, the victim desires only to squat down and is unable even to lower his head. If the skin around the eyes and on the forehead has taken on a slightly virid hue, the lips have turned virid, and the face yellow, treatment is still possible. One hundred moxa-cauterizations should be performed immediately on the transportation [holes associated with the] liver. If, however, the color is a deeply virid or even black and if the face is sometimes yellow and sometimes white, the liver has already suffered irreparable harm. The victim dies after several days.

When the spleen has been attacked by wind, the victim crouches with feelings of repletion. The body is yellow throughout. If [such a] victim vomits a salty liquid, treatment is still possible. One hundred moxa-cauterizations should be performed immediately on the transportation [holes associated with the] spleen. But if the hands and feet have turned virid, a cure is no longer possible.

When the kidneys have been attacked by wind, the victim crouches with pain in the hips. The left and right sides of the body should be examined for the appearance of any yellow discolorations. If such patches are the size of millet cakes, treatment is still possible. One hundred moxa-cauterizations should be performed immediately on the transportation [holes associated with the] kidneys. But if the teeth have turned yellowish-red, the hair stands on end, and if head and face have taken on an earthen cast, a cure is impossible.

When the lung has been attacked by wind, the victim desires only to lie down. A feeling of repletion seizes the breast and the [respiration-] influence is short; the victim is apprehensive and breaks out in a sweat. Examine the area under the eyes, above and below the nose, as well as both sides down to the mouth. If any white patches are discernible, treatment is possible. One hundred moxa-cauterizations should be performed immediately on the transportation [holes] associated with the lung. If, however, a yellowish discoloration is evident, the lung has already been damaged, and hemorrhage will occur. Recovery is then impossible to achieve. The patient foolishly picks up soil with his bare fingers or he gathers his clothes and searches its seams.

This continues for several days until the victim finally dies. If a weak and depleted [movement in the] vessels has been diagnosed, the wind is also [responsible]. If the [movement in the] vessels is slow yet powerful, this, too, can be traced to the effects of wind, as can a [movement that is] at the surface and depleted. The wind also causes a smooth and dispersed [movement in the] vessels.[55]

3.2. Symptomatology of [the Illness Caused by] Wind-Evil (Feng-hsieh hou) (excerpt)

"Wind-evil" means that someone has been harmed by wind-influence. Inside the body men have blood and influences as normal [phenomena]; from outside, wind [attacks the body] as an evil influence. He who is excessively lazy and does not eat and drink at the appropriate times, so that the inner palaces and depots are impaired and depletion of blood [and protective] influences develops outside [of the depots and palaces], enables wind-evil to unfold its injurious effects.

Illnesses are caused by five evil [influences]. The first is to be hit by wind; the second is injury caused by heat; the third is excessive eating and drinking; the fourth is to be hit by cold; and the fifth is to be hit by humidity. The manner in which each of these illnesses arises, however, is different. When wind-evil breaks out [in the body], the victim is no longer himself; he is befuddled and babbles insanely. Anger and joy go completely out of control. [For treatment] there is, in addition to boiled potions, hot compresses, needles, and stones, a procedure to replenish the normal [influences in the body] and restore their flow [by means of gymnastic exercise and massage].[56]

3.3. Symptomatology of [the Illness Caused by] Malevolent Wind (O-feng hou)

There are a total of 404 illnesses caused by wind. All of these, however, can be grouped into five categories, according to the kind of wind responsible for the attack. The first is caused by yellow wind; the second by virid wind; the third by red wind; the fourth by white wind; and the fifth by black wind. Each person has 80,000 worms in his body. Together these worms constitute the complete human body. But if 80,000 worms are not present in the body, it is incomplete and unable to stand upright. Such a [deficiency] leads to various illnesses caused by [the influence of the] Malevolent, and numerous winds harm the human body.

The so-called five kinds of wind engender five kinds of worms that are harmful to man. Black wind engenders black worms. Yellow wind engenders yellow worms. Virid wind engenders virid worms. Red wind engenders red worms. White wind engenders white worms. All five kinds of wind are evil and can damage the human body. They are called violent winds. They invade the five depots and consume both the depots and the victim. The worms, in turn, engender more of their own kind, producing an innumerable amount in the body. They penetrate into the bone marrow and can come and go unhindered. As soon as they consume the liver, the eyebrows fall out. If the worms consume the lungs, the nose collapses. The victim loses his voice if the spleen is consumed. If the kidneys are consumed, sounds resembling the cry of children or the roll of thunder are perceived in the ear. If the worms consume the heart, its impulses are stilled and death follows.

If the [movement in the] vessels approaches slowly and recedes quickly, if depletion exists in the upper [body] while a repletion [of influences] prevails in the lower body, a malevolent wind is present.[57]

3.4. Symptomatology of Ascending Influences (Shang-ch'i hou) (excerpt)

The hundred illnesses have their origin in the influences. Anger causes the influences to rise [in the body]. Joy slows [the flow] of influences. Fear causes the influences to descend [in the body]. Vexation reduces the influences. Cold causes the influences to collect together. Heat opens the skin, allowing the influences to flow out. Grief brings the influences into confusion. Exhaustion reduces the influences to a minimum. Contemplation binds the influences together. In all nine of these situations the influences react differently. Anger reverses the normal flow of the influences. In severe cases the victims cough up blood and food, i.e., the influences ascend. Joy occasions harmony [among the influences]. The constructive and defensive influences flow unobstructed, bestowing their benefits throughout the entire body. This, in turn, diminishes the flow of the [remaining] influences. Vexation causes the large vessels that flow from the heart to contract, and the lobes of the lung begin to rise. This blocks the conduits flowing through the upper burner, preventing dispersal of the constructive and defensive influences and causing heat-influences to accumulate within [the body]. The influences begin to diminish. Fear reduces the essence. A reduction of essence causes the upper burner to close. When this occurs, the influences are forced to reverse their flow, causing swelling in the lower burner and the influences are unable to proceed. Exposure to cold generates unevenness in the conduits, causing the influences to collect. Exposure to heat opens the skin. The constructive and defensive influences are able to flow freely, causing profuse sweating. When someone grieves, the senses have no place to rest, the spirit has no place to withdraw to, and the mind is confused. As a result, the influences fall into disarray. Exhaustion causes the victim to gasp and sweat. Influences rapidly [leave] the inner and outer body, reducing them to a minimum. Contemplation seizes both body and mind. The influences cease to flow and are therefore bound.[58]

3.5. Symptomatology of Sudden [Abdominal-Intestinal] Distress Caused by Being Hit by the Malevolent (Chung-o huo-luan hou)

When someone is exposed to excessive heat or cold and neglects to eat and drink at regular intervals, a conflict arises between the yin and yang influences as well as between the clear and turbid influences [in the body], which ultimately leads to distress in the stomach and intestinal region. This is the cause of sudden unrests [cholera]. When it is therefore said that the cause is being hit by the Malevolent, this means that the victim has been affected totally unexpectedly by demonic influences [kuei-ch'i]. The symptoms are sudden, suffocating pains in the heart and abdomen. The invading evil attacks inside the body, clashing there with the cold [influences] of food and drink. Yin and yang influences finally turn against each other, adding to the unrest. When the stomach and intestines have been emptied, their [influences] are transformed to vomit, diarrhea, and nausea. This, then, is sudden [abdominal-intestinal] distress caused by being hit by the Malevolent.[59]

3.6. Symptomatology of [the Illness] "Hit-by-the-Malevolent" (Chung-o hou)

"Hit-by-the-Malevolent" means that someone whose essence and spirit had been exhausted and weakened has been hit suddenly by the influences of demonic spirits. If the yin and yang [influences] in man correspond to the ideal, if the constructive and defensive influences are present in a harmonious and desirable proportion, and if man's own spirit is preserved, evil cannot gain any foothold. If, however, man neglects the proper assimilation [of influences of both categories], thereby exhausting and weakening the essence and his own spirit, he shall suffer from the poisonous influences of demons. The symptoms include sudden, sharp pains in the heart and abdomen, accompanied by a sensation of tightness in the chest and [intestinal] distress; the victim has but one desire—to die. Whenever someone is hit suddenly by the Malevolent and thus has a swollen and full abdomen, he shall die if the [movement in the] vessels is strong but near the surface. He shall survive, however, if the [movement in the] vessels is fine and weak. The victim will also succumb if, after being hit by the Malevolent, he coughs up several bushels of blood and the [movement in the] vessels is deep, rapid, and fine. But he will recover if the [movement in the] vessels flickers hurriedly, like a flame.

If the victim is cured of the illness "Hit-by-the-Malevolent," but some of [the evil demonic influences] remain [in the body], [the illness] is transformed into possession if these forces are able to break out anew.[60]

3.7. Symptomatology of a Demon Attack (Kuei-chi hou)

Demon attack means that a person has been harmed by the influence of a demonic evil. The attack is completely unexpected, with no gradual development of indications. It is as if the victim has been stabbed with a knife or spear in the stomach or ribs; a sudden, suffocating pain is felt that cannot be stilled. Some [of the victims] cough up blood, while others bleed through the nose or through the lower [digestive openings of the body]. Another name [for this affliction] is demonic stroke, which signifies that someone has been struck by a demon.

If the [protective] influences and the blood are weakened and depleted, if essence and the *hun*-soul are exhausted and weary, and if, in this condition, [the victim] unexpectedly encounters a demonic spirit, a clash erupts that can result in a blow. Mild cases produce indisposition and are curable; more severe cases are frequently fatal.[61]

3.8. Symptomatology of Evil Possession (Hsieh-chu hou)

Possession signifies settlement, namely, that an affliction has settled down permanently. After [the victim] succumbs, the possession moves to someone close by, possessing this person. Evil refers to irregular influences. Thus, the blood and the [protective] influences in man's palaces and depots are the proper influences; wind, cold, heat, humidity, apparitions, trolls, goblins, and demons are all evil [influences].

Whenever someone has been possessed by evil, it is because his body suffered from depletion and weaknesses and was harmed in this state by evil influences. These influences seize the conduits, spreading into the palaces and depots. The mind and spirit lose their stability; sometimes [the victim] is annoyed, at other times he is paralyzed by fear. The illness is therefore called evil possession.[62]

3.9. Symptomatology of Nosebleeding (Pi-niu hou) (excerpt)

In the scripture it is written: "When the spleen transmits heat to the liver, fear and nosebleeding are the consequences." The spleen is soil; the liver is wood. Wood generally overcomes soil. In this case, heat in the spleen signifies an abundance of influences of the soil. When these influences then flow in the wrong direction and overcome wood, this is the result of a depletion [of influences] of wood, which takes from wood its ability to control soil. Thus [the liver] absorbs the heat transmitted by the spleen. The spirit of the liver is the *hun*-soul; the liver also stores blood. If a depletion [of blood] develops and is then followed by heat transmitted [from the spleen], the spirit of the *hun*-soul is not secured and fear is the result.

The blood and [protective] influences fill the palaces and depots within the body; farther out they flow through the conduits, following one another, and thus making their way throughout the body. After one circuit has been completed, they begin their journey anew. When the blood is affected by cold, it thickens and its flow is obstructed. When the blood is affected by heat, it grows thin and disperses. The lung generates the influences and the nose is the orifice of the lung. When heat overpowers the blood, the influences [of the lung] also grow hot. If both the blood and the influences [that flow from the lung] become heated, the blood follows the influences [of the lung] as they are dispersed. The blood exits through the nose, causing nosebleeding.[63]

3.10. Symptomatology of Harelip (T'u-ch'üeh hou)

Some persons are born with a fissure on the lip that resembles the lip of a hare, thus the name harelip. It is said that it is caused by women looking at a hare or consuming hare flesh during pregnancy.[64]

4. *Ch'ien-chin i-fang*
(Additions to the Thousandfold Golden Prescriptions)
Written in the seventh century
AUTHOR: Sun Ssu-miao (581–682?)

4.1. Section Five, The Classic of Interdictions:
Techniques of Gesticulative Magic (Chang-chüeh fa) (excerpt)

Whenever one wishes to perform an [exorcistic] ritual, it is first imperative to assimilate the influences of the three emitters and to do the steps of Yü.[65] If a ritual is then carried out, it will be successful.

The three emitters are the sun, the moon, and the stars. The steps of Yü involve three, seven, or nine steps; the number is not fixed.

To assimilate the influence of the three emitters, go outside on an extremely clear day and face the sun, so that both feet are placed next to each other. The request is then invoked, informally at first, so that each individual determines how much he desires to express at this time. This is then followed by the three steps of Yü. To begin, raise the head and gaze into the blazing sun. Open the mouth, inhale the sun's rays, and then close the mouth again. While holding the breath, proceed now with the three steps, and then exhale immediately.

Each of the three steps taken from the starting position consists of two individual steps, one by each foot. Thus a total of six individual paces are required for the three steps. When the steps of Yü are taken toward the sun, they begin with the left foot, followed by the right foot. When the steps of Yü are taken in the direction of the moon or stars, they begin with the right foot, followed by the left foot. In addition, the number of steps is not always the same. If the steps of Yü are taken toward the stars, for instance, nine steps must be completed: this is six more steps than are taken in the direction of the sun. Three times three steps yields a total of nine. The stars referred to here are the seven stars of the Great Bear. Great care must be exercised in connection with these stars; thus nine steps are necessary. For the sun and the moon either three or seven steps are suitable. The techniques of invocation and breath control remain the same, however, as those used for the sun.

The assimilation of the [influences of the] three emitters requires a clear and bright day.

The sun is yang; the moon and stars are yin. Left is yang and right is yin. Therefore to absorb the influence of the sun, the left foot must be moved first; to absorb the influence of the moon and stars, the right foot must be moved first.

Nine steps are to be taken in the direction of the stars. This requires a considerable amount of time, perhaps too much for a single breath. Therefore, the breath is then held for only three steps at a time, meaning that for the nine steps the breath is held a total of three times. Of course, the desired objective must also be repeated three times. In addition, one should be able to identify the three lowest stars in the group of the Great Bear. In men, the result is the ability to avoid the dangers of incarceration; in women, the ability to eliminate the dangers accompanying childbirth.

Someone might ask the following question: When it is stated that both feet must each be moved twice in order to complete one step, I still do not understand how this is to be accomplished! The explanation is as follows: Both feet must first be placed parallel to each other. The left foot is then raised and moved forward. The right foot is then raised and follows the left foot, so that one is now standing upright once more with both feet parallel. But this does not yet constitute one step; the second part is yet to come. The left foot must again be raised and moved ahead, to be followed once more by the right foot. Only after halting at this point has one step been completed. Repeating this double movement of both feet six times yields three steps. So much for the techniques of the steps [of Yü].[66]

5. *Wai-t'ai pi-yao* (Mysterious and Vital Information from the Outer Tower)
Written in the eighth century
AUTHOR: Wang T'ao (fl. 752)

5.1. Eight Prescriptions against an Exchange of *Yin* or *Yang* [Influences] Following a Cold-Induced Injury (Shang-han yin yang i fang pa shou) (excerpt)

[In the *Chu] ping yüan [hou lun* it is written:] The exchange of yin or yang [influences] after a cold-caused injury has the following significance. When a man or woman, having just barely recovered from an illness caused by cold, has not yet reestablished the ideal proportions [among the body's influences] but is already engaging in sexual relations, the resulting affliction is called "exchange of yin or yang [influences]." When a man has just recovered from his illness but has not yet achieved the ideal harmony [among his body's influences], it is called an exchange of yang [influences] if the woman falls ill after sexual relations with him. When a woman has just recently been cured from her [cold-induced] illness but has not yet reestablished the ideal harmony [among her body's influences], it is called an exchange of yin [influences] if the man falls ill after sexual relations with her. It is impossible for such an exchange to occur between two men or between two women. "Exchange" here refers to the interaction of yin and yang [influences]. The transfer of poison from one person to the other resembles the exchange of goods.

The symptoms of this illness are as follows: the body grows oppressively heavy; cramps are felt in the lower abdomen. In some cases there are vaginal cramps. Heat rises into the chest. The head grows heavy and cannot be raised; the eyes become cloudy. All four limbs are afflicted with cramps; pain fills the lower abdomen. Hands and feet are crippled. In all such cases, death is inevitable.

But there are also other kinds of cases that do not end in death. Here, too, the victim suffers from cramps in the lower abdomen. Heat rises into the chest. The head grows heavy and cannot be lifted. All joints disintegrate. The conduits and blood vessels are slack and weak; the blood and the [protective] influences suffer from depletion. The bones and marrow wither and dry out. Breathing becomes labored; the strength of the influences [i.e., of breath] grows progressively weaker. Finally, [the victim] lies immobile in bed and is able to stand only with the assistance of others. In some of these cases the victim also dies within a few months or a year. Quoted from the eighth chapter [of the *Chu-ping yüan hou lun*].

When Master Shen treated women suffering from warmth-illnesses, he forbade any sexual intercourse after their recovery and restoration of the ideal harmony [among the influences] until one hundred days had passed. If someone has intercourse [during this interval, the partner] will suffer from the exchange of yin [influences]. The hands and feet of the victim grow twisted and death is unavoidable. If the man was ill originally and transmits his [influences] to the woman, it is called an exchange of yang [influences]. If treatment is carried out promptly, a cure is possible. But if four days pass, any treatment is futile. The following prescriptions should be taken for this affliction.

Dried ginger—four *liang*
This drug is pulverized and then boiled. The entire amount is to be taken in one dose. A sensation of warmth and recurrent sweating will result, followed by a relaxation of the cramps. When the hands and feet can once more be stretched out, the cure has been effected. Quoted from chapter 14 of Fan Wang's [prescription work].[67]

(Additional prescriptions follow.)
In the *Ch'ien-chin* (*fang*)[68] it is written: In earlier times there once lived a man who had fallen ill from cold. He had already recovered from his affliction but was not yet completely well. This man then visited Hua Fu, so that the latter could feel his pulse. Fu told him that he had overcome his illness, but that a condition of deficiency was still present, so that it was not yet possible to speak of a complete recovery. Fu told him that his yang influences in particular were not yet present in sufficient quantities and that he was not permitted to engage in any strenuous activities [which would exacerbate the deficiency of yang influences]. Other activities were allowed; sexual relations, however, would spell certain death. If he were to engage in such activities, Fu warned, his tongue would protrude several inches shortly before his death. When the man's wife learned that he had recovered from his illness, she traveled over one hundred miles to see him. They spent only one night together as man and wife. After three days the man fell ill; his tongue protruded several inches from his mouth before he succumbed. Scarcely anyone who has sexual relations before one hundred days have passed after his recovery from an illness, when he still suffers from an imbalance among his vital influences, can escape death.

There once lived a scholar named Kai Cheng. Sixty days after overcoming his illness, he was already able to shoot a bow and hunt. Because he also started to have sexual relations at the same time, he began to cough up phlegm and then died. A heat-illness that arises after sexual intercourse is called the "exchange of yin or yang [influences]." All such illnesses are difficult to cure and are frequently fatal.

There recently lived a scholar-official who suffered from a minor illness caused by cold. Ten days after he recovered he was already able to ride a horse. He then concluded that [his influences] were present in a state of ideal harmony. After resuming sexual intercourse, he began to feel sharp pains in the lower abdomen. His hands and feet grew twisted and he died.

The physician Chang Miao reported: A servant woman fell ill. Only several days later she had sexual relations with six men, all of whom then died. When a woman falls ill she passes [her illness] to the husband, and when a man falls ill, he, too, can pass his illness to the wife. The "burnt undergarment remedy" should be administered; it cures both warmth-illnesses and the exchange of yin [influences].

Take the part of a woman's clothing that has covered her genitals, burn it, and use the ashes.
This drug should be prepared into a powder. Take a square-inch spoonful three times daily. This will cause urine to flow and the glans to swell slightly. This indicates that a cure has been effected. When women fall ill, they can utilize the garments of a man in the same way; the drug is taken with wine or water.

This is originally a prescription from [Chang] Chung-ching. The same instructions are also found in the *Chou-hou [pei-chi fang]*.[69]

5.2. Forty-two Prescriptions against Illnesses Caused by Natural [Influences], Resulting in Sweating or Similar Symptoms (T'ien-hsing ping fa-han teng fang ssu-shih-erh shou) (excerpt)

A therapeutic exercise [recommended by the] *Yang-sheng fang* is as follows: After arising for the first time on a clear morning, cross the left and right hands over the head, grasp the ears firmly, and pull upward. [Both hands] should then immediately be run through the hair. This prevents the head from growing white and the ears from becoming deaf. Next, the palms of the hands should be rubbed together until hot and then used to wipe the face. After twenty-seven downward strokes, remove the sweat. This imparts a glow to the face. Rub the palms together once again until they are hot and then stroke the body with them from top to bottom: this procedure is called "dry washing" and protects man from wind, cold, and the influences of the four seasons. Hot and cold fits, headaches, and various other illnesses are also cured by [this exercise].[70]

5.3. Four Prescriptions against Sexual Intercourse with Spirits and
     Demons (Kuei shen chiao-t'ung fang ssu shou) (excerpt)

Prescriptions of Mr. Ts'ui for the treatment of sexual intercourse
with demons and spirits in dreams.
     wild fox testicles—roast
     leopard testicles—roast
       seven of each
     fox skull—one, also roasted
     realgar; seal; demon-arrow-feather [herb]; bee honeycomb—roast;
     atractylode rhizome, tiger skull—roast;
       one *liang* of each
     asa foetida—two *liang*, roast
     donkey, horse, dog, camel, and cow hair—four *fen* of each, charred
If the symptom of steaming bones is evident, add the brain-bone
of a deceased person to the prescription—one *liang*, roasted
The fifteen drugs listed above are weighed together on a large scale
and then crushed into powder through a sieve. A smooth mixture
should be obtained by stirring. Before this, pine resin is heated to the
melting point in a water bath. Add the resin to the powder. Do not
use the hands to mix, but rather a tiger claw. Prepare pills into small
balls, using them to fumigate the patient. During fumigation cover
[the patient] with his clothes and coverlet, taking care that none of
the medicinal smoke escapes outside. Additional realgar should be
crushed to increase the flammability of the medicine. Regarding frequency and duration of treatment: follow the procedures for aromatic
fumigation. To achieve excellent success, burn part of the medication
under the bed [of the patient]. Peaches, plums, and sparrow flesh are
to be avoided.
     Quoted from chapter seven.[71]

5.4. Three Techniques to Ward Off Snakes (P'i-she fa san shou)
     (excerpt)

Prescription from the *Chi-yen*[72] to ward off all snakes when traveling
in the mountains or through the grass.
     Dried ginger; fresh musk aroma; realgar
Pulverize an equal amount of these three ingredients and fill a small
red pouch, to be carried by the man on the left side of the sash and
by the woman on the right side. This will ward off any snakes that
may wish to attack. If someone is bitten by a snake, immediately use
[this remedy] for treatment. If musk aroma is unavailable, carry [the

two remaining ingredients of the prescription] [mixed] with thickened aconite sap while traveling. [This medicine] is effective against all poisons.[73]

6. Taishō Tripitaka: Canon of Buddhist Writings in Chinese

6.1. Sutra Containing Pronouncements of Buddha on Buddhist Medicine; (Fo-shuo fo-i ching); translated from the Sanskrit into Chinese in A.D. 203

From the time of its very inception, the human body contains four [potential sources of] illness. These are: first, earth; second, water; third, fire; fourth, wind. If wind increases, the influences ascend. If fire increases, heat rises. If water increases, cold rises. An increase of earth signals that strength is present in abundance. These four [primal agents of] illness can generate a total of 404 illnesses.

Earth is associated with the body. Water is associated with the mouth. Fire is associated with the eyes. Wind is associated with the ears. A lack of fire accompanied by violent cold diminishes the eyesight.

The first, second, and third months constitute spring, a time of frequent cold. The fourth, fifth, and sixth months constitute summer, a time of frequent wind. The seventh, eighth, and ninth months constitute autumn, a time of frequent heat. The tenth, eleventh, and twelfth months constitute winter, a time of wind and cold. What is the reason for this? Spring is the time of frequent cold, for it is the time of all creation. [As things are created,] cold departs from them; thus cold prevails in spring. Why is summer a time of frequent wind? In summer all things blossom forth and yin and yang flourish and come together. Thus wind prevails in summer. Why is autumn a time of frequent heat? During autumn all things reach maturity; thus heat prevails in autumn. Why is winter a time of wind and cold? In winter all things die and decay, and all heat leaves them; thus winter is a time of wind and cold.

During the third, fourth, fifth, sixth, and seventh months, man is able to sleep. Why is this so? It is a time of much wind and the body is therefore relaxed. In the eighth, ninth, tenth, eleventh, twelfth, first, and second months, man is unable to sleep. Why is this so? It is often cold, thus the body is tense and tight.

Cold prevails during the three months of spring; thus wheat and beans may not be consumed. The correct foods are late rice and butter-oil, as well as other hot things. The three months of summer are marked by wind; thus it is forbidden to eat aron, beans, and wheat. The correct foods are late rice and curds. Heat prevails during the three months of autumn; thus late rice and butter-oil may not be consumed. The correct foods are fine rice, roasted grain, honey, paddy rice, and millet. Wind and cold mark the three months of winter. Yang and yin [influences] come together. The proper foods are late rice, foreign-bean soup, and butter-oil. While man sleeps the wind sometimes rises and sometimes dies down. While man sleeps fire sometimes flares up and sometimes dies down. Cold sometimes increases and sometimes decreases.

Ten causes are responsible for the illnesses of man. First, sitting too long without eating; second, immoderate eating; third, worry and fright; fourth, excessive exertion; fifth, immoderate sexual cravings; sixth, anger and vexation; seventh, suppression of bowel movements; eighth, intentional retention of urine; ninth, suppression of rising winds; tenth, suppression of descending winds. These are the ten causes of illness.

Buddha says: There are nine causes for the premature, unexpected end to human life. First, eating what should not be eaten; second, immoderate eating; third, eating contrary to custom; fourth, failure to discharge the old before the arrival of the new; fifth, intentional retention of digested foods; sixth, disregard for the principles of proper conduct; seventh, cultivation of bad acquaintances; eighth, untimely appearance and unseemly behavior in the streets; ninth, failure to avoid that which should be avoided. These are the nine causes that bring human life to an unexpected conclusion.

"Eating what should not be eaten" means the consumption of those things that are repugnant to the senses. It also means consumption not in accord with the four seasons, and starting to eat again immediately after the conclusion of a meal. All this is "eating what should not be eaten."

"Immoderate eating" means consumption in excess of one's needs, with no thought to certain limits. This is what is meant by "immoderate eating."

"Eating contrary to custom" means eating at unusual hours. If, while traveling in a distant land where the local foods are unfamiliar, one eats that which he is not used to without first sampling a small amount, this is what is meant by "unusual eating habits."

"Failure to discharge the old before the arrival of the new" means heaping more food on food still undigested. If, for example, an emetic or purgative is taken and the patient eats before the medication's effect is complete, this is "failure to discharge the old before the arrival of the new."

"Intentional retention of digested foods" means preventing the normal release of stools and urine, or suppressing a natural belch, vomit, or the release of wind. This is the meaning of "intentional retention of digested foods."

"Disregard for the principles of proper conduct" means violating the five precepts of proper behavior.[74] Robbers and such persons who act indecently toward the wives of others are today handed over to district magistrates. They are then dismembered, executed, clubbed to death, or starved to death. Some are able to escape and are then slain by the enraged relatives of the victims. Some die because they are frightened, worried or because of fear. This is the meaning of "disregard for the principles of proper conduct."

"Cultivation of bad acquaintances" means that when someone commits a crime, it influences others as well. Why is this so? The reason is that one does not leave bad acquaintances. Since bad people are not counted, one is taken in their place. This is what is meant by "cultivation of bad acquaintances."

"Untimely appearance and unseemly behavior in the streets" means going out during the early hours of the morning or late at night when apparitions clash; or when one allows oneself to be sought and arrested by police officials; or if one enters a strange house and observes that which he should not, hears that which he should not, behaves indecently where he should not, and, finally, if one contemplates that which should not be considered. All this is what is meant by "untimely appearance and unseemly behavior in the streets."

"Failure to avoid that which should be avoided" refers to sick oxen and horses, rabid dogs, poisonous snakes and worms, pools of water, fire, pits, swift carriages and galloping horses, drunks or malicious persons holding a knife, and so forth. This is what is meant by "failure to avoid that which should be avoided."

These are the nine causes for the unexpected and premature end to human life. Attentive persons should therefore take heed. By avoiding that which should be avoided, there are two fortunate consequences for man. First, a long life; second, the ability to comprehend the law and beneficial sayings, having been granted a long time to live according to the law.

Buddha says: There are four foods. First, the food of the son; second, the food that injures man like three hundred spear thrusts;

third, the food that causes worms to crawl out of skin and fur; fourth, the food of misfortune.

"The food of the son" has the following significance: while devouring meat to satisfy a craving for its flavor, a man ponders the fact that this food represents his fathers and mothers, brothers, wives, children, and relatives from earlier life and that this consumption does not free him from the eternal cycle of life and death. If, on the basis of such considerations, the man now renounces his cravings, this signifies the "food of the son."

"The food that injures man like three hundred spear thrusts" has the following significance: someone eats according to his inclinations, pondering the fact that untold misfortune arises for him [from such foods], for only he whose thoughts remain untouched by such desires shall escape the eternal cycle of life and death. This is like the thrust of a spear that separates man from his body. One is forced to meditate continuously on the suffering that still lies ahead in life. This is what is meant by "the food that injures man like three hundred spear thrusts."

"The food that causes worms to crawl out of skin and fur" has the following significance: A person has on his mind that which tastes good and many other things. He is concerned about matters in his household. All this burrows into his thoughts. Such considerations multiply into ten thousand forms, finding expression in one way or another. This is the meaning of "the food that causes worms to crawl out of skin and fur."

"The food of misfortune" has the following significance: Birth, death, and life-conduct are all "foods of misfortune." Fire, for instance, burns many things. In the same manner, man's entire existence consumes his body. Since a parallel exists here to fire, which burns all things, we speak of "misfortune." But why do we also speak of "food"? The reason for this is that man can seek being human [just as he seeks foods]. For this reason we speak here of "foods."

When a person consumes meat, it is as though he is consuming his own son. Each animal that is born is to me father, mother, brother, wife, and child, with no limit of number. There are six cases when man should not consume meat:

1. If he killed it himself.
2. If he authorizes another to kill [for him].
3. If he looks favorably upon the act of killing.
4. If he has seen the killing.
5. If he has heard the killing.

6. If one has doubts about whether he himself was the reason for the killing.

If these six considerations are not a factor, meat may be consumed. He who eats no meat harbors these doubts. He who is able to renounce all meat completely shall enjoy the good fortune of fearlessness.

Buddha says: Immoderate consumption is connected to five evils. First, excessive sleep; second, frequent illness; third, frequent sexual cravings; fourth, inability to recite the words of Buddha; fifth, preoccupation with worldly things. Why is this so? A man driven by sexual desires knows the pleasures of lust. An angry man knows the taste of violence. An ignorant man knows the pleasures of eating. In the rules and sayings it is written: when someone desires a particular flavor, this flavor always brings forth more flavor, but in the next life, this person shall no longer experience the desired flavor.

Buddha says: A single daily meal is proper for those desiring to escape the eternal cycle of life and death. He who falls victim to his own appetites is incapable of moral conduct and of achieving the celestial eyes of self-understanding which reveal the origin of one's own life and where it shall lead. Those who give no thought to dying, consume immoderately, and frequently covet women, commit 140 transgressions. They shall suffer premature death, and the reason for this lies in their foods. He who commits the 10 transgressions[75] shall lose his human form in the next life and be reborn among the animals. Should he nonetheless be reborn in human form, hunger, thirst, and bleeding are his certain destiny. Anger arises together with passions and lusts.

Buddha says: It is of great benefit to fast voluntarily and give one's food to others, so that these persons may continue their life. This is of enormous value. In the following life one is then assured of an abundance of food and drink; anger and vexation shall be unknown. He who bestows nothing of value shall therefore receive nothing. But he who is marked only by passion and avarice has nothing to give and consequently shall experience only passions in the next life. I myself possess nothing, not even a single coin, because I have taken nothing. He who allows avarice and desires to develop unchecked shall suffer in vain and commit transgressions. The man of the law knows neither care nor sorrow. Care arises out of vexation; sorrow arises out of lust. We all have a year, month, day, and hour for death. He who is ignorant of this fact and does not fear it, he who does not live according to the law and ignores the dictates of proper conduct, he who runs to and fro aimlessly, seeks copper and iron, he who is preoccupied with his fields, house, and servants, spreads only sorrow and suffering among mankind and shall be reborn as an animal.

Buddha says: People order their lives as bees prepare honey. Bees remove honey from all blossoms, working hard and diligently the entire day until their task is completed. Someone who just seizes a thing, takes it, and then departs with it shall reap only suffering and be given nothing. A man who pursues such thoughts and concerns shall also be burdened with these cares. He struggles diligently, without thought to hunger or thirst, to accumulate riches; yet even before his death he must occupy himself with the five fates that can befall a family: water, fire, robbers, district officials, and the pain of illness. Frequently they strike unexpectedly. When the victim has died, others come into possession of his goods, and he himself is rewarded only with inexpressible agony. The five fates are: first, fire; second, water; third, robbers; fourth, district officials; fifth, avaricious siblings.

What is the meaning of "no concern for possessions"? If someone disregards the five destinies he shall be unable to escape suffering. Such concern and such suffering can assume ten thousand forms; whenever they collect in the body they lead one away from the correct path, shunting the law into the distance. Man [should] conduct himself within the law as in trade. If he makes profit, it shall not be a source of joy. If he does not achieve a profit, it should not be a source of concern, for this is only the consequence of conduct during a previous life. He who was greedy [in a previous existence] shall achieve no gain in this life. Even if he were to gather together all of the riches on earth, he would be unable to use them freely. He shall be unable to follow those who leave [the world of life and death], but shall only increase his human bonds and his suffering, sowing only the foundation for a future existence. This foundation is like fire, in that it consumes all. Yet we are unaware of this and dare not eliminate our illusions. We [should] know that it increases suffering and sows the seeds of transgressions.[76]

6.2. Sutra of the Thousand-Handed, Thousand-Eyed Avalokitesvara Bodhisattva on the Treatment of Illnesses and the Preparation of Drugs (Ch'ien-shou ch'ien-yen Kuan-shih-yin p'u-sa chih-ping ho-yao ching); translated between A.D. 625 and 650.

At that time Buddha spoke to Ananda: The comprehensive, complete, highly compassionate spell recited by the Bodhisattva Avalokitesvara, which encounters no resistance, is genuine and truly not without substance. Should there be those desiring to make some appeal to Avalokitesvara Isvara Bodhisattva Mahasattva, they must obtain *guggulu* incense and recite the spell three times while burning the incense. The Bodhisattva Avalokitesvara will then immediately hasten to come.

When someone has been possessed by demons, he should burn a cat skull,[77] combine the ashes with pure clay, and then fashion an image of the evil demon. He should then place this before a likeness of the thousand-eyed one, take an iron knife and cut [the image] into 108 pieces while reciting the spell 108 times. When the victim then recites the name [of this demon], the exorcism is completed. The [demon] will now be expelled for all time and shall never return.

When someone has been harmed by ku, he should first combine equal amounts of *karpura* incense and *guggulu* incense, adding to this mixture a bushel of well water that has been drawn in the gray light of dawn. The mixture should then be heated and reduced to one-half bushel. Discard the sediment and drink the liquid. At the same time, while standing before a likeness of the thousand-eyed one, repeat the spell one hundred times, and the exorcism is finished.

When someone has been bitten by a venomous snake or by a scorpion, he should prepare a somewhat coarse powder from dried ginger and recite the spell seventeen times while applying the ginger to the wound. This immediately removes [the poison] and recovery is complete.

If someone should be harmed by evil spells cast by a malevolent enemy, the victim must fashion an image of this evil person out of pure earth, dough, or wax. He then must take a knife fashioned from iron, step before a likeness of the thousand-eyed one, and recite the spell 108 times. During each recitation of the spell he cuts a piece [from the image of the enemy], and finally burns all 108 pieces. The enemy will thereupon become extremely friendly, and the relationship between the two will be marked by mutual love and respect. This person shall no longer feel any hate.

When someone's sight has been damaged, either to the point of complete blindness or so that a white mist or red membrane clouds the eyes, the victim must crush one kernel of harītakī, āmalakī, and vibhītaka each and press out the oil. It is imperative that during this procedure one is protected from any contamination, that is, neither any woman who has recently given birth nor a dog may watch. While reciting the name of Buddha with closed mouth, apply the [oil] mixed with white honey or with human milk to the eyes. The human milk must come from a mother who is nursing a male child. If only mother's milk from a woman nursing a female child is available, [the spell] must be repeated 1,008 times before a likeness of the thousand-eyed one after preparation of the medication. The remedy should remain on the eyes for seven full days. During this time the victim must remain always in a secluded room and protect himself against wind, sexual intercourse, the five acrid spices, as well as against all impure things. This shall restore eyesight to its former glory.

Someone suffering from fever-demon illness should take the fur of a tiger, leopard, jackal, or wolf and cover his entire body with it while reciting the spell twenty-one times. This will exorcise the illness. Lion skins are best suited to this purpose.

When someone is bitten by a snake, remove ear fat from the victim and, while reciting the spell twenty-one times, rub it into the wound. This will effect the cure.[78]

When someone suffers from severe oppression of the heart and wishes to die, take a lump of peach-tree resin approximately the size of a peach and heat it together with one *sheng* of clear water, until the liquid has been reduced to one-half sheng. Recite the spell seven times and take the entire amount of the liquid in a single dose. This exorcises the illness. The medication must not be prepared by a woman, for the process must be free of any contamination. Drugs prepared by women are ineffectual.

When someone suffers from corpse-illness, caused by the influence of the demon of a deceased person, he should burn guggulu incense and inhale the fumes through the nose while reciting the spell twenty-one times. He must then take seven pills the size of hare droppings, swallowing these while reciting the spell fourteen times. This effects the exorcism. The victim must take care to guard against wine, meat, and the five acrid spices and refrain from giving offense to anyone. In addition, combine realgar with white mustard seeds and Indian salt and burn this mixture beneath the victim's bed while reciting the spell twenty-one times. This shatters the body of the demon that has caused the illness, and it flees, not daring to remain.

When someone suffers from wind-influence in half of his body, so that his ears and nose are clogged and he is unable to move his hands and feet, boil a mixture of sesame oil and beaver root and rub the liquid, while reciting the spell twenty-one times, over the victim's body for an extended period of time. The body should also be rubbed, accompanied by reciting the spell twenty-one times, with pure butter-oil from cow's milk. This procedure is very effective.

When a woman experiences a difficult birth, rub sesame oil around the navel and into the jade gate of the victim. Birth will also be facilitated by the consumption [of the oil].

When a woman carries a dead child within her body, take one large *liang* of *apamarga* herb, boil it together with two sheng of water, drain the liquid and discard the sediment. The victim then takes one sheng of the liquid while reciting the spell twenty-one times. The child will then be expelled with no pain whatsoever. This drug should also be taken when the afterbirth fails to appear; it, too, will be expelled promptly.

When someone suffers from sudden, unbearable heart pains, it is because he has become possessed by the demon of a corpse lying by the wayside. In such a case the victim must, while reciting the spell twenty-one times, chew and swallow *kunduru* incense in an amount the size of the female nipple; the exact amount, however, is not absolutely critical. The [drug] causes vomiting, thus expelling the demon. The victim must take care to guard against the five acrid spices, wine, meat, and oily substances, and all unclean things, and refrain from sexual intercourse.

When someone has been severely burned, rub the affected areas with hot dung of black oxen while reciting the spell twenty-one times. This will effect a cure.

When someone suffers heart pains caused by the bite of internal worms, he must consume one-half sheng of the dung from white horses and recite the spell twenty-one times. This will effect the exorcism. In severe cases the dose is one whole sheng. The worms will be expelled in the form of a dark-green rope.

When someone suffers from sores on the lower [body openings], he must consume the liquid pressed from water chestnuts, recite the spell twenty-one times, and at night, while lying down, apply the liquid to the eyes. This produces the exorcism. [This is followed by a short, garbled passage.]

When someone suffers from abdominal pain, he should take one-half sheng of two grains of Indian salt dissolved in well water drawn in the early light of dawn and recite at the same time the spell twenty-one times. This effects a cure.

When someone suffers from reddening of the eyes, or when growths or a white veil form in the eyes, he should consume the liquid pressed from green *sami* leaves, recite the spell seven times, place a coin [in the liquid] overnight, recite the spell an additional seven times, and they apply [the liquid] to the eyes. This effects the exorcism.

When someone is frightened at night and cannot calm down, or when someone is afraid to go in or out, prepare a cord from white threads, recite the spell twenty-one times, tie twenty-one knots, and place the cord around the neck. This will effect a cure. Not only does this technique eliminate fears, it also brings about a contented existence, erases all transgressions, and leads to a long life.

When someone's home is unexpectedly struck by misfortune and hardships, the victim must cut the branches of a pomegranate tree into 1,008 pieces[79] and rub both ends [of all pieces] with butter, curds, and honey. He then recites the spell once each time as he burns the individual pieces. This will eliminate all misfortune and hardships. The procedure should be carried out before a likeness of the thousand-eyed one.

[Seven directions for nonmedical purposes follow.]

When someone has been possessed by demons, so that he remains silent, foams at the mouth, no longer recognizes anyone, and lies near death, give him finely ground amber mixed with wine while reciting the spell 108 times. Following this, press the liquid from the dung of white horses and give this [to the victim] while reciting the spell fourteen times. A likeness of the demon should be drawn on the forehead of the victim and the spell repeated an additional 108 times. This exorcises the demon.

When someone has burned himself with hot liquid, combine wood ashes with water and apply this mixture to the burned areas three times daily while reciting the spell twenty-one times. Hot cow dung can also be applied to the affected areas, accompanied by twenty-one recitations of the spell. This effects a cure.

When someone is poisoned after consuming raw flesh and suffers from such severe oppression of the heart that he desires to die, boil a mixture of one sheng pure earth and three sheng water, reducing it to one sheng, and give it to the victim while reciting the spell twenty-one times. This effects a cure.

When someone suffers from sudden swellings and boils, crush onion leaves and combine with wine; while reciting the spell twenty-one times apply this mixture to the swelling. This effects a cure.

When someone suffers from such severe swelling throughout his body that he desires to die, combine cow dung with wine, applying the mixture to the swellings while reciting the spell twenty-one times. In addition, [the victim] should also consume this medication. This effects a cure.

When someone suffers from such severe nosebleeding that he wishes to die, boil fresh *p'eng-lai* leaves and have the victim consume this while reciting the spell twenty-one times. The amount of the drug [taken] is unimportant; he will survive.

When someone has bloody stools, have him swallow an egg-sized amount of peach-tree resin and recite the spell twenty-one times. This effects a cure.

For coughing, take one sheng peach pits heated over fire, combined with sugar—all taken as one dose after the victim has recited the spell 108 times. After three or four such treatments, he is cured.

When someone suffers from anal itching, prepare a hot [potion] of finely ground *ts'ao-chien-lo* fruit, add sugar, recite the spell 108 times, and rub [the liquid] on the anus three times daily. This relieves the symptoms.

When someone suffers from constipation, boil two sheng of k'uei seeds with four sheng water until it is reduced to one sheng. Taking this liquid while reciting the spell twenty-one times will restore regular bowel movement.

For urinary retention, take the liquid pressed from cow dung while reciting the spell twenty-one times. This produces a cure.

For urinary retention, use three fingers to remove dust from ceiling beams and, after pressing through a sieve, mix with clear water. The victim should drink this while reciting the spell twenty-one times. This effects a cure.

When someone suffers from frequent and sudden forced urination, during which one *tou* is passed each time, boil one *liang kua-lou* root with three sheng clear water; remove the liquid after it has been reduced by one-half, and have [the victim] take the entire amount at one time while reciting the spell 21 times or 108 times. This effects a cure.

When a woman suddenly falls ill during pregnancy, boil five sheng small beans and three sheng salt beans [?] with one *tou* clear water, reducing the mixture to three sheng. The liquid is then divided into two portions, which [the victim] takes after reciting the spell 108 times. This exorcises the illness. The birth proceeds peacefully and successfully.

When a woman experiences a difficult delivery due to breech presentation, and comes close to death, boil one *sheng p'eng-lai* with three sheng water until it is reduced to one sheng; the victim should then take the entire amount while reciting the spell twenty-one times. Delivery will take place without complications.

When a small child cries and is unable to sleep at night, write the character for demon under his eyes, recite the spell twenty-one times, and spit three times. This exorcises the demon and calms the child.

When a small child has sores on his head, combine charred cow horn with pig fat and spread the mixture on the sores while reciting the spell twenty-one times. This effects a cure.

When a small child suffers from a swollen tongue and is unable to drink the mother's milk, rub the sap from the eastern mulberry tree on the tongue while reciting the spell 108 times. Recovery will occur immediately.

When a small child has sores in the mouth and is unable to eat, combine finely ground and sifted *huang-lien* root with the milk of a mother nursing a small boy. Spread [this mixture] on the sores in the mouth while reciting the spell twenty-one times. This effects a cure.

At that time Avalokitesvara Bodhisattva Mahasattva spoke to a large crowd: After the final passage of Tathagata into nirvana, all men will decline in wanton existence as the end of the world approaches. Innumerable illnesses will therefore be inevitable. For this reason I shall today reveal several therapeutic techniques in order to render assistance. If there are now monks and nuns, lay brothers and lay sisters, good men and good women who can learn and pass on these techniques in order to relieve the suffering of others, they shall now hear that I have assumed this human body with great compassion to help all mankind. I myself must appear here so that all these techniques achieve their highest possible efficacy. He who comprehends and passes on the miraculous words of this compassionate and profound spell, which faces no obstacles, in order to heal the suffering of the world, shall be like me; between this person and myself there is no difference.

When men and women of pure faith, who accept, preserve, and also recite this spell for the relief of suffering, treat illnesses using obscure worldly techniques, they should nonetheless recite [the spell] 108 times out of compassion and with an upright mind. All shall then receive the power of the Avalokitesvara. When all men shall be able to carry on my techniques, they shall immediately be received by me when their destiny is complete. I shall journey with them in unbounded joy in the bejeweled celestial carriage and assist them to rebirth in the world of peace and happiness. After a short time they shall rise again in the lotus blossom and attain perfection as Buddha.

Thereupon Shakyamuni praised the Bodhisattva Avalokitesvara and spoke: "Praise the Great Master! It is so! It is so! Exactly as you have spoken! If there be good men and women who give but a small portion of such remedies to a sick person, their happiness shall be assured and every transgression in their present existence be forgiven. In future worlds inexhaustible happiness shall be their reward. In every world in which they are reborn, they shall receive a body free from illness and every fortune shall be bestowed upon them. Both in heaven and among men, every success will be theirs. Both in heaven and among men, their destiny shall be immortality. They shall achieve the Tao in just a short time."

When the tremendous gathering of bodhisattvas, mahasattvas, brahmans, the four kings, devas, nagas, and yaksas, as well as all spirits, demons, kings, humans, and nonhumans had heard the words of Buddha, there was great rejoicing among them. Devoutly they perceived his words, showed him their reverence, and then departed to carry out his instructions.[80]

7. *Ju-men shih-ch'in*
   (How a Confucian Scholar Serves his Parents)
   Written ca. 1200
   AUTHOR: Chang Ts'ung-cheng

7.1. Madness (Huang)

A man of sixty became enraged when the state forced him into labor, and he was suddenly struck by madness. It felt to him as though worms were crawling through his nose and mouth; he scratched with both hands. His condition remained unchanged for several years. Tai-jen examined the victim's hands. The [movement in his] vessels was vast and strong, resembling a strong rope. His diagnosis was as follows: "The mouth is *fei-men* (winged gate), the stomach is the *pen-men* (gate of strength). It is said the mouth is the upper source of the stomach. As for the nose, the foot-yang-brilliance conduit originates at the point where nose and forehead merge, and touches the great-yang [conduit] as well. It then proceeds downward along the ridge of the nose, passing through the "human center,"[81] circumvents the lips downward, and passes through the *cheng-chiang* [hole]. The illness in question here came about in the following manner. Anger over being conscripted is nothing more than a fire-transformation. Fire has seized the yang-brilliance conduit, thus generating the madness. In the scripture it is written: victims of illnesses of the yang-brilliance conduit climb to high altitudes and then sing; they remove their clothing and run around; they utter degrading words with no regard for whether they affect strangers or relatives. The liver is responsible for planning; the gall makes decisions. When someone is angry at being forced into labor, it is as if he has money that cannot be spent. This means that the liver is continually forging plans, while the gall has no opportunity to make a decision. [It is as if one were] bent, unable to stretch out; one is enraged, yet has no opportunity to release his anger. The fire in the heart flares up powerfully and takes over the metal of the yang-brilliance conduit. Originally the stomach belongs to the soil, and the liver to wood, while the gall belongs to the minister-fire. In this case, the fire has followed the influences of wood and has penetrated into the stomach. This was the cause of the sudden madness." [Tai-jen] then directed the old man to enter a warm room to vomit and sweat there three times. In the *Nei-ching* it is written: "If [the influences associated with the phase] wood are depressed, allow them to spread; if the [influences associated with the phase] fire are depressed, allow them to develop." That is well said! [Hence Tai-jen], in addition, reduced one-half *chin* of the "decoction that harmonizes the stomach and supports the influences"—to which he had added five sheng of water—through boiling by one half, and divided [the remaining amount] into three doses. This produced twenty violent occurrences of diarrhea. Blood, water, and clotted blood became separated, and several *sheng* [of these substances] were discharged. As a result, [the patient] recovered. With the "powder to communicate with the sages" [Tai-jen finally] harmonized [the old man's] behind.[82]

7.2. Fetid Breath (K'ou-ch'ou)

A twenty-odd-years-old son from the family of Chao P'ing-shan was afflicted with influences flowing from his mouth whose odor resembled the stench from latrines. Even his own relatives could no longer stand to speak with him. Tai-jen spoke: "The lungs [correspond to] metal [and are generally] responsible for frowzy odor. The metal is melted by fire. The fire is responsible for burned odors. This is the cause of this [affliction]. If the condition persists for an extended period of time, decay will result. The kidneys are [the depot] that will decay, because extreme heat will cause transformations in water in contrast [to what is usual, namely, that water destroys fire]. Since the illness is located in the upper part of the body, it must be purged by vomiting."

[Tai-jen first] administered the "powder to harmonize with tea," causing [the patient] to vomit, and eliminated in this manner 70 percent [of the illness]. At night he then administered the "boat and carriage pills" and the "deep-river powder," thereby emptying the intestines five to seven times. By the next morning, the fetid breath was eliminated.[83]

7.3. Noises during Knee Bends (Ch'ü-hsi yu sheng)

Li Wen-ch'ing from Ling-pei was afflicted with a creaking noise from both kneecaps whenever he stretched or bent his legs. Someone believed this to be the sound of bones, but Tai-jen had the following to say: "This is not so. The bones are not struck—how could they ring out! In this case the muscles are affected by humidity. When the muscles are humid they become tense. The only [thing to do is] to relax [the muscles again]. When they are relaxed they will not produce any sounds; tense [muscles] produce sounds. If [the patient] uses my medication, which will cause him to vomit and to defecate once, his water will be discharged both upward and downward. Once the water has been eliminated, the noises will cease." Li Wen-ch'ing followed these words, and the result [of the treatment] corresponded to the prediction.[84]

7.4. Conception of a Child following Purgative Therapy (Hsieh erh)

A thirty-four-year-old woman dreamt at night of having sexual intercourse with demons and spirits. She lived in fear of strange things, and the hall of the spirits and the palaces of the departed appeared to her in visions; she also saw boat paddles and bridge beams. All of this had continued for some fifteen years, and during the entire period she had never once been with a child. She sought help in the prayers of shamans and supplications of sorcerers—there was nobody to whom she had not turned already. The wounds where needles had pierced her muscles and where her flesh had been cauterized numbered in the tens of thousands. She grew increasingly yellow and emaciated, she developed hot spells, and refused to drink. Her abdomen grew full and her feet were swollen. She herself had already placed her destiny into the hands of heaven. One day she sought aid for her suffering from Tai-jen. Tai-jen spoke: "An excess of yang fire manifests itself in the upper [part of the body], an excess of yin fire in the lower [part of the body]. Demons and spirits are yin forces; the hall of the spirits is a yin place. Boat paddles and bridge beams are used in the water. The [movement in the] vessels at the 'inch[-openings]' of both hands is deep and subdued. All this reveals that the chest is filled with phlegm." After three repetitions of vomiting, purgation, and sweating, all of the woman's dreams disappeared in fewer than ten days. After one month she was already pregnant. Tai-jen spoke: "I have restored life to a woman and enabled her to become pregnant. This technique cannot be wrong!"[85]

8. *Ku-chin i-t'ung ta-ch'üan*
(Comprehensive System of Medicine of All Times)
Compiled around 1556 by Hsü Ch'un-fu

8.1. The Origins of Illnesses (Ping chih suo yu)

Illnesses have many causes, yet they are all related to [something] evil; evil is the ultimate cause [of all illnesses]. This is to say that everything that is not a part of the normal order in the human body, that is, wind, cold, heat, dampness, hunger, surfeit, exhaustion, and idleness, is evil and not solely the influences of spirits and epidemics, [as some authorities claim].

Just as the fish in water, man lives surrounded by influences. If the water is turbid, the fish waste away; if the influences are irregular, man falls ill. The most severe harm to man is caused by evil influences. These influences are absorbed by the transportation channels, which transport them into the depots and palaces. Here, as a result of [already existing] depletion or repletion, or as a consequence of [irregular] heat or cold, [the evil influences may] accumulate and illnesses develop. These illnesses, in turn, may cause additional illnesses, which then spread in all directions [throughout the body].

Essence and spirit are present in the body from its very inception; [the body] constitutes the material manifestation [of essence and the spirit]. When the body assimilates evil influences, essence and spirit will also be confused. When the spirit is confused, demons and foreign spirits are able to enter the body. If [in such a situation the intruding] demons are quite strong, while the ability of [one's own] spirit to protect [the body] decreases continuously, how is it then possible to avoid death?

In ancient times men compared this process to the planting of a willow tree: the underlying principle is precisely the same.[86]

There are some illnesses, however, whose primary cause is the action of demons and alien spirits. Prayers are suitable for expelling these [creatures]. Li Tzu-yü with his red pills, however, offers an example where the possibility of an exorcism was discussed, but where successful therapy was the result of using drugs.[87] An example of a case where drugs were ineffective and exorcism impossible is the *kao-huang* illness of Duke Ching of Chin.[88]

In general, we may conclude that injuries caused by spirits and demons are diverse, and some of the various causes of illness may be regarded as minor, while some are serious. [Quotation from the] *San-shuo pen-ts'ao.*[89]

8.2. On Injuries Caused by Evil (Hsieh-sui hsü-lun)

In the *Nei-ching* it is written: when evil is present in abundance, repletions occur. If the correct influences are dissipated, depletions arise. Thus the so-called evil discussed in the scripture concerns such excess evil as wind, cold, heat, warmth, dryness, and fire, but not— as is generally claimed—demonic or spectral apparitions![90]

When someone is afflicted by a depletion [of correct influences] in the heart and therefore is tormented by fear and anxiety, the symptoms may resemble drunkenness, madness, or even demonic possession. Or someone [suffers from a] repletion in the yang-brilliance [conduit] and climbs to high elevations or sings, tears off his clothing, and runs away. Such repletions are always caused by phlegm and fire [in the organism], and are never a result of disturbances engendered by an injury from some strange evil. In ancient times exorcisms were a specialty, as were the [Buddhist] invocation techniques of Nāgārjuna, but these were techniques for treating the loss of [the body's] essence and for the transformation of influences.[91] The same therapy, however, can also be used to eliminate doubts and rectify delusions, thereby causing the senses and the mind to return to a correct [condition]. But how could these [techniques] be used to eliminate injuries caused by evil?[92]

8.3. All Injuries Caused by Evil Originate in the Senses
   (Hsieh-sui chieh tzu hsin sheng)

In mountain valleys and in dark and obscure places, there are either demons, spirits, elves, or fox-specters. Even among fowl and dogs who have been with humans many years, occasionally a spook may occur!

Although it is then claimed that these apparitions are able to confuse the mind, it appears that this is nothing other than that some people have come close to a condition of depletion of their [body] influences and blood and in which their correct influences have been weakened. When the correct influences have been weakened, evil [influences seize control] of the senses, and when evil [influences have taken control of the] senses, the victim begins to hear, see, and speak nonsense and races madly to and fro. All this is "evil." It is only because [someone, whose senses have been affected by] evil perceives evil, that [the evil of demons] exists. No one in his right mind, who is free of all illness, is able to perceive [such evil]. Taking this fact into consideration, we reach the following conclusion. If one's senses are in the proper condition, one is protected from all evil. How could any doubts then remain regarding injuries caused by evil?[93]

8.4. Integrated Treatment Using Spells and Drugs (Chin-chu fu-yao chien-chih)

For the treatment of illnesses arising from the harmful effects of evil there are both spells, which eliminate all uncertainty [as to a possibly demonic origin of the affliction], and drugs, which require a careful investigation of depletions and surpluses, an examination of phlegm and fire [in the organism], as well as a consideration of the severity [of the individual case]. When both therapeutic approaches are combined, inner and outer [elements] are unified, and a rapid recovery from the illness is assured.

He who consults only a shaman and utilizes no drugs of any kind shall not recover from his illness, for there is no underlying principle to bring about the cure. He who takes only drugs and does not consult a shaman to eliminate all uncertainty, shall be cured, but the recovery will be slow. Therefore both inner and outer elements must be treated simultaneously, as this will produce a rapid success. This is the justification for the introduction of the "exorcism of the cause" [chu-yu].[94]

Drug prescriptions.

Boiled potion for the correction of the senses. The prescription is contained in the section "[Impairment of] the senses by wind." Cures injuries caused by evil, demonic visions, and unconsciousness.

Storax pills. The prescription is found in the section "Wind."
   Heals any illness arising from evil.
Tan-preparation,[95] which returns the hun-soul.
   Prevents unexpected death caused by being struck by the
   malevolent.
Ephedra [herb], three *ch'ien*, Cassia-twigs, two ch'ien, apricot, 12
   kernels; to be boiled in water, force [the patient] to drink. He
   will then come back to life.
Li Tzu-yü's red pills with eight effective ingredients.
   Heals demonic possession and all injuries caused by evil. Taking
   these pills brings immediate relief.
Realgar, cinnabar, arsenic, roasted aconite roots, black hellebore,
   tree peony, and croton seed, one *liang* of each; centipede, one
   animal.

Pulverize all ingredients and heat together with honey; form into
pills the size of small beans. Take five or seven pills; the time of day
is unimportant. Swallow [the pills] with cold water.

In the *Wei-sheng pao-chien*[96] it is written: The Vice-Consul Hsü
K'o-tao came to Hsiung-chou and requested that I examine his pulse.
I examined the pulse and determined that the beat was alternately
strong, weak, prolonged, and brief. This indicated that the blood and
influences had been disturbed and that an evil influence had injured
the proper [influence]. The official told me that he had spent the night
in the government hostel in Han-tan, where a woman in a virid robe
had appeared to him in a dream; he had been unable to recognize her
face and eyes, and with her hand she had delivered a blow to his ribs.
A pain subsequently developed at this spot and did not subside. At
the same time, he began to suffer from hot and cold fits and was
unable to eat. [He concluded that] he had been attacked by a demon.
I told the man: "For this affliction take the red pills with the eight
potent ingredients." The official had already read the Records of Renowned Medical Men and thus knew that, according to Li Tzu-yü,
the red pills with eight potent ingredients were used to kill demons.
He therefore entrusted himself to my care, and I gave him three of
these pills, which he took upon retiring for the night. On the next
morning he discharged two *tou* of clear water and the treatment was
successful.[97]
   In the autumn of the year *wu-wu*, I encountered a woman of thirty
in an inn in Hang-ch'eng. She had burned incense in a temple and

had become too warm. While underway, she had then drunk a bowl
of cold water. Upon her return, her abdomen began to swell, and she
was unable to eat. Gradually, her mind grew confused and she suffered
from sensations of oppression. The condition became so grave that
she began to speak incoherently and to suffer from hallucinations. All
agreed that she was possessed by evil! Shamans carried out their prayers but without success. On my belt I carried with me the red pills
with the eight potent ingredients, from which I gave the woman seven.
After [taking these] she passed an entire vessel of black fluid, grew
noticeably weaker, and lay down to sleep, without having uttered a
single word. She later took one dose of Master Shih-chün's boiled
potion and was healed.[98]

9. *Chang-shih lei-ching* (The Scripture, Arranged According
    to Topics by Mr. Chang)
    Written in the seventeenth century
AUTHOR: Chang Chieh-pin (ca. 1624)

9.1. Commentary of Chang Chieh-pin on Statements in the
    Huang-ti nei-ching Pertaining to the Techniques "Exorcism of
    the Causes" (*chu-yu*)[99]

"Exorcism of the causes" refers to techniques of inscribing an amulet,
invocation, casting of spells and sacrificial rites. But how can amulets
and invocations be employed [for illnesses] that are not caused by
demons and spirits? This is why the following is recorded in the section
"Destroyer-Wind" ["Tsei-feng" of the *Huang-ti nei-ching ling-shu*]:
The Emperor spoke: "When someone suddenly falls ill, without having
been struck by evil influences and without having been frightened,
what is the reason for this? Is this not a condition that is due solely
to [the actions of] demons and spirits?" Ch'i Po replied to this: "This,
too, is the result of evil [influences], but of those that slumbered [in
the body] and had not yet manifested themselves. When the mind
loathes or desires something, this causes unrest in the blood and body
influences, and they turn against each other.[100] The cause of such
affliction is very subtle. If one tries to observe it, he will recognize
nothing; if one tries to hear it, he will perceive nothing. Demons and
spirits therefore appear to be responsible." The Emperor then asked
the following: "But how, then, is it possible for an invocation to

provide a cure [in such cases]?" Ch'i Po replied: "The wu shamans in ancient times knew how one is overcome by all illnesses. Thus, once they knew the origin of an illness, they needed only to perform an invocation and a cure was effected."[101]

These words illustrate the general meaning of "exorcism of the cause" and "demons and spirits." I would now like to elucidate the sense [of these statements] in detail. When it is stated above that "demons and spirits appear to be responsible," this means that this appears to be the case, but in fact is not connected [with demons or spirits] at all. When it is stated above that "when the mind loathes or desires something," this means that the demons are [an illusion] created by the mind. When it is written that "the [wu shamans] knew how one is overcome by all illnesses; once they knew the origin of an illness, they needed only to perform an invocation and a cure was effected," this means that they discovered the cause of the illness in question and then expelled the demon from the senses.

How, then, were they able to accomplish this? All seven emotions of man spring from either affection or aversion. If affection or aversion is one-sided, this leads to disruptions among the [body's] influences. Such imbalances cause [some influences] to be suppressed while others gain the upper hand. This, in turn, confuses the spirit and the senses. But disharmony in the spirit and senses allows evil to penetrate and establish itself. As a consequence, demons are created in one's mind. Thus when someone desires something, he will be able to see only the object of this desire. When someone has only doubts about something, then he will be able to see only the object of his uncertainty. When someone has a fear of something, he will see only the object of this fear. This situation not only manifests itself in illnesses but also leads to visions in dreams. This is [the significance of the statement of Ch'i Po above]: "when the mind despises or desires something, this upsets the equilibrium of blood and influences within the body. It therefore appears that demons and spirits are responsible."

When the spirit and influences are not protected, evil is able to enter the body. Thus it is written, for example, in the "Directions for Restoring Losses by Means of Acupuncture," that when someone suffers from a depletion, he loses his spirit, for it has not been preserved; this enables evil demons to attack the body from outside. When someone falls ill from a depletion in the liver and then encounters a seasonally insufficient development of ceasing-*yin* influences, he is attacked by the white corpse-demons. When a person falls ill from a depletion in the heart and then encounters an insufficient development of the two fire-influences in the seasonal progression, he is attacked by black corpse-demons. When a person falls ill from a depletion in the spleen and is then afflicted with an insufficient development of great-yin influences in the seasonal progression, he will be attacked by virid corpse-demons. When a person suffers from a depletion in the lung and then encounters an insufficient development of yang-brilliance influences in the seasonal progression, he will be attacked by red corpse-demons. When a person suffers from a depletion in the kidneys and then encounters an insufficient development of great-yang influences in the seasonal progression, he will be attacked by yellow corpse-demons. Not only the attacks of corpse-demons but the attacks of all kinds of evil result from the fact that the spirit has lost its protected position. In other words, when a depletion occurs among the proper influences, enabling evil to seize control [of the conduits and depots normally filled by these proper influences], this allows the five demons to arise. This is the significance of the words [of Ch'i Po]: "This, too, is due to evil [influences]," and also of his remark "they knew how one is overcome by all illnesses."

Furthermore, in *Kuan Yin-tzu* it is stated: "Should the heart harbor thoughts of fortune and misfortune, the demon of magic power shall seize control. Should the heart harbor thoughts of man or woman, it shall fall to the demon of lust. Should the heart harbor thoughts of darkness or fear, it shall fall to the demon of the depths. Should the heart harbor thoughts of release or retreat, it shall fall to the demon of madness. Should the heart harbor thoughts of oaths and curses, it shall fall to the demon of strangeness.[102] Should the heart harbor thoughts of drugs and diet, it shall fall to the demon of the material." Thus, when the heart concentrates on something, the spirit has something which it reveres. When this reverence is inappropriate, evil demons arise. This is what is meant by the above statement: "understand first of all the origin of an illness."

After first having recognized in this manner the origin, there are then specific techniques for the treatment [of each illness]. One must therefore seek to understand what [the patient] abhors, what he desires, which [of these two emotions] has gained the upper hand, and how this situation occurred. When an invocation is then performed, it shall be successful in every case. The following case illustrates this.

Wang Chung-yang once treated a woman who had gone mad because she suspected her husband had a lover. The taking of drugs brought little improvement. Finally, [Wang Chung-yang came to the conclusion that the woman] was incurable with this kind [of a treat-ment]. Secretly, he requested that someone, so as to be overheard [by the patient], say that the lover had died and what a misfortune this was. The woman [heard these words and] thereupon experienced great joy and was cured. [Wang Chung-yang] is no wu-shaman, but it can be said that he adopted the methods [of the shamans] in order to eliminate the source of this [patient's] aversion.

Another example: Han Shih-liang had been treating a woman who, as a child, had lived with her mother in a relationship of great mutual affection. She had later married and the mother had died. [The young woman] subsequently thought frequently [of her mother] and fell ill. Numerous drugs remained completely without effect. Han [Shih-liang] spoke: "[The woman is] ill because she thinks constantly [of her mother]; it is therefore difficult to cure her with drugs. One must utilize the art [of the *wu*-shamans] in order to treat her." He then paid a wu-priestess and instructed her confidentially what she was to say. One day the husband said to his wife: "I wonder whether that [woman] under the earth thinks of you in the same way [as you of her]. I have to go somewhere else; you should consult a *wu*-priestess who will perform a divination for you!" The woman gladly agreed to this and then consulted the wu-priestess. After the woman arrived, [the en-chantress] burned incense, prayed, and invoked the spirit of the mother to descend. The spirit spoke for a time and was silent for a time, so that it was as if the mother was still among the living. The young woman thereupon began to cry bitterly, but the mother reproached her, saying: "Stop crying! Your life destroyed my own! I therefore had to die. My death is your work alone! Now I inhabit the underworld and wish to achieve retribution for this hostility. That you have fallen ill is indeed my doing! When I still lived, my relationship with you was that of mother and child. Now that I am dead, I am your ruthless enemy!" Thereupon a violent anger erupted in the young woman and she replied: "It is because of my mother, then, that I fell ill! My mother was the source of my injury. What pleasure can there be for me to continue to think of her!" From this moment, her illness was healed.

It can be said that this is a case of eliminating that which was loved. In the section "Yin yang ying-hsiang ta-lun" [of the *Huang-ti nei-ching su-wen*] it is recorded: "Anger harms the liver. Compassion overcomes anger. Joy harms the heart. Fear overcomes joy. Remembrance harms the spleen. Anger overcomes remembrance. Grief harms the lung. Joy overcomes grief. Fear harms the kidneys. Remembrance overcomes fear." This fact—that some emotions overcome others—constitutes the basis of the technique of establishing which emotions overcome prevailing ones, so that the latter can be brought under control. . . .

A further example: I myself was once treating a young bride. A hot evil had seized her stomach, giving the impression that she was possessed by demons and spirits. She flailed about with her arms, cursed, was easily frightened, and out of her senses. Her entire family was deeply concerned and wished to consult a wu-shaman for treatment. I was asked for my view and I said to them that such a step was unnecessary, that I could help the woman. I then had myself announced by a herald in a loud voice, so that her influences could first be calmed. I then made my sudden entrance in highly elegant attire. The woman's garments were threadbare and she treated me with no respect. We stared at each other, and I adopted a furious countenance in order to subdue her. After gazing upon her for a long period, I noticed how she began to blush and grow modest. All of a sudden she desired to conceal herself. I then directed someone to bind her, and she, in a desolate mood, no longer tried to leave. I then administered to her one dose of white-tiger potion, and all evil [influences] retreated. In this way I was able to overcome her neglected condition through dignity and to overcome her evil fire by means of a cold and cooling [medication].

A further example: I once was treating a Confucian. Because he had suffered an injury caused by cold, his two depots of metal and water were unable to fulfill their functions sufficiently. One day at noon, he suddenly said to me with a great sigh: "For my entire life I have continually cultivated Confucianism. Never have I done harm to anyone. Why, then, has this white-haired old man, clothed in white mourning and carrying a fan, suddenly appeared. He has been watching me for three days now and has not left. I suspect that his appearance is connected with some sort of grievance. What is the meaning of this?" I laughed and told him: "He is probably holding in his hands a fan made of white paper!" Frightened, he replied, "So you see him as well?" I replied that this was not the case, and then elucidated to him the meaning of the "Discussion of the Techniques of Acupuncture"[103] [of the *Huang-ti nei-ching su-wen*], which concerns the attack of the five demons from outside when the human spirit loses its protection. I then explained: "Since a deficiency of influences is present in your lungs, white flowers [arise] frequently in your eyes. Therefore you perceive white demons. When there is an insufficiency of water in the kidneys, black flowers frequently [arise] in the eyes, and you consequently perceive black demons. The cause of this is always that the correct influences are not present in sufficient quantities, and that the spirit as well as the *hun*-soul therefore do not remain bound in the body. One then perceives outside the color of the affected depot. What grievance could possibly be involved here?" The man was overjoyed at my words and exclaimed: "It is so! That was a miraculous explanation. There is indeed a black demon beside my bed. Although there is no fear of him in my heart, only a great aversion, I could not bring myself to speak of it. Today I have received your instructions and can therefore now undertake to disperse these [apparitions]." The man then took a drug combination that influenced the depots of both the metal and the water and was healed.

These were examples of how an illness, once the origin is understood, can be relieved with just a few words. In all these cases the demons were a product of the senses [literally: the heart]; but in reality, the effects were totally unrelated to the actions of demons or spirits. Therefore, [in the words of Ch'i Po] cited above: "Demons and spirits appear to be responsible." Since these demons have established themselves in the senses, it is extremely difficult to achieve any results with plant or mineral drugs. Only an exorcism of the cause is effective in such cases. Thus experts in the exorcism of the cause, using the words of Ch'i Po, are able to carry out their miracles. None of their successes remains disregarded, and each application of their art reveals a supranatural power. Is it therefore any wonder, that they are regarded as one of the thirteen specialties of medicine?[104]

10. *Shih-shih mi-lu*
   (Secret Records from the Mountain Cavern)
   Written in the seventeenth century
AUTHOR: Ch'en Shih-to (ca. 1687)

10.1. Direct Therapy (Cheng-i fa) (excerpt)

Ch'i, the Celestial Master, spoke the following words: Whenever a person suffers greatly from ascending air and coughing, it is due to a lung illness. The lung is the depot of metal; it is also the depot of beauty and is located above the heart. Its structure resembles that of the lotus blossom. It is red and surrounded by a purple ring. The lung conduit leads downward from the throat, controlling the entrance and exit of the [breath-]influences while permitting no food to pass. At the upper end of the throat is the stomach flap, which resembles a small tongue. The stomach flap seals the opening to the throat. Food is then able to enter the esophagus directly and travels down into the stomach. If a person talks too much, however, while eating or drinking, the stomach flap does not seal completely and thus rice, for example, can enter the air passage. This inevitably leads to an incessant coughing fit. From this we can see that the air passage does not admit any matter and, consequently, drugs are unable to enter directly. It is therefore extremely difficult to treat the lung by means of direct therapy. A [medicinal] therapy must thus proceed indirectly through the spleen. When the influences that are transmitted from the spleen are filled, the soil will engender metal from itself, and the coughing will cease.

With the exception of the conduit leading to the lung, all five depots can be treated directly. Only the lung conduit cannot be utilized for direct therapy. When, however, an ulcer develops in the lung conduit, what therapy is then possible? Boil one *liang yüan-shen*, one *liang* fresh *kan-ts'ao*, eight *liang chin-yin-hua*, and one *liang tang-kuei* in water and then consume this [medication]. Following this, take one *liang mai-teng*. Among all these ingredients, only *mai-teng* cleanses the fire in the lungs. All of the remaining drugs enter the spleen, the liver, and the heart. Why, then, are these substances used at all? When they penetrate the liver, they then smooth the wood there, and, consequently, the metal knife of the lung need not act to cut [the wood]. As a result, metal in the lung is given the opportunity to restore and replenish itself. When [these drugs] enter the spleen, the soil of the spleen can engender additional metal of the lung, thereby also leading to a restoration of metal in the lung. When [these drugs] penetrate into the heart conduit, the fire of the heart will not consume the metal of the lung, thereby assisting the metal of the lung to replenish itself. Although the indicated drugs are means for treating the heart, spleen, and liver, and although it thus appears that they are techniques that are once, twice, and three times removed,[105] they are, in reality, a direct therapy of the metal of the lung.

Chang Chung-ching, the supervisor from Ch'ang-sha, spoke the following words: It is indeed the case that the metal of the lung is the repository of beauty; this depot is unable to assimilate matter of any kind. Only [breath-]influences are absorbed here. There once lived a man who had long suffered from a cough that seemed to continue without end. He took many kinds of lung-strengthening drugs to restore his lung, but all were without effect. It was only with the method of the Celestial Master Ch'i that a cure was effected.

If, however, drug potions are taken without [breath-]influences also passing through the throat entrance, it will be extremely difficult to achieve a prompt cure of lung illness. In such cases, the method requires that a thirteen-year-old girl exhale her [breath-]influences so that [the victim] can inhale them. Each day, at the time of the fifth watch of the night, instruct the girl to exhale with her entire strength her [breath-]influences from below the diaphragm into the mouth of the victim. The girl should then move away [from the patient]. It is forbidden that an embrace occur, for it might lead to a stimulation of mutual emotions. The [breath-]influences should be expelled once daily in this manner. If drugs are then taken in addition to this, the result will be successful. Great care must be taken to prevent the least stirring of passions at the moment of exhalation of the [breath-]influences. Otherwise, not only will the result be of no benefit, but it is possible that there might be actual harm! Only one or two mouthfuls are required, as there is the danger that the girl herself will be stricken.[106]

10.2. Reverse Therapy (Ni-i fa) (excerpt)

The Celestial Master spoke the following: There are many symptoms that indicate [influences in the body] are flowing in the false direction; sudden mental disturbances are only one example of many. When, for instance, a person's [breath-]influences gasp and ascend, this is the result of reversed [influences]. One may then suspect a repletion of influences, without knowing that the supposed repletion is in reality to be viewed as a depletion of influences. An excess should be perceived as the insufficient [presence of influences].

When, for example, a repletion of influences in the lung is falsely diagnosed, and *su-yeh, chieh-keng, pai-pu,* and *shan-tou-ken* are mistakenly administered, life is endangered. Instead, a boiled potion of one *liang* ginseng, three *ch'ien niu-hsi,* five *ch'ien shou-ti,* four *ch'ien shan-chu-yü,* one *ch'ien kou-ch'i-tzu,* five *ch'ien mai-teng,* one *ch'ien pei-wu-wei,* five walnuts, and five slices of fresh ginger should be taken. The [drugs in this] prescription do not enter the conduit leading to the lung, and yet they are suited for therapy. Influences are engendered by man in the lung. At night, while he sleeps, [these influences] withdraw into the kidneys. This corresponds to the refuge that a mother finds in the dwelling of her son. Suppose that as a result of excessive sexual lust, a great exhaustion of the water of the kidneys has occurred. It is only natural that the metal of the lung will then strive to create this [water] anew. If [the exhaustion of the water of the kidneys] extends over a long period of time, [the metal of the lung is eventually] no longer able to maintain [the continuing production of new water]. Consequently, both the water of the kidneys as well as the metal of the lung are exhausted. An illustration of this is a family with a wasteful son who spends one thousand pieces of gold each day. His mother gives to the son something from her own savings each day. Gradually her own pockets and purses are depleted. If she continues to give away in this fashion, both the son as well as the mother will become impoverished. How, then, can the demands made by others be met? When threats are made by others, [the mother] will flee to her son's dwelling to escape her tormenters. But even in the house of the son there is nothing for the mother, and she must once again seek another refuge to avoid the shame of [unfulfilled] demands from others. Under such lamentable circumstances, death will eventually offer the sole escape. In our case, the water of the kidneys was exhausted and the metal of the lung already affected by deficiency. Injury from outside was inflicted by the fire of the heart and attacks by the wood of the liver. Even the soil of the spleen was unable to assist by producing water. [The few remaining water-influences] start moving here and there and it is difficult to keep them stored. When, as a result of such conditions, the influences begin to ascend in a gasping manner contrary to their normal flow, death might be avoided solely because, fortunately, a strand of original yang [influences] has not yet been severed. It is now imperative to assist the kidneys with a large contribution as quickly as possible and induce the destitute son to accept this [gift]. For how else could the metal of the lung replenish itself. In addition, not only will the house of the mother grow prosperous through the sudden wealth of the son, but the creditors shall no longer venture to continue their insults. Thus, the lung itself has not been treated, and yet it was a proper treatment of the lung.

Someone may still harbor doubts and maintain that for restoring the [influences in the] kidneys only a small amount of ginseng should be used, since ginseng is a drug for the lung and spleen. But such a person would probably not know that during a severe lack of water in the kidneys there is suddenly a point where the vital life-[influences] can no longer be retained. If the influences of the [kidneys] are not replenished immediately at this time, the final thread of the original yang [influences] shall itself tear. Moreover, when only a small amount of ginseng is used, [the effect] remains superficial. Only in large doses does [the drug] penetrate downward into the body. Approximately one liang is the most effective amount. In this manner one can ensure that [the drug] reaches the point of origin of the illness and replenishes influences here, so that water for the kidneys is once again produced.

The other drugs in this prescription, such as *shou-ti* and *shan-chu-yü*, transmit all similar influences and support one another in directly entering the Gate of Life. How could [a person] ever suffer from an excess [of these drugs]! Those victims who are severely ill must increase [the amount of medication]. For them, even one *liang* would be too little! It should be noted, however, that there are different kinds of coughing fits. Some are due to a depletion, others to an excess. Acute coughing often results from an excess of evil [influences]. When someone suffers from chronic coughing, the cause is frequently a lack of influences. If someone coughs because he has absorbed an excess of evil [influences], it will lead to a raising of the eyebrows. If, however, a depletion of influences has occurred, exhalation will be rapid, but in very small amounts. In my discussion I have been concerned with chronic coughing. For acute coughing, simply give the patient one dose of *ssu-mo* or *ssu-ch'i* potion and [the attacks] shall cease immediately.[107]

These illnesses are therefore a result of [influences] flowing [in the direction opposite to their normal passage]; through the use of drugs, a reversal of this flow is achieved.[108]

11. *Hsü Ling-t'ai i-shu ch'üan-chi*
   (Complete Medical Works of Hsü Ling-t'ai)
   Compiled in the eighteenth century by Hsü Ta-ch'un
   (1693–1771)

11.1. On Illnesses Caused By Demons and Spirits (Ping yu kuei shen lun), from *On the Origin and Development of Medicine (I-hsüeh yüan liu lun)*

For a person to absorb something evil, there must be a place [in the body] where this assimilation can occur. If [the evil] has been engendered by a specific condition, it corresponds [to this call] and establishes itself at this [location].

If a person's essence and spirit are firmly established, no evil outside of [the body] will venture an assault. But whenever that which protects [essence and spirit] fails, the harmful agents will collect in its place. Whenever illnesses were caused by demons and spirits, the uneducated claim that demons and spirits truly possess the ability to bring misfortune to man. Educated persons, however, maintain that although the specific characteristics of some illnesses may give the impression, demons and spirits, in reality, do not exist. Both of these views are false. Demons and spirits are evil [forces] similar to wind, cold, summer heat, and dampness. Whenever there is a depletion of defensive influences, [the body] then absorbs cold. When there is a lack of constructive influences, [the body] will absorb heat. If there is a depletion of influences of the spirit, [the body] then absorbs demons. The [human] spirit, of course, belongs to the yang category. When the yang [influences] have been depleted, demons take control of them. The *Nei-ching* speaks of the illnesses of the five depots and the demons that appear in the corresponding five colors. In the *Nan-ching*[109] it is recorded that he who loses yang [influences] shall see demons. Thus, among the openings of the conduits, for instance, are the "demon bed" and the "demon chamber." In all cases, one must rely on influences of the spirit to fill and seal these openings. If, however, the influences of the spirit fail, demons and [alien] spirits seize control of these [openings]. This resembles the injuries to man that are caused by wind and cold. Therefore, in treating a cold [injury], it is necessary to replenish the yang [influences]; in treating a heat [injury], it is necessary to replenish the yin [influences]. In treating [an injury caused by] demons, one need only strengthen the spirit [of the victim]. Since fluid, rumination, or fear can also cause [depletion of the spirit] in such cases, one must first investigate such a possibility before undertaking any therapy.

Scholars aware of [these] principles must therefore make every effort to discover the cause [of an injury due to demons and spirits]. Only this will remove all doubts and produce concrete results. Otherwise, one remains bound to a one-sided view that only obscures the underlying principles, producing only utter confusion.

Other than the [possibilities] already mentioned, there are also illnesses that result [directly] from an attack by demons and [alien] spirits. In such cases prayers are effective. In addition, there are also numerous demons that arise from deceased persons who have suffered an unavenged wrong. It also occurs that someone himself commits a transgression, thus provoking a bitter, inextinguishable hostility. There are some cases involving an ancestor, or even where [demons have] falsely caused harm to some person. Irrefutable evidence exists for all these occurrences. It appears that the Confucians had no understanding for such things. But examples in ancient scriptures and historical writing, like Kung-tzu P'eng and Sheng-po, are plentiful. Not a few of them I witnessed with my own eyes. Such [attacks] cannot be averted with drugs, stones, or prayers.[110]

11.2. Illnesses Resulting from [Demon-Caused] Injuries (Sui-ping), from *Medical Cases of Hui-hsi* (*Hui-hsi i-an*)[111]

Old Mr. Chu Yüan-liang, who was originally a neighbor of mine, was once staying in the prefectual city. At the beginning of the year, the widow of his nephew set out to visit her uncle there. While passing the Lou Gate in a boat, she saw on the city wall the temple of the Serpent King, of which it was commonly believed that burning incense there would prevent the formation of ulcers and swellings. For this reason she then visited the temple. Upon her return, she had gone mad, speaking deliriously. Her tongue moved like that of a snake, and she reported that the Serpent King had sent one male and two female slaves to receive her. I was asked to examine the woman and establish a diagnosis. I thereupon gave to an old woman one of the "pills of supreme value," so that she, in turn, could present it to the patient. The sick woman declared that the pill was poisonous and refused to take it under any circumstances. She took the pill into her mouth and then spit it out at the old woman. The old woman immediately fell to the ground; she was unable to recognize anyone; she stuck her tongue far out of her mouth and twisted her head back and forth. She resembled a snake. I then bid someone else to give the medication [to the victim] until it had been entirely consumed. The patient then stated that a female servant had been consumed by flames, and all of the demons had stoked the fire with cinnabar. The next day I prepared medication with the drug "demon-arrow-feathers." [After taking this,] the patient reported that a manservant had been killed by an arrow; demons had used the "demon-arrows" as a weapon. Thereupon she gradually grew calm, and I was able to harmonize her with expectorants and other means to soothe her spirit. After approximately one month, she was healed. Her illness belonged to the group of possession by a guest-[demon]. Successful therapy in such cases is possible only with minerals and those drugs that are effective against demons.[112]

11.3. Demon-Caused Pregnancies (Kuei-t'ai men), from *Medical Cases from Gynecology* (*Nü-k'o i-an*)

In a woman of more than thirty years, the monthly flow had been interrupted for eight or nine months. Her abdomen had slowly swollen day by day. The color of her face alternated between virid and yellow. She took medication for pregnancy complaints, but they provided no relief. I examined the woman. Her pulse was irregular and the face virid. She suffered from alternating hot and cold spells. This indicated an illness of the liver and gall bladder. Her face then turned yellow and her abdomen became greatly extended. She was greatly fatigued and refused all nourishment. This could indicate an illness of the spleen and stomach. This case, however, was not a true pregnancy. Depression had damaged the spleen and liver; the gall bladder and stomach were unable to transform [foods] into clear influences. A demon had [taken advantage of this condition] and harmed the woman, an illness called "demon pregnancy." I boiled a drug to restore the functions of the spleen together with a soothing tea, and had the patient swallow three *ch'ien* "demon-killing pills" with it. Thereupon [the woman] discharged a great amount of blood and turbid water, in which I discovered an afterbirth. The afterbirth contained a bloody clump that closely resembled a demon. I have related this incident here to make such unusual occurrences better known.[113]

12. *Tzu-jan pien-cheng fa* (Nature-Dialectic). Journal of the Shanghai People's Publishing House, four volumes, 1973–1976.

12.1. The Struggle for and against a Belief in Fate in the Medicine of Our Land (Wo-kuo i-hsüeh-shang fan-t'ien-ming yü tsun-t'ien-ming ti tou-cheng)
AUTHOR: Historical Museum for Medicine of the Shanghai Academy of Chinese Medicine

From their long experience in the struggle against disease, our workers in antiquity created our fatherland's medicine and pharmacy which are unique in the entire world. The history of the genesis and development of our fatherland's medical and pharmaceutical teachings did not proceed without complications. The reform-minded and progressive political course, as well as the materialist view of nature of the Legalists, spurred on the development of the medicine of our fatherland, while the reactionary political line and the idealistic fate concept of the Confucians inhibited the progress of the medicine of our fatherland. Therefore, it is now of paramount importance to enlist the pointed and keen weapon of Marxism to eradicate the inherited venom of the principles of Confucius and Mencius and analyze, using the proper approach and techniques, both the progressive tendencies and the restrictions that Legalist thought exerted on medical history, so that we may critically adopt our native medical tradition and pursue the integration of Chinese and Western medicine as well as the further development of the medicine of our land!

Illness or Fate

How is it possible that illnesses arise in men? In response to this question two different courses of understanding evolved over the course of history. The Confucians and the Legalists found themselves diametrically opposed in their approach to this problem as well.

The members of primitive society were not yet able to understand diseases properly. Frequently, they attributed the causes of illness to metaphysical principles. As Lenin stated, primitive peoples, who did not yet possess the power to undertake the struggle with natural forces, inevitably had to develop "a belief in a god, demons, and unusual phenomena" (*Socialism and Religion*). Following the rise of a slave society, the class of slaveholders systematized the primitive superstitious notions of demons and spirits, making them the intellectual cornerstones of their efforts to deceive the slave majority while maintaining their own reactionary dominance. They propagated the view that man's birth, aging, illness, and death were, from beginning to end, "divinely ordered" with "divine significance," and that the origin of disease was a punishment inflicted upon man by heaven, demons, or spirits. In some records that reflect conditions prevailing in the slave society, the question of why a person is stricken with an illness, harmed, survives, or succumbs, is consistently explained as the consequence of decisions deriving from the impenetrable mysteries of heaven. Should fate determine that someone is to live, spirits and mountain hermits were able to raise the individual, even though he had already succumbed, and restore him to the world of the living; if fate decreed that someone must die, spirits and mountain hermits led the victim away, even though he was in full possession of his powers, vital spirit, and ethereal soul.

Toward the end of the spring and autumn period, the spokesman of the declining class of slaveholders, the second-born son of the family K'ung,[114] made the fate concept the theoretical foundation with which he hoped to advance the reactionary course of "self-transcendence and the reestablishment of morality." The works of the second-born son of the family K'ung represent the ultimate development of the fate concept in the slave society of the Yin and Chou periods. From legends [recounting] the mysterious metamorphoses of celestial spirits and men as well, he invented a heaven that determined all existence on heaven and earth, the god on high [shang-ti]. He maintained that the "death and life [of all existence] was the result of fate; happiness and wealth are determined in heaven." Birth, aging, illness, and death are "fixed by celestial destiny"; man has no choice but "to fear divine fate" and willingly submit to the directives of the venerable father in heaven. When his disciple Po-niu fell ill, the second-born son of the family K'ung pulled his hand through a window and lamented helplessly: "You must soon die; your fate wills it thus! What sorrow that a man such as you must suffer from such an affliction!"[115] This episode is revealing proof that the second-born son of the family K'ung was himself a slave who had surrendered to providence!

If, then, diseases are sent down from heaven, and if fate is predetermined by heaven, what reason would men then have to strive to understand more about illnesses and initiate the struggle against these afflictions. Does not such a perspective signify the complete rejection of all medicine? It is obvious that Confucian thought and scientific medicine are as mutually exclusive as fire and water.

But why would Confucians seek to link illness and divine fate so forcefully? Because the slaveholders have been destined by fate to be god's deputies among men. Thus when the Confucians concluded that the source of illness in the human body was "divine fate," and when they required that man passively submit to such divine intervention, their intention in reality was to illustrate that whether someone was born rich or poor, of a high or low station, and so forth, was always determined by fate, and that consequently man must obey divine dictates, seek to accept his fate, and tolerate the repressive rule of the slaveholders. All this, however, was intended to facilitate survival of the seriously threatened existence of slavery itself.

The Legalists, who reflected the interests of the newly emerging class of landed gentry, confronted the fate concept of the Confucians with a diametrically opposed materialist view of nature, channeling all of their efforts into explaining the causes of illness from a materialist perspective. The working population of antiquity had, over the course of their struggle with illness, already accumulated numerous insights, which attributed the origin of illnesses to the actions of certain objects lying outside of the human body. That numerous herbs, trees, and other plants could heal illnesses, that stones and needles provided effective therapy, and that certain cooked foods were able to relieve bodily suffering are just some of these discoveries that were also con-

nected with the struggle against disease. Even the pictographic significance of certain written characters reveals the genuine knowledge of
the ancient masses regarding illness. The character *chi*, in the term
chi-ping ["illness"] on incised oracle bones and carapaces, conveys the
sense that someone has been struck below the ribs by an arrow.[116]
The character *yung* symbolizes a resting patient who is suffering from
sores or a festering infection following some injury. The Legalists
adopted such knowledge, revealing the origin of illness to be unrelated
to divine fate. When Tzu-ch'an, a forerunner of the Legalists, revealed
to the Duke of Chin the source of his illness, he argued that it had
been due to irregularity in "eating and drinking, in joy and sorrow."[117]
Such insights are not only materialist, they also contain elements of
a primitive dialectic, for "food and drink," which lie outside of the
organism, are brought into conjunction with the emotions "joy and
sorrow," which are found within the organism. Hsün-tzu had once
said: "He who ensures that vital things are present in sufficient quantities and takes heed that corresponding efforts are made at the appropriate time will not be allowed to fall ill by heaven."[118] In other
words, when clothing and food are sufficient, and if one conducts
one's life in accordance with the demands of [daily and seasonal]
occurrences, heaven has no opportunity to allow illness to arise within
the body. Han Fei also recognized the close connection between illness
and food and drink. In discussing the epoch of primal man he declared:
"The people ate the fruits of trees and herbs, as well as oysters and
other shellfish. If [these foods] had spoiled, body and stomach were
harmed and many fell ill."[119] In discussing the era of slaveholders, he
perceptively pointed out that the tainted existence of the slaveholders,
with their insatiable and wasteful character, was the primary cause of
the "form that their illnesses took."

The ideological orientation of the Legalists thus led to the strengthening and development of the tradition of a primitive materialism,
which marks the beginnings of our native medicine. Toward the end
of the spring and autumn period, a renowned medical practitioner of
the Ch'in state, the physician Ho, introduced the theory of the "six
influences" [*liu-ch'i*] as an explanation for the causes of illness. He
had recognized that the six natural phenomena "yin, yang, wind, rain,
darkness, and light" were able to induce pathological changes that
were in accord with neither the structure nor the nature of man: "An
excess of yin [influences] leads to cold-illnesses. An excess of yang
[influences] leads to heat-illnesses. An excess of wind leads to illnesses
in the limbs. An excess of rain leads to illnesses of the body. An excess

of darkness leads to emotional illnesses. An excess of light leads to an affliction of the heart."[120] Another man, Chiao, also underlined the fact that illnesses "are caused neither by heaven nor by demons," but rather are the result of "imbalances in [the influence of the body by] cold and heat, excessive deficiencies or surpluses, hunger, surfeit, lusts, and desires, as well as disturbances of the spirit."[121]

The oldest surviving medical-theoretical work of our land, the *Nei-ching,* was written during the period of the Warring States, when the conflict between the Confucians and Legalists had reached its zenith, and exhibits an obviously pro-Legalist and anti-Confucian tendency. On the basis of an analysis of both the objective influences in the natural world as well as the changes in the human body, a discussion of illness in the *Nei-ching* concludes: "If a person is struck by evil, it is because he lacks [bodily] influences." "Wind, rain, cold, and heat are by themselves unable to harm men unless a depletion is already present. When a person is suddenly struck by a violent storm, searing heat, or heavy rain, and nonetheless is not taken ill, this is because the individual had no depletion." Thus the evil influences in the natural world and numerous other pathogenic factors can indeed generate illnesses, but when the body is totally healthy and its defensive forces are strong, it is able to repulse any onslaught of evil influences. Therefore the claim "whenever the correct influences are present in the body, evil [influences] are unable to attack" represents a direct criticism of the Confucian perspective of a divine fate.

Faith in the Medical Practitioner or in the Wu-Shaman?

The Confucians and Legalists not only possessed a different understanding of the [nature] of illness, they developed two completely opposed courses of therapy, namely faith in a wu-shaman or in a medical practitioner. Slaveholders believed that illness was determined by divine decree and that it was therefore necessary to appeal to heaven to heal such afflictions. But how is this appeal to heaven to be carried out? Only the wu-shaman, it was believed, was able to establish contact with the divine will and thereby facilitate divine mercy. Wu-shamans are parasites who emerged from the slaveholding class, devoting themselves in particular to supplication, sacrifice, and divination. Inscriptions on the oracle bones and carapaces, as well as cultural artifacts removed from the tombs dating from the Yin dynasty indicate that the wu-shaman flourished in the slave society. Whenever slaveowners were stricken with illness, they always instructed the wu-conjurers to intercede on their behalf with demons and spirits and keep watch for favorable or inauspicious portents.

The second-born son of the family K'ung was a great Confucian, but he was also a great wu-shaman. Yet even this political swindler, who claimed that he "understood divine fate" and that "heaven has bestowed upon me powers that arise from morally correct behavior," was unable, in his rashness and loud clamoring for the interests of the slaveowner class, to escape the natural laws of birth, aging, illness, and death. It was therefore inevitable that he, too, fall ill and therein lies a splendid irony of the concept of fate! Was it not so that you, the second-born son of the family K'ung, understood divine fate? If the venerable father in heaven blessed you so favorably, why, then, should he desire to punish you? There is only one explanation for this: this so-called divine fate is nothing more than unadulterated nonsense, with which one deludes both oneself and others. When the second-born son of the family K'ung finally fell ill, not only did he himself perform sacrifices and prayers, but his pupils also carried out such actions for their master day and night. But of what benefit were sacrifices and prayers? The illness worsened unabated, and the second-born son of the family K'ung could do nought but console himself with the words: "He who transgresses against heaven has no one left to whom he can turn!"[122] At another time, when the second-born son of the family K'ung had once again been stricken with illness, Chi K'ang,[123] who belongs to the reform movement, sent him medications, to which the former replied: "I do not yet understand [drugs] sufficiently and therefore cannot venture to accept your offer."[124] He feared, then, that the taking of drugs might possibly represent an even greater transgression in the eyes of the venerable Celestial Father. This true incident reveals in absolute clarity the visage of the second-born son of the family K'ung to have been polluted by a blind faith in divine fate and by a hostility toward medicine.

The Legalists required science and medicine to promote their political course, and thus propagated, in opposition to the Confucians, the concept of faith not in the wu-shaman, but in the medical practitioner. Hsün-tzu explained that all sacrifices, supplications, consultation of oracles, and all similar [forms of quackery] were nothing more than tricks intended to deceive the people, that wu-shamans had no ability to communicate with spirits and that men should not conduct their lives as slaves to a divine fate, but rather strive "to seize control of divine fate and use it for their own purposes."[125] According to Hsün-tzu, it was therefore useless to rely on wu-conjurers for treating illnesses; instead, one should turn to medical practitioners on such occasions. Hen Fei went one step further, perceptively pointing out that unquestioning belief in divine fate and the conjurations of the wu-shamans were a symptom of the approaching downfall of the political system based on slavery: "Anyone who passively waits for good fortune, serves demons and spirits, believes in prophecy, and gladly performs sacrifices, shall himself perish."[126] It is indeed the truth that belief in religion and superstition, as well as the invocation of nonhuman forces for subjugating man, revealed the corruption and impending collapse of the slaveholders and represented an early sign of their imminent end. Moreover, Han Fei unmasked the true countenance of the swindlers who roamed throughout the countryside with incantations on their lips, concluding: "Today the conjurers promise the people that their spells will assure them [a life] that will encompass a thousand autumns and ten thousand years. A thousand autumns and ten thousand years, so goes their nonsense, and yet they are incapable of adding even one day to the length of human existence. For this reason the people do not hold spells of the shamans in high esteem."[127] When the conjurers' bubbles of lies had burst and it was obvious that they were unable to prolong human life for even one day, should not the people have despised these swindlers? But the ensuing struggle involving whether one was to place faith in the wu-shamans or in medical practitioners was bitter. At the time of the Warring States, there lived a renowned physician named Pien Ch'io. His view was that "anyone who places his trust in a wu-shaman, but not in a physician,"[128] cannot be helped. For this reason, the masses welcomed Pien Ch'io without reservation, placing complete faith in him. Since the doomed slaveowner class despised him, he journeyed from place to place; he was underway day and night. First he provoked the anger of the ruler of Wei; he was then driven from Ch'i by the nobility. Finally, he reached the state of Ch'in, where the chief court physician, Li Hsi, a representative of the condemned slaveholding class, had Pien Ch'io ruthlessly murdered. "If, one day, the principles of mathematics were to damage the interests of men, or more precisely, the class interests in the class struggle, these principles shall also encounter bitter opposition" (*Lenin's Collected Works,* chap. 20, p. 194). Is the hardship that Pien Ch'io was forced to suffer not clear proof of this truth? The fields of science and technology in class society are certainly not marked by a calm wind and tranquil sea!

Evil is unable to overcome that which is correct. No matter what pressure the slaveowners exerted or what destruction they carried out, the medicine that had its roots in the rich practical experiences of the folk masses could not be destroyed. Instead, the art of the wu-shaman, which violated all objective natural laws, was unable to escape its impending collapse. The appearance of the *Nei-ching* is a consequence of the victory of medical science over wu-shamanism and underlines the fact that the theoretical system of our native medicine assumed its initial forms in this struggle. As if emblazoned upon a banner, the *Nei-ching* proclaims: "It is impossible to discuss the supreme morality with someone who believes in demons and spirits. It is impossible to discuss the utmost skills with someone who maintains an aversion to needles and stones!"[129] This aggressive message is nothing but a sharp dagger flung at the fortress of Confucianism.

The Legalists, of course, represented the attitudes of the landed class, and their struggle against witchcraft and superstition was not radical in every sense. Hsün-tzu maintained, on the one hand, that wu-shamans were swindlers, but, on the other hand, he also argued that the use of sacrificial rites and supplications for the embellishment of state business was helpful for securing control over the ignorant masses. Han Fei advocated medicine, yet at the same time he also believed that when misfortune struck, the demons were to be feared. This restriction of the Legalists regarding their class [affiliation] and historical [situation] also had a less favorable influence on medicine.

To Reform or Preserve the Old?

After the theoretical system of our native medicine had assumed its initial form, we faced the problem of just exactly how progress and further development was to be achieved: to reform or preserve the old? This question constituted the focal point of the struggle between the Legalists and Confucians in the area of medicine during the historical phase of Chinese feudalism. The conceptual center of this struggle continued to be the opposing perspectives on the notion of fate. After the Confucians had become part of feudal society, they propagated the slogan that Confucianism and medicine should "flow in unison." They developed the reckless plan of restructuring medical therapy using the trap of the fate concept, thereby preventing the further progress of our native medicine. But the Legalists and all progressive medical practitioners with Legalist leanings carried on a stubborn struggle with the declining and decaying Confucians. With all their strength they strove to advance medical science.

Tung Chung-shu[130] was the first to undertake the distortion of our native medicine on the basis of the fate concept. He repeatedly made the blunt assertion that "man's destiny is bestowed upon him by heaven" and "fate is a divine command." Whether in regard to phenomena outside of the body or to organs within, whether concerning body structure or psychological transformations such as grief or joy, he always invoked a mystical-infinite and supreme heaven for the explanation. He wrote: "the two halves heaven and earth and the dualism of yin and yang are bestowed upon the body. The body corresponds to heaven. Both are in harmony in many aspects, and thus [the body's] fate is also dependent upon [heaven]." Even the most important theories of our native medicine, which rested on the doctrines of yin/yang and the Five Phases, did not escape Tung Chung-shu's vile attempt to turn them forcibly upside down by his claim that yin/yang and the Five Phases were "a divine course" and that this divine course was eternally immutable. In this way, the elements of a primitive materialism and primitive dialectic, originally present in these two doctrines, were completely lost, constituting instead an enormous salad of idealism and metaphysics.

Wang Ch'ung, the great materialist from the early Eastern Han, got into a violent conflict with people such as Tung Chung-shu regarding the concept of fate. Wang Ch'ung was relatively close to the great masses and was deeply concerned about medicine, and he utilized medicine as a powerful weapon to oppose the notion of fate. He had come to the conviction that human life arose from finest matter and finest influences; death, he concluded, was due to the deterioration of finest matter and finest influences in the body. After finest matter and influences have passed away and the physical body has decayed into dust, he argued, where, then, were there demons and spirits? Even illnesses have material causes in his view: "Human illnesses are caused in nearly every case by wind and dampness, as well as by food and drink," and "when the blood channels develop an imbalance, man falls ill." This materialist understanding of illness stimulated the advancement of our native medicine.

Chang Chung-ching, a renowned physician of the late Eastern Han period, carried on the progressive medical tradition initiated by the forward-looking medical practitioners of the first Ch'in dynasty. He was not content with the fact that the knowledge of the current ruling class was restricted solely to superstition and wu-sorcery, and that medicine was despised, thereby exacerbating the widespread problem of epidemics. In a preface [to his work] *Shang-han tsa-ping lun* (On the Diverse Illnesses Caused by Cold), he recorded the painful observation that during the course of some ten years, the widespread epidemics had claimed two-thirds of his entire clan, which originally had numbered some 200 persons! This horrible fact convinced him that the notion of fate was a concept harmful to man. With a loud voice he therefore warned: "placing hopes in the spells of the wu-shamans" was a shameful act that "allows the will to sink and the joints to bend," producing but one conclusion—"a declaration of poverty, death, and an acceptance of defeat with bound hands." Chang Chung-ching resisted the malevolent efforts of Tung Chung-shu to reverse completely the significance of the doctrines of yin/yang and the Five Phases. Instead, he clung stubbornly to the primitive-materialist and dialectical perspective of the transformation of yin and yang. By demonstrating the truth of the medical principles of differential therapy, he integrated the theory of our native medicine with clinical practice, thereby making a significant contribution to the further advancement of the medicine of our fatherland.

But the Confucians doggedly pursued a single course of action—leading medicine astray on the search for longevity without aging. Especially after the Wei and Chin [dynasties], the Confucians, Taoists, and Buddhists entered into a reactionary alliance formed on the basis of idealism. Boasting loudly, they maintained that high in the mountains and on islands in the ocean, where spirits and mountain hermits dwelled, there existed a drug that bestowed "longevity without aging." One had only to absorb the finest rays of the sun and moon and heaven and earth, and was then capable of preparing this miraculous medicine, the cinnabar pill of the mountain hermits, utilizing a melting process. This so-called art of "long life without aging" reflected [the efforts] of the feudal ruling class to continue indefinitely their exploitation and oppression of the people; in addition, it mirrored the requirements of a wanton and shameless life and eventually reflected the widespread fashion of the time, to search for the herbs of the mountain hermits, prepare their cinnabar pills through a melting process, and then consume these pills. Among the archaeological relics from the Han, T'ang, and subsequent dynasties are large so-called po-shan-lu kilns. When empty, these ovens resemble the paradise islands of the mountain hermits as they tower up out of the ocean. When heated moderately, the water on the floor of the ovens slowly turns to steam, giving the appearance of a miragelike, misty paradise of spirits and hermits. Before these ovens the bureaucrats and landed gentry bowed down in their idleness, seeking a long life.

The folk masses and all progressive medical practitioners resisted these erroneous tendencies. Li Shih-chen was one of the great medical scientists who opposed efforts to seek out the mountain hermits and take the cinnabar pills. He fiercely criticized the doctrine that one could, by taking the wonder drug prepared from the cinnabar of the mountain hermits, achieve a long life without aging, calling such efforts "fallacious" nonsense and "beneath serious consideration and totally implausible." In this way he revealed the true countenance of those sorcerers [*fang-shih*], whose only result was that "innumerable persons," who took these [drugs], "developed severe illnesses and lost their bodies."[131] In complete contrast to those title-hungry Confucian students and the prescription-masters who were only interested in groveling for financial gain and recognition from the rulers, Li Shih-chen without prejudice sought out instructions from the peasants, boatmen, woodcutters, and hunters, and himself journeyed deep into the wilds of the mountains and into the fields. With both feet planted firmly on the soil of reality, he investigated the effects of all drugs, eventually compiling his discoveries into the world-renowned *Pen-ts'ao kang mu*. This work represented a monumental contribution to the history of medicine in our fatherland.

The Confucians claimed that the medical successes that had been achieved by the working population were simply signs of grace bestowed upon humanity by the venerable divine father through individual "sages," and that medicine must not be allowed to deviate from the therapy of the "sages" who embodied the divine intention. Thus Chu Hsi, for instance, argued that the Yellow Emperor "had received everything from heaven and therefore understood all principles under heaven and was able to regulate all matters." In this view, then, the [writing of the] *Nei-ching* represented the zenith of medicine, and no room remained for further development. This conservative approach of the Confucians concerned with maintaining prevailing conditions constituted a serious obstacle for our native medicine in its objective of eliminating the old and bringing forth the new.

The Legalists, however, did not fall victim to this trick. Shen Kua,[132] a natural scientist who enthusiastically supported the reforms proposed by Wang An-shih, used the opportunity of a discussion of medical problems to criticize severely the conservative philosophy of clinging to old regulations and outmoded doctrines. He believed that these old guidelines and traditional doctrines "by no means represented the last word [on the subject]"; rather, they must be used flexibly in conjunction with the concrete situation of each patient. In reference to the various medicinal forms, he stated that "boiled potions, powders, and pills are each appropriate in specific cases" and that it is "difficult to follow strict rules in such cases."[133] On the question of collecting drugs, Shen Kua pointed out that "according to ancient regulations, only the second and eighth months are appropriate for gathering plant drugs. This is incorrect, however," he claimed, since all herbs and trees are subject to different periods of genesis and growth, and geographic conditions vary greatly. "How is it possible to restrict activity to one specific month?"[134] From these statements it becomes evident that Shen Kua sought to transform our native medicine and pharmacy in order to correspond to new circumstances and new insights. Shen Kua himself wrote a work entitled *Liang-fang* (Effective Prescriptions). Under the influence of the reformist tendencies of the Legalists, the beginnings of a discussion on medicine finally became evident following the Northern Sung dynasty. At this time important medical personalities, who opposed conservative efforts and sought reforms, made renewed contributions to the advancement of our native medicine.

Wu Yu-k'e, who lived during the late Ming and early Ch'ing periods, was another physician who resisted the [concept of] divine fate and ventured to break new ground. He concluded correctly: "The methods of preserving old traditions no longer correspond to illnesses of the present. When one seeks guidance for present-day illnesses in the old writings, there are no words that can throw some light on the [problems of] today. For this reason the drugs are ineffectual, physicians run helplessly to and fro, the patients approach their ruin day by day, illnesses grow worse, the use of drugs is more and more chaotic, and if the affliction itself is not fatal, the actions of the physicians are."[135] This constituted a sharp criticism of the conservative thought of the Confucians. Wu Yu-k'e had observed the circumstances surrounding the epidemic of infectious diseases that took place at the end of the Ming era, studying their characteristics in great detail. He boldly pointed out that the infections were the result of contact with a particularly virulent "evil influence" present in the air and by no means due to wind, cold, dampness, or heat. He explained that infection occurred primarily through the mouth and nose, not through the skin. This insight contains the first conjecture that the cause of infectious diseases was an infection in the air. This was a decisive breakthrough for the theories inherent in our native medicine and laid the foundation for the doctrine of warmth-illnesses.

The struggle between Confucians and Legalists in the field of medicine teaches us that science in class society continues to be subject to the influences of the class struggle, and that even the scientists themselves are unable to rise above this class struggle. "No matter what approach natural scientists adopt, they are always dependent upon philosophy" (*Nature-Dialectic*). We must distinguish in the medicine of our fatherland between the clear and the turbid. If, like certain ethnonihilists, we deny the whole of our native medicine, this is nothing less than a denial of the contributions to this medicine made by the masses of the people and the Legalists and represents a gross distortion of history. It is imperative, of course, to recognize and criticize the harmful venom which the Confucians added to the medicine of our fatherland and thereby eliminate the obfuscations created by Confucian thought. But we must also differentiate among the Legalists and medical practitioners with Legalist tendencies, and although we affirm their contributions, we must also understand the limitations that grew out of their class [consciousness] and historical [situation].

Today, the tendency of medical circles to look down upon our native medicine and embrace Western medicine with blind faith is widespread and constitutes an obstacle to the further development of medicine in this land. We desire to criticize in detail those ideological trends in the realm of medicine that revere Confucian medical thought and oppose Legalism, and thereby carry on critically the tradition of our native medicine. Let us therefore carry on the fight to build China's new medicine and new pharmacy![136]

13. *Tsen-yang chan-sheng man-hsing chi-ping*
   (How to Overcome Chronic Illnesses)
   Published in 1978
AUTHOR: Tuan Chen-li

13.1. How to Recognize Illnesses of the Human Body
   (Tsen-yang jenpshih jen-t'i chi-ping) (excerpt)

The human body is an integrated whole.

Research in astronomy seeks to initiate us into the infinite expanse of space; astronomical numbers cause men to shudder and also stimulate inexhaustible fantasies within us. The recent successes of nuclear physics have opened up the microcosmos; the atom itself—which in earlier times was regarded as the most elementary of particles—is now known to contain a diverse kingdom [of particles]. The study of the human body itself, beginning with observations by the naked eye and then aided by the microscope, has since progressed to the stage of the electron microscope. The development of molecular biology, in turn, has enabled our knowledge of the human body to penetrate, for the first time, to the level of molecules.

Spaceships travel through the cosmos, venturing into the vastness of nature. The investigation of elementary particles probes into the depths of nature. The study of the human body seeks to unlock its inner secrets, helping us to conquer disease and maintain well-being. Of course in a class society all scientific research serves to further the interests of those classes that control the financial capital.

Our own native medicine and modern medicine arose and developed under two different sociohistorical conditions; both are the result of the experiences gathered by the working classes and the medical practitioners of previous generations in their struggle with disease. Although these two dissimilar medical systems exhibit significant disparities in their physiological and pathological insights, they are nonetheless in accord in their view of the human body as an integrated whole.

Our native medicine takes the view that the inner human organism contains the five depots and six palaces, the finest influences, blood, and the aqueous fluids, while the outer portion consists of the four extremities, the one hundred different bones, the five sense organs, and the nine body openings. All of these internal and external elements are then linked with one another through a system of conduits and together form an integrated whole, in which the normal activities, that is, the so-called physiological functions of the human body, proceed ceaselessly.

Modern medicine views the human organism as composed of some one hundred billion cells. Many cells together form tissue; various kinds of tissue together form an organ, while several organs in mutual dependence form a system. Inside the human body, according to this approach, are the motor system, blood system, circulatory system, respiratory system, digestive system, urinary system, reproductive system, nerve system, sensory system, and the system of inner secretions. Together, these systems constitute the human organism. [These systems,] however, are not linked mechanically but rather organically. The human organism is not a federation of individual cell-states, but rather an integral whole. This organic union is accomplished by means of the nervous and body-fluid systems. It is the mechanisms of the nerves and body fluids that make the human body into an organic, integrated whole, enabling the systems of organs to perform their respective functions.

The perception of the human body as "the simple sum of its cells" and of illnesses as "anomalous activities of locally restricted cells" is a false one, but one which is reflected in clinical therapy to such an extent that for a headache the head is treated and for foot pain the foot. In other words, one sees only individual trees while missing the forest; one sees only individual illnesses but misses the whole person. In so doing, one fails to mobilize the patient's own subjective forces for therapy.

The perception of man as an integral whole finds expression in the view that he is a whole composed of parts. These parts, in turn, reflect the whole, for the whole and the individual parts are closely linked. Every pathological deviation in one of these parts, no matter how limited the affected area or how minor the extent of this change, can influence other parts of the body by means of the nervous system and body fluids; conversely, the condition of the organism as a whole, by means of these same channels and pathways, also brings about pathological changes in individual parts of the body. Therefore each pathological transformation in any individual area must be regarded as a problem of the entire organism. Taking as an example an infection in one part, we see that it is not restricted to reddening, swelling, heat, and pain in the affected area, but is inevitably accompanied by changes in the entire body. Either through a nerve impulse or the absorption of some substance from the affected area into the bone marrow and its subsequent irritation, the marrow is stimulated to increased production, evidenced by a rise in the number of neutrophilic leucocytes. As the infection progresses, the absorption of waste products from the tissue or of the products of metabolism frequently leads to fevers of varying intensity, as well as to swelling and pain in nearby lymph glands. Heart rhythm is accelerated and the pulse grows rapid. Changes also occur in the central nervous system; the patient becomes easily agitated at the most minor irritant, and his sensitivity to pain in the affected area is increased. These changes involving the entire body become especially evident when the infection in one part of the body enters a particularly grave phase. When, conversely, the infection passes through a phase of only minor significance, these changes [in the entire body] are not particularly noticeable. Despite this, the indicated changes are nonetheless objectively present. The treatment of any illness, therefore, requires a holistic standpoint. Especially in the case of complex illnesses, it is imperative to discover the primary contradiction, investigate the situation from all angles and act accordingly, destroy the core of the illness, demonstrate the proper course of therapy using the holistic approach of dialectical materialism, sufficiently release the patient's own subjective powers, and thereby stimulate the powerful defensive capabilities that are inherent in the body of the victim himself. This is the only way to overcome an affliction quickly and thoroughly.

The stability of the inner environment is a cardinal requirement for the preservation of well-being.

All mountain and seas, the air and sunlight, wind, rain, thunder and lightning, living creatures and minerals, indeed every aspect of nature in the entire world exert a highly specific influence on human life. But mankind by no means stands solely under the influence of the natural world, for man's social environment is of even greater significance. Man is already no longer a natural creature but a social one. The detrimental consequences of the "three types of waste products"[137] in the capitalistic and social-imperialistic[138] countries have produced a serious contamination of the air, rivers, and seas, posing a critical threat to the health of the people there. This means, therefore, that the quality of the social system not only determines the quality of the natural environment, but what is even more important, influences the progress of mankind.

The social and physical surroundings together constitute the external environment of human existence. In addition to this external world is the inner environment within the human organism.

If we view the earth in its entirety, we see that water covers most of the surface, a situation expressed in the well-known saying: "three parts mountains, six parts water, one part fields." In the human organism as well, water constitutes 60 to 70 percent of the total substance. Of this, 70 percent is located within the cells and is termed cell fluid; 30 percent is located outside of the cells and is known as extracellular fluid. Blood plasma is contained in the blood vessels and is a constituent of the blood fluid. Tissue fluid is distributed among the tissue cells and is also known as intertissue fluid. This means that the one hundred billion cells in the human organism are submerged, so to speak, in the extracellular fluid. Thus we call the extracellular fluid the inner environment of the organism.

The inner environment is the indispensable medium of metabolism. Aqueous and nutritive substances from the external world first enter the blood plasma and are subsequently distributed into the tissue fluid, until they finally reach the tissue cells. The products of metabolism produced in these cells are then transported from the tissue fluid to the blood plasma and then eliminated from the body.

The human body is an organism with extraordinarily complex and subtle functions. Scientists believe that life arose in the sea, progressing over the course of some four billion years from single-celled creatures to man's present form. Four billion years ago the water in the ocean formed the ideal environment for life processes. This still applies to single-celled creatures of the present day, which exist in a state of constant osmosis with their fluid environment. Saltwater thus constitutes their external environment; they possess no inner environment. In the relatively more complex multicelled beings the structure of the organism became closed, and only then could an inner environment arise. But the inner world of primitive living creatures, as well as the formation and nature of their extracellular fluid, generally change in accordance with the transformations to which their respective external environments are subjected. At this stage it is still impossible to speak of a stable inner environment. Only with the appearance of birds and mammals, whose inner body mechanisms are increasingly favorably differentiated, did the structure and characteristics of the inner environment achieve virtual permanence. And finally in man, whose complex nervous and bodily fluid system had continually progressed toward mutual adaptation of all possible functions, the inner environment developed even greater stability. Of extraordinary interest is the fact that this stable inner environment resembles the seawater upon which the existence of the primordial life-forms depended.

The preservation of the structure and function of the cells depends largely on the relative constancy of the inner environment within which these cells are located. This includes [constancy] of temperature, pH, osmotic pressure, and all chemical elements. All changes within the inner environment that exceed certain values help to create a favorable climate for the genesis of illness. Changes in the temperature, for instance, can give rise to fever but can also prevent body temperature from rising [sufficiently]. Changes in the pH can lead to acid or alkaline poisonings. Changes in osmotic pressure can produce edemas or dehydration. Changes in body electrolytes can produce similar effects; the concentration of these elements directly affects metabolism and numerous other physiological processes. Let us take the potassium ions as an example. A normal blood serum potassium level is 4–5m eq./l (16–22 ml %). If the concentration drops below a certain minimum, dropping below 3 m eq./l, heart muscle damage as well as enervation usually occur. This is a case of potassium deficiency. In contrast, if the concentration exceeds certain limits, reaching a level above 7 m eq./l, the result may be nerve disturbances in the heart. Higher concentrations can produce irregular heartbeats and, eventually, death.

In clinical practice the results of chemical blood analyses frequently enable us to understand the circumstances surrounding changes in the inner environment, to diagnose the illnesses, determine a suitable course of therapy, such as the type, amount, and concentration of fluids to be administered, and thereby restore a condition of normalcy to the inner environment and achieve the therapeutic objective.

In summary, we see that a normal inner environment is essential if the organism is to adjust to continually changing external conditions. Changing circumstances in the external environment can therefore present a genuine threat to the life of an organism and lead to disease when they have destroyed the normal condition of the inner world. In other words, external conditions can exert their effects solely through inner conditions. Thus a normal condition in the inner environment is a necessary condition for the preservation of well-being.

Using the Concept of the Unity of Opposites to Recognize Illnesses[139]

When the pulse is regular, each beat consists of one systolic and one diastolic beat. If no systolic beat occurs, a diastolic beat is impossible; if no diastolic beat occurs, a systolic beat is also not possible. Systolic and diastolic therefore represent a contradiction; they are opposites and yet together they constitute a whole. The situation in the lungs is the same. Inhalation and exhalation ensure the continuation of respiration in the body. Innumerable similar examples could be listed here; stimulation and inhibition, absorption and excretion, assimilation and dissimilation, and an infinite number of other contradictions and processes in the human body constitute the living integrated organism—life itself.

But this is not yet the entire story—the human body is similarly engaged with the external world in a state of opposition and struggle. This opposition and struggle ensure that the organism and the external world maintain a relative equilibrium and a relative unity. The unity in this contradiction is relative; the struggle in this contradiction is absolute.

The life of mankind in nature is constantly exposed to the ongoing onslaught of pathogenic factors. Unusual climatic conditions, bacteria and viruses, venomous snakes and wild animals, as well as changes in the external environment strive to exert an effect on the human body. How are these factors able to induce illness? How is it possible that they cause no illness? Numerous factors play a role, but the most important element lies in the inner circumstances of the human body.

A section of the *Ling-shu,* entitled "The Genesis of all Illnesses," contains the following passage: "Wind, rain, cold, and heat are evil [influences] and harm man only if he already suffers from some depletion. Thus, if a person is unexpectedly struck by a violent wind or a rainstorm and does not fall ill, it means that he was not suffering from any depletion, for evil [influences] are by themselves incapable of harming man. An evil wind can establish itself in the body only if two depletions are present simultaneously—namely, evil winds that can penetrate a condition of depletion and a depletion in the body of [correct influences]." Thus evil influences alone cannot induce illness; only when two depletions are present in the human body can evil influences generate illnesses. If no depletion is present in the body, a violent wind or a rainstorm presents no threat whatsoever.

These conclusions of our native medicine, recorded more than two thousand years ago, are in accord with dialectical materialism.

In the years 1918 and 1919, an epidemic of influenza gripped the entire world, striking a quarter of the entire population. Twenty million died—a tremendous catastrophe! Yet what must also be noted is that three-quarters of the people remained untouched. Why did these people not fall ill, although they were subject to the same pathogenic conditions as the victims? The key lies in the defensive forces of the organism.

Some bacteria and viruses are always present in the nose and throat of people. But because of the powerful defensive forces of man, as well as a number of protective organs and functions, and because the organism and the outer environment exist in a state of relative equilibrium, these people do not fall ill. This is health.

When, however, someone is chilled by wind or drenched by rain, or exhausted by excessive exertion, the defensive forces of the organism and the protective functions of the nose and throat are diminished. Bacteria and viruses are now able to gain the upper hand, breaking through the body's lines of defense, penetrating deeply into the human body, where they bring about the breakdown of physiological functions. In other words, the equilibrium that existed between the organism and its external environment is destroyed. Under such conditions, illnesses such as influenza or respiratory infections can arise.

From this we can see that well-being and illness are two different manifestations of the opposition and struggle that exist within the human body. So-called good health is nothing more than a relative equilibrium in the normal relations between the organism and its surrounding world. Illness is nothing more than the collapse of these normal relationships between the organism and its environment. Whenever man suffers from an illness, this relationship between the organism and its surroundings undergoes a change that is manifested in a series of clinical symptoms, such as the decline or loss of one's capacity for work.

The course of an illness is also replete with contradictions. On the one hand, the pathogenic factor damages the organism, while on the other hand, a physiological defensive reaction of the organism occurs in its opposition to this injury. If, at such a moment, the effects of the factors that give rise to the illness are relatively weak and the resisting forces of the organism relatively strong, the condition of the victim, after the organism has overcome the pathogenic factors, improves, he is eventually healed, and well-being is reestablished in the individual. It is also possible, however, that the pathogenic factors are relatively strong while the defensive powers of the organism are relatively weak. If this is the case, the illness may progress, taking a turn for the worse, and eventually result in death.

Our native medicine utilizes the both understandable and highly important [concepts] "correct" and "evil" to designate the defensive forces of the organism and the pathogenic factors. These terms clearly and unmistakably underlined the fact that "if the correct influences are present within [the body], the evil [influences] are unable to carry out any assault" and that "whenever evil [influences] accumulate, a deficiency of [correct] influences is the cause." In the struggle with disease, one must therefore not concentrate solely on driving out evil; it is even more important to strengthen and support that which is correct."[140]

13.2. Some Insights Regarding the Use of Drugs
(Yu-kuan yung-yao i-hsieh chih-shih) (excerpt)

Medicinal drugs are, in the final analysis, an external cause.
The human body possesses a variety of means to maintain the equilibrium existing between the organism and the external world, and so-called health is nothing more than the preservation of this equilibrium. Whenever the balance is destroyed, illnesses can arise. In a

certain sense, the effect of drugs consists of helping the organism maintain this balance. Thus drugs are ultimately an external cause; they are unable to replace the organism's own inner forces for overcoming illness.

Thus in treating illnesses, great care must be taken to ensure that measures are adopted to strengthen the organism's internal functions for resisting disease. This encompasses an appropriate diet, proper physical exercise and active relaxation, as well as the establishment of an attitude of revolutionary optimism and the creation of a determination to fight the illness, so as to mobilize the abundant functions of each organ in the organism and strengthen the capabilities of resistance. This is the sole way to ensure predictable success with the aid of practical drug therapy.[141]

14. *Wen-hui pao* (Chinese newspaper of October 22, 1980)

14.1. The Evaluation of Acupuncture Anesthesia Must Seek Truth from Facts by Keng Hsi-chen and T'ao Nai-huang

Editor's Comment: Acupuncture therapy is a peculiar ancient medical technique of our country. The application of acupuncture in surgery certainly has pain-suppressing effects. But to assess the exact size of the effects of acupuncture anesthesia one must adopt a scientific approach of "seeking truth from facts." With this, these effects cannot be easily denied but they also will not be willfully exaggerated. Over the past years, acupuncture was raised to an inappropriate position. This was unrealistic. Comrades Keng Hsi-chen and T'ao Nai-huang offer their personal opinion regarding acupuncture anesthesia, based on their own practice and fact finding research.

What are the exact effects of acupuncture anesthesia? What are its exact functions in therapy? These are questions worth inquiring into. At public occasions we have, during a ten-year period of turmoil, filled newspapers and magazines with compliments stating things like "the application of acupuncture anesthesia is a new chapter in the history of anesthesia; it represents a milestone," "it is a leap forward in the history of the development of anesthesia," "acupuncture anesthesia is something new," and so forth. But, at the same time, there occurred some phenomena that caused some deep thoughts: Why is such a "good method" not seen applied with delight by even the majority of those medical personnel and patients who praise it? Why are there some people who even resort to "going through the back door" [that means: to seek advantages through influence] only to reach their goal of not being subjected to acupuncture anesthesia? Why haven't the basic technical problems been resolved yet despite the employment of such a tremendous amount of manpower, despite the spending of so much time and financial resources and despite the carrying out of millions of surgical operations with acupuncture anesthesia? When we talk about basic problems here, we have in mind that an anesthesia method must achieve a condition of no pain, or of anesthesia. If, at the time of the application of an anesthesia method, it is still necessary to apply simultaneously such techniques as deep-breathing exercises, suggestion therapy, and hypnosis, then this cannot be called an ideal anesthesia method. For this reason we believe that acupuncture an-esthesia should be evaluated on the basis of seeking truth through facts.

It Is Not Yet a Mature Anesthesia Method

As is commonly known, appraisal and selection of any anesthesia method is based on several principles: (1) safety, (2) no pain, (3) it must create the conditions for surgery, (4) interference with and in-fluence on the patient's physiology must be small, (5) anesthesia ac-cidents must be rare, (6) the effects and side effects of the anesthesia must be known beforehand and must be assessable. Furthermore, during the operation it should be easily applicable. These standards have been set, since anesthesia has become an academic discipline, in accordance with the development of medicine, with the benefit of the patients and with the requirements of surgery. Any anesthesia method, be it excellent or not, must be judged and tested according to these standards, and every effort must be undertaken to conform to them. If we apply these standards to an assessment of acupuncture anesthesia then, first of all, it cannot achieve absence of pain or basic absence of pain. This is acknowledged in all the treatises dealing with acupuncture anesthesia; stated in common language, the suppression of pain is incomplete. As has been published already in some relevant materials, in some surgeries where the application of acupuncture anesthesia is appropriate acupuncture anesthesia reaches excellent results in at the most merely 60 to 85 percent [of the cases], while in 15 to 40 percent the results are not good or are even a failure. Now there are people who offer a new concept concerning anesthesia, namely, "the sense of pain slows down but does not disappear." This is nothing else than raising the quality of acupuncture anesthesia by way of changing the concept. We take exception to this way of changing the concept. Second, the conditions for surgery created by acupuncture anesthesia are not ideal. Things in surgery that formerly could be achieved without any difficulty can often not be inquired into further and thus golden opportunities slip away because [acupuncture anesthesia] leads to pain. On the surface, the effects of acupuncture anesthesia on the physiology of the patient are not as strong as those of drug anesthesia, but this is at the expense of mental and physical suffering by the patient. The patient undergoes surgery in a state of full consciousness. Because the suppression of pain remains incomplete and because he develops a tense mood, he has difficulties of enduring [this type of surgery]. Would it not be better, then, to apply conduction blockade anesthesia or general anesthesia which already have been practiced effectively earlier, in order to ensure smooth progress of the operation? With regard to both physicians and patients, this would not be a bad thing. Furthermore, in contrast to drug anesthesia, acupuncture anesthesia allegedly penetrates the human body's nerves, liquids or, as some say, the meridians to suppress pain. Because every individual body is different, the effects [of acupuncture anesthesia] vary, and only after a complete psychological and physiological analysis of the patient can it be determined whether or not this method is appropriate. But sometimes, even though these efforts have been made, it is still difficult to achieve an effect with acupuncture anesthesia. It is a common occurrence in the clinical application of acupuncture anesthesia that one has to switch to an application of drug anesthesia because the effects of the former are not satisfactory.

Of course, in some sections of surgery, acupuncture anesthesia is still effective, such as in surgery on thyroid glands or in ligation surgery for family planning or in cranial surgery where pain sensitivity is relatively low. Here one can avoid those mishaps of injuring nerves as they can easily appear under conditions of general anesthesia. But, after all, there are not many kinds of diseases suitable for acupuncture anesthesia, and it cannot be denied that in some respects drug anesthesia is better than acupuncture anesthesia. For instance, in ophthalmological surgery one drop of an anesthetic drug is easily administered, has disinfecting functions and anesthetic effects. If, in contrast, acupuncture anesthesia is used, the patient risks infection and he may suffer from pain. In the past it was assumed that acupuncture anesthesia, although not perfect, would be profitable in preparations for war because of its simple operation. In fact, however, in the most recent war the rate of utilization of acupuncture anesthesia did not reach one percent of the cases. Practice has already proven, under the tense conditions of warfare, acupuncture anesthesia is definitely not an anesthesia method that can effectively be used to handle large quantities of war injuries.

It Is Not Suitable for Large-Scale Clinical Practice

The large amount of practice carried out so far enables us to determine that surgery with acupuncture anesthesia is successful as a result of the following four reasons: first, where there is a definite pain-suppressing function achievable through the application of needles; second, where drug anesthesia provides the basis [that is to say, if simultaneously with the application of the needles a certain amount of drugs is injected as, for instance, Du-leng-ding]; third, where there is proficient skill of the physician; and fourth, where the patient has an ability to endure pain. If he holds out, this means success; if he doesn't hold out, this means a failure. Thus, acupuncture anesthesia is not yet sufficiently developed for an anesthesia method.

Now, because acupuncture anesthesia does not yet represent a fully developed anesthesia method, it is not suitable to extend it to large-scale clinical practice. In other words, to make acupuncture anesthesia a practicable anesthesia method, there is no other way than to have, in practice, the physician and the patient decide what to select for optimal usage. It is absolutely impossible to work out an administrative order, or to stipulate a rate of utilization for acupuncture anesthesia in order to enforce its practice. Any therapeutic technique or drug must serve the patient, and it shouldn't be that the patient serves the technique or the drug. But there was a period when we subjected acupuncture anesthesia to administrative orders to push it toward clinical use even though it was a problem still waiting for more research. Not only did we entirely neglect the procedures and methods of scientific research, we also blindly increased the amount of the practice of acupuncture anesthesia. Up to now there are already more than one hundred surgical operations where acupuncture anesthesia is put to use, resulting in more than two million cases treated. At peak times the rate of acupuncture anesthesia utilization reached 80 percent in some hospitals. One may say there was virtually no area of surgery where acupuncture anesthesia was not applied. To spread an insufficiently developed medical technique to such an extent is obviously inappropriate. According to the objective rules of scientific research, with such a tremendous practice it should be possible to see those things which should be seen. If there should be a breakthrough in acupuncture anesthesia in the future, there must first be important advances on the theoretical level; one should not rely on further increases of the number of surgical operations.

The pushing of acupuncture anesthesia into large areas of clinical application cannot be separated from the peculiar historical conditions in our country of that time. During the period of the "Cultural Revolution," acupuncture anesthesia served politically as a standard to judge progress or backwardness, revolution or nonrevolution. Physicians and patients were under the pressure of the political requirements of that time. They had no choice but to have exceptional courage in order to carry out or undergo surgery, especially as the patients who felt pain could not cry out. Some resorted to shouting political slogans during surgery in a loud voice. At one place, the chairman of ophthalmology was enthusiastic about acupuncture anesthesia, and he tried the knife at his own eyelid. Finally he reached the conclusion: the effects are not good, it should not be extended. He wrote a report to higher authorities and as a result he was labeled one with three hats [i.e., an intellectual not interested in practice] and met the criticism of the masses. Under this type of political pressure, not a few people made statements against their will and acted against their conscience. Thus, in some hospitals the rate of acupuncture anesthesia utilization reached 20 percent, but among these, 80 percent were ligation operations. In other hospitals before clinical application of acupuncture anesthesia, the patients were given already sufficient amounts of anesthetic drugs through injection and then, in addition, needles were pierced into their ears pretending acupuncture anesthesia. Only joy was reported but not sorrow; one did not dare to tell the facts. This of course had decisive influence on how the concerned leadership department passed correct decisions regarding the real situation of acupuncture anesthesia.

The Scientific Attitude of Seeking Truth through Facts Should Be Adopted

To push acupuncture anesthesia blindly in clinical usage has blocked the development of the anesthetic cause and the training of personnel. The contents of anesthesiology are very complex; in today's world anesthetic physiology, anesthetic drugs and pharmacology, as well as emergency treatment and resuscitation of critically ill patients are important problems in anesthesiology—they are subjected to attention and research by various people. In addition, there are speedy progressive developments day by day in some areas, and advanced levels comparable with the treatment of diseases have been reached already. Acupuncture anesthesia is only one immature method among many anesthesia methods; its functions are limited. By unduly emphasizing the functions of acupuncture anesthesia and by using excessive force, it [anesthesiology] was unnecessarily thrown into this type of research with unpredictable perspectives. It goes without saying that there are not many specialized anesthesia personnel in our country; because of these circumstances, there will certainly be an influence on the development of other areas of anesthesia in our country. And, at the same time, there was an influence on the development of acupuncture itself.

In conclusion, our opinion is as follows. Up to now acupuncture anesthesia represents a not yet fully developed anesthesia method. It has effects but it also has limits. In clinical use it should be selected on the basis of what is best for the patient and physician. It should not be spread extensively and, even more, it should not be set against other acupuncture methods and there should be no application of administrative policies to enforce its practice. If acupuncture anesthesia is to become scientific, there is no alternative except bringing it into the realm of science, to probing into it, and to having it undergo practical trials. If, in the future, there are no major breakthroughs on its theoretical level [i.e., understanding the theory of acupuncture], acupuncture anesthesia may finally [very well], following the fading away of the enthusiasm of its advocates, disappear from the great majority of areas of [its current] clinical application. To assess acupuncture anesthesia by seeking truth through facts does in no way weaken the splendor of our country's traditional medicine, and it will have no bearing on the progress of research on the theory of acupuncture anesthesia. There is a well-known saying: "Those who fall are at least on solid ground"; to have one's feet planted on solid ground, to seek truth through facts, this is exactly a scientific attitude.

There is one thing here which needs special explanation. Our opinions expressed here are not taken out of thin air. We, the authors, have in the past, from 1969 through 1977, as part of our work in the hospital, conducted more than thirty thousand surgical operations under acupuncture anesthesia as an exploratory practice in order to warmheartedly promote acupuncture anesthesia. This represents about 1.5 percent of all cases of surgery under acupuncture anesthesia in our country. This tremendous amount of practice has led us to publish the opinions offered above. Also, these opinions are not really our own original ideas, they are extensively discussed and acknowledged among medical personnel of anesthetics and surgery. It is just that due to the political pressure of the past period, nobody dared to state them openly. In raising this issue now we hope that it will receive attention from the medical world and the leadership, so that they provide acupuncture anesthesia with an evaluation of seeking truth through facts, of science. We certainly do not oppose scientific research, nor do we oppose clinical use of acupuncture anesthesia if this happens under circumstances allowing patients and physicians to make the best choice. But as far as the academic issues are concerned, we must carry out the policy of having a hundred schools of thought contend and talk it over in order to benefit the development of scientific techniques in medicine.

Notes

Introduction

1. Among the earliest Chinese medical and pharmaceutical books brought to Europe were (fragmentary?) copies of the *Wan-ping hui-ch'un,* a comprehensive book on prescriptions first published in 1587, and copies of the herbal *Cheng-ho pen-ts'ao,* first published in 1116. Both these works came into the hands of European physicians some time between 1605 and 1611. See Hintzsche 1960. For an account of the westward spread of acupuncture techniques, and their reception in Europe, see Lu and Needham 1980, pp. 269–302.

2. Edelstein 1967, pp. 205–207.

3. Cf. Ackerknecht 1942.

1: Illness and Healing in the Shang Culture

1. Franke and Trauzettel 1968, p. 27.

2. Ibid., p. 34.

3. Keightley 1975, p. 4; Keightley 1978.

4. Keightley 1975, p. 3; Franke and Trauzettel 1968, p. 32.

5. Hu Hou-hsüan 1944, pp. 2a–3a; see further: Ting Shan 1928, pp. 243–245.

6. Yen I-p'ing 1951, p. 20.

7. Hu Hou-hsüan 1944, p. 2a.

8. Chang Tsung-Tung 1970, pp. 6, 17.

9. Hu Hou-hsüan 1944, pp. 2a–3a.

10. Ibid., p. 6b.

11. Ibid., p. 3a.

12. Chang Tsung-Tung 1970, p. 34.

13. Hu Hou-hsüan 1944, p. 7a.

14. Ibid.

15. Ibid.

16. Chang Tsung-Tung 1970, p. 41.

17. Yen I-p'ing 1951, p. 14.

18. Ibid., p. 22.

19. Ibid.
20. Chang Tsung-Tung 1970, p. 34.
21. Ibid., p. 36.
22. Ibid., p. 15.
23. Hu Hou-hsüan 1944, p. 11a.
24. Yen I-p'ing 1951, p. 14.
25. Chang Tsung-Tung 1970, p. 69.
26. Yen I-p'ing 1951, p. 17.
27. See appendix 2.6, and appendix 9.
28. Yen I-p'ing 1951, p. 17; Ma Chi-hsing 1979.
29. Foster 1965, pp. 293–315; see further: Schoeck 1974, pp. 83–112.
30. Ardener 1970, p. 146.
31. Franke and Trauzettel 1968, p. 35.
32. Keightley 1975, p. 4.
33. Granet 1976, pp. 31, 67.
34. Ibid., p. 34.
35. Ibid., p. 36.
36. Yen I-p'ing 1951, p. 15.
37. Chang Tsung-Tung 1970, p. 45.
38. Akatsuka Tadashi quoted in Kanō Yoshimitsu 1980, p. 283.
39. Hu Hou-hsüan 1944, pp. 12a–b.
40. Keightley 1975, p. 4.
41. Ibid., p. 10.
42. Ibid., pp. 9–10.
43. For further details see Ahern 1973 and Jordan 1972.

2: The Chou Period and Demonic Medicine

1. Levenson and Schurmann 1969, pp. 28–30; Franke and Trauzettel 1968, p. 38.
2. Levenson and Schurmann 1969, pp. 31–33; Franke and Trauzettel 1968, p. 40.
3. Franke 1930, 1:153.
4. Franke and Trauzettel 1968, p. 40.
5. Ibid., pp. 70–73.
6. Granet 1976, p. 86.
7. Ibid., p. 146.
8. Franke and Trauzettel 1968, pp. 66–73.
9. Ibid., pp. 74–76.
10. Ibid., pp. 78–79.
11. For an example of the application of the tortoise oracle in a therapeutic context see Legge 1960, 3:351–356.
12. Eichhorn 1976, p. 17.
13. Ibid., pp. 17–19.
14. Ibid., pp. 34–35.
15. Ibid., pp. 23–25.

16. Ibid., p. 27.

17. Ibid., p. 22.

18. Wilhelm 1930, pp. 32–33.

19. *Han Fei-tzu,* 1966, chap. 6, p. 6*b*.

20. Eichhorn 1976, p. 34; Wilhelm 1930, p. 34.

21. De Groot 1892–1910, 6:973–974.

22. *Wu-shih-erh ping fang,* 1979, p. 129. Harper 1982, pp. 226–228. In an earlier publication I had tentatively accepted an interpretation of the ailment concerned here (*ch'ao*) that had been offered by the Chinese editors of the *Wu-shih-erh ping fang,* namely, "body odor." (Unschuld 1982*a*, p. 17) Harper's analysis is convincing.

23. Harper 1982, p. 227.

24. Ibid., p. 80.

25. Ibid., pp. 85–86.

26. Ibid., pp. 104–105.

27. Ibid., pp. 105–106.

28. Ibid., p. 103.

29. Dubs 1955, pp. 537–539.

30. Ibid.

31. Eichhorn 1955, p. 310.

32. Doré 1966, vols. III/I–XXII.

33. Harper 1982, pp. 30–33.

34. Cf. *Tso-chuan,* Bk 8, 10th year.

35. De Groot 1892–1910, 5:679–680.

36. *Wai-t'ai pi-yao,* 1964, p. 362.

37. Sivin 1968, pp. 208–209.

38. De Groot 1892–1910, 6:1078–1082.

39. *Ch'ien-chin i-fang,* 1965, p. 8.

40. Ibid., p. 341.

41. Granet 1976, pp. 54–57; Eberhard 1942, pp. 50–60; Harper 1982, pp. 98–101.

42. *Ch'ien-chin i-fang,* 1965, p. 347.

43. Ibid., p. 348.

44. Ibid., p. 327.

45. Cf. Keupers 1977 and Hou 1979 for detailed accounts of specific demonological concepts and their respective application in actual contemporary exorcistic therapy.

46. Feng and Shryock 1935; De Groot 1892–1910, 5:826–869; *Pei-k'ao shih-wu pen-ts'ao kang mu,* "Chih ku lun fang" appendix to chap. 22 (cf. *Medicine in China: A History of Pharmaceutics,* p. 228).

47. Legge 1960, 5:164, 574.

48. Feng and Shryock 1935, pp. 7–8.

49. Ibid., p. 9–10.

50. Ibid., p. 23.

51. Ibid., p. 16.

3: Unification of the Empire, Confucianism, and the Medicine of Systematic Correspondence

1. Frazer 1926, 1:52ff.
2. *T'ai-p'ing yü-lan,* 1968, pp. 3398–3399.
3. *Shan-hai ching chien-shu,* 1974, p. 44.
4. Ibid., p. 6.
5. *Ch'ung-chi hsin-hsiu pen-ts'ao,* 1964, p. 262.
6. Read 1931, p. 650.
7. Eichhorn 1976, p. 17.
8. Kranz 1958, pp. 20, 22.
9. Granet 1963, pp. 87–88.
10. Granet 1976, p. 51.
11. Eberhard 1933; Needham 1956, pp. 253–259.
12. Legge 1960, 5:531.
13. Ibid., p. 242.
14. Ibid., 3:56.
15. *Shih-chi,* 1969, p. 1368.
16. *Lun-heng,* 1974, pp. 48–49; Needham 1956, p. 266.
17. Franke and Trauzettel 1968, p. 51.
18. Ibid.
19. Yamada 1979.
20. *Hsün-tzu chi-chieh,* 1971, p. 27.
21. *Huang-ti nei-ching su-wen,* 1971, chap. 1, p. 14*b.* It might be of interest to quote here, for comparison, the Greek physician Erasistratos (ca. 304–240 B.C.) who, only slightly earlier had suggested similar insights, resorting, though, to a different analogy: "It is after all, better not to let people get sick than to cure their diseases; similarly, the helmsman of a ship will be more eager to reach port before encountering a storm than finally to arrive in port after being buffeted by the storm and enduring many perils." (Quoted by Edelstein 1967, pp. 307–308.)
22. Watson 1963, pp. 2–6.
23. *Hsün-tzu chi-chieh,* 1971, pp. 13–14.
24. Ibid., p. 205.
25. Ibid., p. 211.
26. Needham 1956, p. 238; translation slightly modified.
27. See below p. 76.
28. Yamada 1980; P. Unschuld 1982*a.*
29. Yamada 1980, p. 219; Kanō Yoshimitsu 1980, pp. 282–283.
30. *Huang-ti nei-ching t'ai-su,* 1981, p. 532.
31. Edelstein 1967, p. 116.
32. Cf. P. Unschuld 1983.
33. The Chinese term for "vessel" is *mo* in the *Yin yang shih-i mo chiu ching,* and *wen* (?) in the *Tsu pi shih-i mo chiu-ching.* The latter term appears in no other ancient source. I have chosen the English term "vessel" in order

to convey the notion that these entities appear to have been considered as "containing" some contents. In contrast, in the *Huang-ti nei-ching* texts we should regard the term *mo* as an abbreviation of the term *ching-mo* ("conduit vessel"). The contents of "conduits" are generally considered to be in constant flow; they do not stagnate, except in case of obstructions, that is, in case of illness.

34. *Wu-shih-erh ping fang,* 1979, pp. 1–20.

35. Ibid., pp. 21–23.

36. *Huang-ti nei-ching su-wen,* 1971, chap. 39, p. 1*b*. Usually only the first sentence of Ch'i Po's remarkable statement is quoted (as a Western example see, for instance, Lu and Needham 1980, p. 29) to demonstrate that the Chinese awareness of blood circulation predates Harvey's findings by about sixteen centuries. The full extent of the statement and the context of its origin, to be illustrated below, suggest, however, that it is questionable whether the Chinese and the European concepts of circulation are comparable at all. One should hesitate, especially in a history of ideas, to isolate statements from their conceptual environment and to set them against insights that may appear similar on first glance but in reality are fundamentally different.

37. Epler 1980.

38. See, for instance, *Li-yang chi-yao,* a work on leprosy from the sixteenth century, chap. 1, pp. 1*a–b*.

39. See, for instance, *Huang-ti nei-ching,* treatises 9 ("Liu chieh tsang hsiang lun"), 10 ("Wu tsang sheng ch'eng lun"), and 44 ("Wei lun").

40. The argumentation of Lu and Needham (1980, p. 31) that conveys the notion that the concept of the heart as a bellow may date back to the *Huang-ti nei-ching* texts is noteworthy. It may serve as an example of the approach not unfrequently employed by these authors when they cut out short statements with a particular meaning from longer passages conveying, as a whole, a rather different meaning, and also when they confuse the ideas conveyed by commentaries added many centuries later with the concepts conveyed by an original source, in this case the *Huang-ti nei-ching.* Lu and Needham write: "We also find it in the *Su-wen:* 'Asthma (*chia*) will occur if there is no drumming in the vessel of the heart,' on which Wang Ping comments that 'if there is no working of the bellows [lit. drumming, *ku*] then the blood will not flow round.' It seems likely, in view of all that has so far been said, that the heart must have been thought of through the centuries as a pump of some kind, working in systole to propel the blood through its system of tubes." This argumentation appears to be convincing; in reality, however, the *Su-wen* passage reads as follows: "If the [movement in the] vessels of the kidneys is weak and speedy, if the [movement in the] vessels of the liver is weak and speedy, and if the [movement in the] vessels of the heart is weak and speedy, and if there is no drumming, all this indicates a *chia*-illness." Wang Ping's commentary from the eighth century reads as follows: "[A movement that is] 'weak and speedy' indicates [the presence of] abundant cold. In case there is 'no drumming,' the blood does not flow. When the blood does not flow and

when it meets with the cold, the blood will, as a result, congeal inside [the body] and this is a *chia*-illness." The term *drumming* was used to describe the throbbing movement felt in the vessels. The causal twist given to this term by Lu and Needham's translating it as "working of the bellows" is not supported by the texts quoted. A few lines further down in the same paragraph Wang Ping commented again on the term *drumming*. Here the *Huang-ti nei-ching* speaks of "external drumming"; Wang Ping remarked: "'External drumming' means that a drumming and beating does not occur exactly in the 'foot' and 'inch' [sections at the wrist] but at the outer sides of the forearms." Also, the first commentary of Wang Ping does not speak of "flow round," but says simply "flow." Seen as a whole, neither the passage quoted from the *Huang-ti nei-ching*, nor the commentary added by Wang Ping, appear to convey the idea of the heart pumping, like a bellow, the blood through the vessels (cf. *Huang-ti nei-ching su-wen*, 1971, chap. 48, p. 7*b*). It should also be pointed out, in this context, that the term *chia* refers—in the *Huang-ti nei-ching*—to accumulations of stagnant influences in yang conduits; Wang Ping employed the term to designate illnesses resulting from accumulations of congealed blood. In any case, the term *chia* should not be rendered, from a historical text, as "asthma." Lu and Needham close their argument with the following statement: "It seems likely . . . that the heart must have been thought of through the centuries as a pump of some kind . . . and we can find at least one clear analogy with a forge-bellows in pre-Harveian times. For in the *Lei-Ching,* Chang Chieh-Pin wrote: 'The heart and pulse (mo) is not itself either *chhi* or blood (*hsüeh*), but rather it is the bellows of the *chhi* and the *hsüeh*.'" Unfortunately, even this "clear analogy" does not survive closer scrutiny; the Chinese text of the *Lei-ching,* in all editions I could consult, says only *mai* (or *mo*) *che fei ch'i fei hsüeh* . . . ("The vessels are neither *ch'i* nor blood, they are the bellows of *ch'i* and blood"). The reference to the heart was added by Lu and Needham. See Chang Chieh-Pin 1975, p. 192.

41. Ku Te-tao 1979, p. 22.

42. For details see *Medicine in China: Nan-ching—The Classic of Difficult Issues.*

43. Watanabe Kōzō 1956.

44. Quite similar findings were recorded for early Greek medicine by Ludwig Edelstein in his "History of Anatomy in Antiquity" written in 1932: "Their [i.e., the pre-Socratics'] investigation of the invisible, and this term includes the internal organs of the human body, rests on analogies. And therefore, even physiology, like all explorations of nature, was tied to the method of analogy. Nor did the Hippocratics proceed differently: they too explained the unknown by comparison to the known. . . . It was only in Alexandria that conclusions by analogy were replaced by the method of dissecting. If one asks what is the principle difference between such analogical study of the human body and its study through human dissection, the answer would seem to be that dissection, through the very renunciation of such

analogies, centers the investigation on the object itself. Thus the study replaces conclusions drawn from other empirical knowledge. Or, to put it differently, the one method is linked to extraneous data, while the other is not. (Reprinted in Edelstein 1967, pp. 292–293.)

45. Granet 1976, p. 260.

46. Needham 1961, pp. 107, 109.

47. Granet 1976, p. 265.

48. Ibid., pp. 266–268.

49. Needham 1970, p. 81.

50. This allegory was outlined explicitly in the treatise "Shih-erh shui" (The Twelve Waters) of the *Huang-ti nei-ching t'ai-su*. Cf. *Huang-ti nei-ching t'ai-su*, 1981, pp. 63–69.

51. *Kuan-tzu*, "Tu-ti p'ien," in *Kuan-tzu chiao-cheng*, 1954, p. 303.

52. *Lü-shih ch'un-ch'iu*, chap. 3, "Chin-shu," in *Lü-shih ch'un-ch'iu chi-shih*, 1969, chap. 3, p. 7.

53. Lu and Needham (1980, p. 115) deny the *Nan-ching* its innovative character when they characterize it as follows: "Covering no really new ground, it brings out many subtleties of theory and practice."

54. *Medicine in China: Nan-ching—The Classic of Difficult Issues,* "The Fiftieth Difficult Issue."

55. Ibid., "The Second Difficult Issue," commentary by Liao P'ing.

56. Ibid., "The Fourth Difficult Issue."

57. Ibid., "The Fifth Difficult Issue."

58. Ibid., "The Second Difficult Issue."

59. Ibid., "The Third Difficult Issue."

60. Ibid., "The Eighteenth Difficult Issue."

61. Ibid., "The Thirteenth Difficult Issue."

62. In contrast to Shun-yü I, Pien Ch'io, a semilegendary physician of the Chou era, is presented by Ssu-ma Ch'ien in the *Shih-chi* as a man who argues in terms of yin and yang vessels, who knows that yang influences may enter the yin system, and who is aware of the fact that the flow of the influences may be interrupted, in which case a sharpened needle brings about the cure. No supporting evidence exists, though, to prove that Ssu-ma Ch'ien recorded here ideas other than of his own time.

63. Akahori 1979, 1981; P. Unschuld 1982a; *Wu-shih-erh ping fang,* 1979, pp. 187–191.

64. I find it rather difficult to accept two early incidents documented in the *Tso-chuan* (a historical work relating events of the Chou era), quoted by Lu and Needham (1980, pp. 78–79), as indications of acupuncture practice in China prior to Han times. The first incident concerns the Physician Huan who told the Prince of Chin: "Nothing can be done about [your] illness. It has settled in the region between the heart and the diaphragm. It cannot be attacked, and it cannot be reached, because drugs will not get there!" (Or: "to attack it is impossible, to reach it will not succeed, and drugs will not get

there!") The former version of the translation would refer to drugs only; the latter does not indicate what could be the means to "attack" or to "reach" the illness, that is, the demons in the patient's body. Lu and Needham's rendering of the last sentence as "No [needle] can penetrate to it, no drug can reach it" is based on a conjecture which, if true, would support the very argument refuted by the authors a few lines later, namely, that of a possible demonological origin of needling therapy. In the course of the second incident quoted as evidence, from the *Tso-chuan,* for the pre-Han practice of acupuncture, Tsang Sun told his charioteer: "Chi Sun's loving me made me suffer from a fever; Meng Sun's hatred [had the effect of a] medicinal mineral [or: "of drugs and stones"]. Still, a nice fever is not as good as a bad mineral [or: stone], because [the effects of] a mineral [or: stone] are like bringing me to life again, while even a nice fever spreads its poison to many [places]. Meng Sun is dead. My own end will come soon!" (Cf. Legge 1960, 5:499). From the second and third reference to a mineral [or: stone] it becomes quite obvious that the rendering of "medicinal mineral" as "drugs and stones" cannot be justified. However, even if one were to split the Chinese term *yao-shih* into two separate components, a reference to acupuncture could still not be read into it. For comparison, the rendering of this passage by Lu and Needham is added: "Chi Sun was attracted to me because my slight recurrent fever gave me a handsome hectic flush. Meng Sun disliked me because I took drugs and acupuncture to cure it. But the most becoming fever is not as good as the worst stone needle, for that could keep me alive instead of spreading poison through me as the fever did. Now Meng Sun is gone I shan't last long."

65. In Western literature see, for example, Lu and Needham 1980, pp. 69–79, and Chow Tse-tsung 1978, pp. 81–83.

66. Chow Tse-tsung 1978, p. 81: "there seems to be no question that one aspect of the ancient wu[-shaman] physicians was acupuncture."

67. Epler 1980.

68. Ibid., pp. 361–362.

69. Liu Tun-yüan 1972. If we follow the arguments offered by Japanese scholars, Pien Ch'io belonged to a group of shamans, roaming through East China dressed like birds. Shantung, the home of Pien Ch'io, was also the region where a belief in bird-spirits controlling the wind existed. (Kano Yoshimitsu 1980, pp. 284–285.) In this context it may not be without significance that the caves in which the phoenix, that is, the wind-spirit of the Shang, resides were called *hsüeh,* a term that reappears in the *Huang-ti nei-ching* as a general designation of the holes in the skin through which influences can pass and where the needles may be inserted. Cf. *Huai-nan-tzu chu,* "Lan-ming hsün," 1968, chap. 6, p. 93.

70. Lu and Needham 1980, p. 87.

71. Occasionally a sixth hole was conceptualized to account for six depots and palaces. See *Nan-ching,* "The Sixty-sixth Difficult Issue."

72. In addition to the holes on the streams located in the body's extremities,

so-called concentration holes and transportation holes were acknowledged by the *Nan-ching* to be located on the front and on the back side of the body, respectively. While the needling of the extremities was integrated primarily into the Five Phases theories of correspondence, the holes on the back and front side of the body were associated with yin and yang. See *Nan-ching*, "The Sixty-seventh Difficult Issue."

73. *Wu-shih-erh ping fang,* 1979; Shang Chih-chün 1980; Li Chung-wen 1980; Harper 1982; P. Unschuld 1982*a*, 1983*a*.

74. *Huang-ti nei-ching su-wen,* 1971, chap. 3, pp. 1*b*–2*a*.

4: Taoism and Pragmatic Drug Therapy

1. *Tao-te ching,* chap. 76.

2. Ibid., chap. 78.

3. Ibid., chap. 59.

4. Wilhelm 1940, p. 76, translation modified.

5. Ibid., p. 70.

6. Needham 1956, pp. 100f.

7. Stinchcombe 1965.

8. *Tao-te ching,* chap. 80; Bauer 1976, p. 34, translation modified.

9. Wilhelm 1940, pp. 46–48, translation modified.

10. Bauer 1976, p. 39.

11. Wilhelm 1940, p. 116.

12. Eichhorn 1973, p. 105.

13. Cf. Chou I-mou 1980 and Kuo Ping-ch'üan and I Fa-yin 1980.

14. Tu Wei-ming 1979, p. 108.

15. Ibid.

16. Bauer 1976, p. 46.

17. Ibid., pp. 100–109.

18. Wilhelm 1948, as quoted by Needham 1956, pp. 143–144.

19. *Huai-nan-tzu chu,* 1968, p. 35.

20. Needham 1956, p. 43.

21. Ibid., p. 44.

22. Ibid., p. 43–44.

23. *Ishimpo,* 1955, pp. 633f.; Ishihara and Levy 1968.

24. Needham 1974, pp. 71–76.

25. Cf. P. Unschuld 1982*a*, pp. 60–61.

26. Needham 1974, pp. 114f.; Wasson 1968.

27. Bauer 1976, pp. 64–65.

28. Eichhorn 1973, pp. 117–118.

29. Needham 1961, p. 111.

30. *Huai-nan-tzu chu,* 1968, p. 331; P. Unschuld 1975, p. 177; the following outline of the early history of drug therapy in China is repeated in greater detail in *Medicine of China: A History of Pharmaceutics.*

31. Bauer 1976, pp. 25–26.

5: Religious Healing: The Foundation of Theocratic Rule

1. Eichhorn 1955, 1973; Welch 1972; Michaud 1958; Stein 1963; Bauer 1976, pp. 113ff.

2. Michaud 1958, pp. 69–72.

3. Ibid., pp. 61–62.

4. Ibid., pp. 63–64.

5. Eichhorn 1955, pp. 295–299.

6. Ibid., p. 304; Michaud 1958, p. 84.

7. Eichhorn 1973, p. 141.

8. Ibid.

9. Michaud 1958, p. 85; Kaltenmark 1979, pp. 19–20, 23.

10. Michaud 1958, p. 103.

11. Bauer 1976, pp. 113–116.

12. Eichhorn 1973, p. 144.

13. Mo Ti: "Against War," trans. Schmidt-Glintzer 1975, pp. 94–95.

14. Ibid., pp. 106–107.

15. Ibid., p. 111.

16. *Lao-tzu Hsiang-erh chu chiao-chien,* 1956, p. 78.

17. *Pao-p'u-tzu,* 1969, p. 27.

18. Ibid.

19. *Lao-tzu Hsiang-erh chu chiao-chien,* 1956, pp. 12, 13; cf. Eichhorn 1973, pp. 144–145.

20. *Lao-tzu Hsiang-erh chu chiao-chien,* 1956, p. 33; cf. Eichhorn 1973, p. 145.

21. *Lao-tzu Hsiang-erh chu chiao-chien,* 1956, pp. 29–30; cf. Eichhorn 1973, pp. 145–146.

22. Eichhorn 1973, p. 140.

23. Ibid., p. 315.

24. Eichhorn 1955, p. 314.

25. Ibid., p. 315.

26. Ibid., p. 323.

27. Eichhorn 1954, pp. 328–329.

28. Ibid., p. 331.

29. Kaltenmark 1979.

30. *Cheng-t'ung tao-tsang,* 1977, chap. 50, Nr. 70–71, pp. 32592–32593.

31. Ibid., chap. 50, Nr. 74, p. 32596.

32. For further examples and literature, see Prunner 1973, pp. 59–67.

6: Buddhism and Indian Medicine

1. Franke and Trauzettel 1968, pp. 115–128.

2. Ibid., p. 133.

3. Ch'en 1964, pp. 3–11.

4. *Nan-Ch'i shu,* n.d., p. 933.

5. Bauer 1976, p. 158.

6. P. Unschuld 1978a pp. 503–510; see section 9.2.1.

7. These include Earth, Water, Fire, Wind, Mind, Perception.

8. These include the six sense organs (eyes, ears, nose, tongue, body, and mind), the six sense dimensions (sight, sound, smell, taste, touch, and thought), and finally the six levels of consciousness.

9. *Hōbōgirin*, 1929, p. 225.

10. Ibid., p. 228.

11. Ibid., p. 229.

12. Ibid., p. 236–239.

13. Ibid., p. 241.

14. As far as we know Buddhism only related its own "four-elements doctrine" to China; the "five-elements doctrine" of the Upanishads, generally identified as underlying Indian (ayurvedic) medical conceptions, does not appear in Buddhist texts translated into Chinese.

15. *Hōbōgirin*, 1929, p. 251.

16. Ibid., p. 250.

17. *Taishō Tripitaka*, 1914–1932, chap. 150, p. 882.

18. *Hōbōgirin*, 1929, p. 257.

19. *Wai-t'ai pi-yao*, 1964, pp. 562–563.

20. Ibid., p. 563.

21. (*Ch'in-ting*) *ch'üan T'ang-shih*, 1887, chap. 13, p. 47*b*.

22. *Ishimpo*, 1955, p. 126.

23. Filliozat 1979.

24. Okanishi Tameto 1969, pp. 1150–1151.

25. *Sheng-chi tsung-lu*, 1978, chap. 111, p. 6*b*.

26. Okanishi Tameto 1969, pp. 1151–1153.

27. *Yen-k'o ta-ch'üan*, n.d., chap. 5, pp. 54*b*–55*a*.

28. Literally the text states "South-sea Kuan-yin Bodhisattva"; *nan-hai* may be a mistake for *nan-wu*.

29. According to the *Huang-ti nei-ching* (see section 3.3.5), the gall was considered to be responsible for judgment and decisions; it was also seen as the seat of bravery.

30. *Yen-k'o ta-ch'üan*, n.d., chap. 5, p. 55*a*.

31. Ibid., p. 55*b*.

32. Wright 1948.

33. Okanishi Tameto 1969, pp. 528–531.

34. Ibid., pp. 567–568.

35. P. Unschuld 1978*a*, pp. 43–53.

36. *Pei-chi ch'ien-chin yao-fang*, 1965, p. 3.

37. Ibid., p. 483.

38. *Hōbōgirin*, 1929, p. 264.

7: Sung Neo-Confucianism and Medical Thought: Progress with an Eye to the Past

1. Ch'en 1964, pp. 204–206.

2. Franke and Trauzettel 1968, p. 152.

3. Eichhorn 1973, p. 176.

4. Ibid., p. 199.

5. Cf. *Medicine in China: A History of Pharmaceutics,* pp. 230–232.

6. Franke and Trauzettel 1968, p. 185.

7. Porkert 1974, p. 59.

8. Ibid.

9. Franke and Trauzettel 1968, p. 165.

10. Ibid., pp. 193–195.

11. Ibid., p. 200.

12. Needham 1970, pp. 309–315.

13. Ch'en 1964, p. 400.

14. Needham 1956, p. 452.

15. Ibid., pp. 444, 471.

16. Ch'en 1964, p. 395.

17. Ibid.

18. Needham 1956, p. 453.

19. Cf. *Medicine in China: A History of Pharmaceutics,* pp. 30–43 and 72–82.

20. U. Unschuld 1972, pp. 88–92.

21. Taki Mototane 1956, p. 830.

22. Peking Academy of Chinese Medicine 1968*a,* pp. 56–58.

23. Ibid., pp. 58–59.

24. *Chin-kuei yao-lüeh,* 1966, chap. 1, p. 1*b.*

25. Cf. *Medicine in China: A History of Pharmaceutics,* pp. 104–106.

26. P. Unschuld 1978*a.*

27. Cf. *Medicine in China: A History of Pharmaceutics,* pp. 104–108.

28. Peking Academy of Chinese Medicine 1968*a,* pp. 59ff.; *P'i-wei lun,* 1975.

29. Yamada Keiji 1979, pp. 68–69; P. Unschuld 1982*b,* p. 93.

30. *Huang-ti nei-ching t'ai-su,* 1981, pp. 14–20.

31. At that time the *T'ai-su* version of the *Huang-ti nei-ching* must have been regarded as completely obsolete in comparison with the *Su-wen;* not surprisingly it was lost in China after the Sung and was not mentioned again in bibliographies. An almost complete manuscript of the *T'ai-su* was discovered in a Japanese library earlier this century. This manuscript appears to be a copy of a Chinese original from the ninth century. *Huang-ti nei-ching t'ai-su,* 1981, preface pp. 1–3.

32. U. Unschuld 1977, pp. 228–229.

33. The following data are based on U. Unschuld 1977.

34. *T'ang-yeh pen-ts'ao,* 1956, p. 14.

35. Ibid., p. 6.

8: Medical Thought during the Ming and Ch'ing Epochs

1. Franke and Trauzettel 1968, pp. 239–243.

2. Bauer 1976, pp. 238–239.

3. Franke and Trauzettel 1968, pp. 266–268.

4. De Bary 1970a, p. 7.

5. De Bary 1970b, p. 173.

6. Sakai 1970, p. 337.

7. Ibid., p. 331.

8. Chan 1970, pp. 29–51.

9. Liu Ts'un-yan 1970, pp. 290–291, 309.

10. Franke and Trauzettel 1969, pp. 272–275.

11. Hummel 1970, pp. 421–425.

12. Bauer 1976, pp. 251–252.

13. Franke and Trauzettel 1968, pp. 311–337.

14. Tang Chun-I 1970, p. 105.

15. De Bary 1970a, p. 20.

16. Jen Yu-wen 1970, pp. 72–76.

17. Ch'en Pang-hsien 1969, p. 177; Peking Academy of Chinese Medicine 1968b, p. 154.

18. *Huang-ti nei-ching su-wen,* 1971, chap. 1, pp. 15b, 18b.

19. Peking Academy of Chinese Medicine 1968b, p. 189.

20. Ibid., pp. 188–192.

21. *Huang-ti nei-ching su-wen,* 1971, chap. 2, p. 11b; *Ling-shu ching,* 1966, chap. 2, p. 1a.

22. *Nan-ching shu-cheng,* 1961, "The Thirty-sixth Difficult Issue," p. 55.

23. Peking Academy of Chinese Medicine 1968b, p. 158.

24. Ibid., p. 159.

25. Ibid.

26. Ibid., pp. 163–165; on the original meaning of *tung-ch'i* see *Huang-ti nei-ching su-wen,* chap. "Chih-chen yao ta-lun."

27. Peking Academy of Chinese Medicine 1968b, pp. 174–176.

28. Ibid., p. 174.

29. P. Unschuld 1978a, pp. 17–18.

30. Taki Mototane 1956, p. 1181.

31. Peking Academy of Chinese Medicine 1968b, p. 212; *Wen-i lun p'ing-chu,* 1977, pp. 10–11.

32. Ch'en Pang-hsien 1969, p. 178.

33. Peking Academy of Chinese Medicine 1968b, pp. 211–213.

34. *Medicine in China: A History of Pharmaceutics,* pp. 181–183.

35. Taki Mototane 1956, pp. 418–420.

36. *Medicine in China: A History of Pharmaceutics,* pp. 183–202.

37. Peking Academy of Chinese Medicine 1978b, p. 256.

38. For further details on this author's work see *Medicine in China: A History of Pharmaceutics,* pp. 101–104.

39. *Hsü Ling-t'ai i-shu ch'üan-chi,* 1969, chap. 1, p. 89; see also *Medicine in China: A History of Pharmaceutics,* pp. 192–196.

40. *Hsü Ling-t'ai i-shu ch'üan-chi,* 1969, chap. 1, p. 123.

41. *Medicine in China: A History of Pharmaceutics,* pp. 164–168.

42. P. Unschuld 1978*b*.

43. Chang Tzu-kao 1962.

44. *Ch'uan-ya nei-wai pien*, 1957; *Ch'uan-ya wai-pien hsüan-chu*, 1977; *Ch'uan-ya nei-pien hsüan-chu*, 1980.

45. *I-lin kai-ts'o*, 1849; *I-lin kai-ts'o p'ing-chu*, 1976; Shang-kuan Liang-fu 1974, pp. 177–179.

46. *I-lin kai-ts'o*, 1849, chap. 1, pp. 9*a*–11*a*.

47. Ibid., pp. 8*b*, 12*a*; Shang-kuan Liang-fu 1974, p. 179.

48. *I-hsüeh ju-men*, 1973, p. 637.

49. Ibid.

50. *Shou-shih pao-yüan*, 1974, chap. 1, p. 38.

51. *I-pu ch'üan-shu* (*Ku-chin t'u-shu chi-ch'eng*), 1958, p. 12157.

52. De Groot 1892–1910, 5:789–790.

53. *Ku-chin i-t'ung ta-ch'üan*, 1570, chap. 65, p. 19*a*.

54. Ibid., chap. 49, pp. 15*b*–16*b*.

55. *Chang-shih lei-ching*, 1975, pp. 246–248.

56. Ibid., p. 247; cf. Steininger 1953, pp. 84–85.

57. *Shih-shih mi-lu*, 1974, p. 159.

58. *I-hsüeh hui-hai*, 1826, chap. 34, pp. 37*a*ff.

59. *I-ku*, 1891, chap. 2, pp. 8*b*–9*a*.

60. Doré 1966.

61. *Mi-ts'ang i-shu chu-yu shih-san k'o*, 1895, chap. 1, p. 4*a*.

62. Ibid., chap 1, p. 4*b*.

63. Ibid., p. 6*a*.

64. Ibid., p. 11*b*.

65. Ibid.

66. Ibid., p. 12*a*.

67. "A Chinese View of the Plague" 1896, p. 55; I am indebted to Dr. M. Topley, Hong Kong, for informing me of this source.

68. Ibid.

9: Medicine in Twentieth-Century China

1. Opitz 1972, p. 9.

2. Ibid., p. 6; Croizier 1968, p. 64; Kwok 1965, p. 12.

3. Bauer 1976, pp. 395–396.

4. Sigerist 1963, p. 706.

5. Mark 9, 17–28; John 5, 14; 9, 3.

6. Harnack 1892, p. 54.

7. Ibid., p. 56.

8. Franz 1909.

9. P. Unschuld 1978*a*, pp. 509ff.

10. White 1897, p. 55.

11. Ibid., p. 58.

12. Ibid., p. 62–63.

13. Kwok 1965, p. 21.

14. ABC Archive Harvard, 8.5, III; Gulick 1973, p. 48.

15. Thomson 1887.

16. *Hsi-i lüeh-lun,* 1857, pp. 1*b*–2*b*.

17. Ibid., pp. 4*a*–4*b*.

18. Gulick 1973, p. 133; Young 1973, p. 254.

19. Gulick 1973, p. 20; Spence 1969, p. 39.

20. Gulick 1973, p. 71.

21. Balme 1921, p. 99.

22. Gulick 1973, pp. 133–137.

23. Young 1973, p. 256.

24. Balme 1921, p. 85.

25. Hume 1922, p. 90.

26. Balme 1921, pp. 72–74.

27. Ibid., p. 98; on ethical conflicts resulting from such views see P. Unschuld, 1983*b*.

28. Young 1973, p. 267.

29. Balme 1921, pp. 104–105.

30. Ibid., p. 102.

31. Spence 1969, p. 165; for details of the circumstances leading to the establishment of another "American transplant in China," the Peking Union Medical College, see Bullock 1980.

32. Opitz 1972, p. 56.

33. In a speech on the occasion of the thirty-fifth Convention of German Scientists in 1860; Schipperges 1977, pp. 320–321.

34. Kwok 1965, p. 135.

35. Ibid., p. 140.

36. Ibid., p. 141.

37. Ibid., p. 145.

38. Ibid., pp. 165–166.

39. Mao Tse-tung 1967, 2:381.

40. Croizier 1968, pp. 60–67.

41. Kwok 1965, p. 65.

42. Balme 1921, p. 181.

43. Croizier 1968, p. 54.

44. Ibid., pp. 72–75.

45. Ibid., pp. 154–155.

46. F. T. Gates in a letter to J. D. Rockefeller, January 31, 1905: "Quite apart from the question of persons converted, the mere commercial results of missionary efforts to our own land is worth, I had almost said, a thousand fold every year of what is spent on missions. . . . Missionary enterprise, viewed solely from a commercial standpoint, is immensely profitable. From the point of view of means of subsistence for Americans, our import trade, traceable mainly to the channels opened up by missionaries, is enormous." Brown 1976, p. 899.

47. Lampton 1974, pp. 49–91.

48. Mao Tse-tung 1967, 1:312.

49. Ch'en Pang-hsien 1920, p. 137b.

50. P. Unschuld 1978a, pp. 37–38, 53, 58, 78.

51. For example, Hsu 1973.

52. Croizier 1968, pp. 81–104.

53. Ibid., pp. 92–93, 129.

54. Ibid., p. 155.

55. Committee of the Department of Hygiene of the Department of Logistics of the Army Unit Canton 1972, p. 7.

56. Cf. Li Lun 1975.

57. Mao Tse-tung 1967, 1:314.

58. Committee of the Department of Hygiene 1972, p. 131.

59. Jen K'ang-t'ung 1974, pp. 63–64.

60. Ibid., p. 78.

61. Committee of the Department of Hygiene 1972, p. 129.

62. Ibid.

63. Ibid., p. 130.

64. Mao Tse-tung 1967, 1:303.

65. Ibid., p. 304.

66. Frontispiece, no pagination.

67. Yung-yao hsin-te shih-chiang, 1978, p. 281.

68. Ibid., p. 282.

69. As one example from a voluminous literature published in Taiwan and Hong Kong, explaining and advocating demonological therapy, see Fu-chou ch'üan-shu ("Complete Compilation of Amulets and Spells"), 1977; see also ethnographic field studies by Ahern, Gould-Martin, and Topley in Kleinman et al., eds., 1978; Topley 1970; Keupers 1977 and Hou Ching-lang 1979.

70. Personal communication by health administration officials in the People's Republic of China; see also Pascoe 1980.

71. For recent contributions to this debate see Chao Kuei-hsin 1982, and Yang Shou-i 1982.

72. This maxim appeared in Mao Tse-tung's definition of China's "new-democratic culture" of 1940; see above p. 246.

Appendix: Primary Texts in Translation

1. The translation of *Huang-ti nei-ching* must remain tentative for the time being. No definite conclusions are possible as to the meaning of *nei-ching* in contrast to *Huang-ti wai-ching*, a title also mentioned by the *Han-shu* but no longer extant. The choice, here, of "scripture of internal [treatment]" should not be confused with the modern concept of "internal medicine," in contrast to surgery or externally applied treatment. "Internal [therapy]" may have referred to treatment of the individual organism as such while the *wai-ching* ("scripture of external [therapy]") may have dealt with questions of govern-

ment politics and state economy. Other hypotheses are equally possible, though, especially because the Han bibliography also mentions a *Pien Ch'io nei-ching* and a *Pien Ch'io wai-ching* and one may assume that the legendary physician Pien Ch'io talked about medicine in both scriptures.

2. For a more detailed philological discussion of the following *T'ai-su* texts see P. Unschuld 1982*a*. The treatise *Pa-cheng feng-hou* was incorporated, in full length and almost literally, into chap. 79 of the *Ling-shu;* it appears also in chap. 1 of the *Chia-i ching,* a third century work.

3. *Huang-ti nei-ching t'ai-su,* 1981, pp. 533–535.

4. This treatise was incorporated, in full length and almost literally, into chap. 77 of the *Ling-shu;* parts of it appear also in chap. 1 of the *Chia-i ching.*

5. *Huang-ti nei-ching t'ai-su,* 1981, pp. 526–530.

6. This treatise was incorporated, in full length and almost literally, into chap. 79 of the *Ling-shu;* parts of it appear also in chap. 1 of the *Chia-i ching.*

7. The meaning of the term *chiao-li* is not clear. Yang Shang-shan, in his commentary, considered it to be an abbreviation of *san-chiao* and *tsou-li* ("Triple Burner" and "Pores"), and interpreted it as a passage-way for the influences sent out by the Triple Burner.

8. This is an indication of health. The body is well-nourished and oily; dust clings to it.

9. *Huang-ti nei-ching t'ai-su,* 1981, pp. 530–533.

10. This paragraph is quoted here from a longer treatise, parts of which appear also in chap. 66 of the *Ling-shu,* in chap. 23 of the *Su-wen,* and in chap. 2 of the *Chia-i ching.*

11. *Huang-ti nei-ching t'ai-su,* 1981, p. 512.

12. This treatise does not appear in the *T'ai-su.* I have quoted it here from the *Ling-shu* to provide an example of the integration of the wind-concept into the concept of yin- and yang-categorization.

13. *Ling-shu ching,* 1966, chap. 2, bk. 6, pp. 3*a*–3*b*.

14. This treatise was incorporated, in full length and almost literally, into chap. 58 of the *Ling-shu;* it appears also in chap. 5 of the *Chia-i ching.*

15. *Huang-ti nei-ching t'ai-su,* 1981, pp. 399–401.

16. This treatise was incorporated, in full length and almost literally, into chap. 58 of the *Ling-shu;* it appears also in chap. 5 of the *Chia-i ching.*

17. In his commentary, Yang Shang-shan interpreted "exorcism" not as a method to expel illness-causing demons but as a diagnostic interrogation of omniscient spirits by the shamans who, in contrast to ordinary men, were able to establish contacts with such beings. Yang Shang-shan did, obviously, not question the existence of spirits and demons; he denied that they cause illness and that illness can be treated by exorcising, that is, driving away, demons.

18. *Huang-ti nei-ching t'ai-su,* 1981, pp. 525–526.

19. This treatise appears with various changes in its wording in chap. 42 of the *Su-wen* and in chap. 2 of the *Chia-i ching.*

20. The exact meaning of the term *fen-jou,* obviously combined here with *tsou-li* to *fen-li,* is not clear. It is sometimes defined as the flesh immediately underneath the skin. The *Su-wen* and the *Chia-i ching* changed the wording to *fen-jou.*

21. The meaning of this sentence is not clear. It was omitted by the *Su-wen,* but it appears—in a different wording—in the respective passage of the *Chia-i ching.*

22. *Huang-ti nei-ching t'ai-su,* 1981, pp. 519–522.

23. This treatise appears with various changes in its wording in chap. 42 of the *Su-wen* and in chap. 2 of the *Chia-i ching.*

24. The lung is categorized as "great-yin." Hence, its illnesses are acute at night.

25. According to the Five Phases theory, each depot is associated with a specific color. White corresponds to the lung, red to the heart, green to the liver, yellow to the spleen, and black to the kidneys.

26. *Ch'ü* is generally interpreted as "bent" by Chinese and Japanese commentators; the entire phrase could, thus, be read "[the extremities] are bent and cannot be moved freely." In the treatise *Yin-yang pieh-lun* of the *Su-wen,* however, *yin-ch'ü* is defined as referring to the discharge of the monthly period in females or of semen in males. These physiological processes are usually seen in relation to the functions of the kidneys. Hence the secondary meaning "sprout," "shoot" of *ch'ü,* as mentioned in the *Shuo-wen,* may be applicable here. Yang Shang-shan commented: "The discharge of stools and urine is interrupted."

27. In the same context the term *ke* appears in the *Su-wen* with the radical flesh, assuming the meaning of "membrane." This may, however, represent not a correct reading of the *T'ai-su* phrase. The original meaning of *ke* (without the radical "flesh") refers to a pot, indicating here, I believe, the stomach or, at least, the region where digestive processes take place. The *Chia-i ching* uses the character of the *T'ai-su* but replaced "closed" by "cold."

28. *Shang-lai* makes little sense here. Both the *Su-wen* and the *Chia-i ching* have different wordings which are equally unclear, though.

29. *Huang-ti nei-ching t'ai-su,* 1981, pp. 522–524.

30. Parts of this treatise appear also in chap. 2 of the *T'ai-su,* in chap. 8 of the *Ling-shu,* and in chap. 6 of the *Chia-i ching.*

31. See above pp. 103–104.

32. *Huang-ti nei-ching su-wen,* 1971, chap. 1, pp. 6a–11a.

33. Compare *T'ai-su,* chap. 2, and *Chia-i ching,* chap. 1, for corresponding treatises.

34. *Huang-ti nei-ching su-wen,* 1971, chap. 1, pp. 11a–14b.

35. The following is an excerpt from a treatise corresponding versions of which appear also in chap. 3 of the *T'ai-su* and in chap. 6 of the *Chia-i ching.*

36. *Huang-ti nei-ching su-wen,* 1971, chap. 2, pp. 1a–3b.

37. Compare *T'ai-su,* chap. 6, and *Chia-i ching,* chap. 1, for corresponding treatises.

38. *Huang-ti nei-ching su-wen,* 1971, chap. 3, pp. 13*b*–15*a*.

39. This treatise appears only in the *Su-wen.*

40. *Huang-ti nei-ching su-wen,* 1971, chap. 4, pp. 1*a*–2*b*.

41. This excerpt appears only in the *Su-wen.*

42. *Huang-ti nei-ching su-wen,* 1971, chap. 4, pp. 2*b*–3*a*.

43. This excerpt appears only in the *Su-wen.*

44. The term *pi* cannot be rendered adequately into English with a colloquial term. Symptoms of *pi* include weakness of limbs, paralysis, closure of passages. The *Ling-shu* (see appendix 1.5) defines certain yang-afflictions as "wind" and certain yin-afflictions as *pi.* I have, tentatively, chosen here the term "rheumatism" because it is a prescientific term indicating that various symptoms are the result of an influx (greek: *rheuma*) of entities like wind or moisture.

45. The term *chüeh* refers to the phenomenon that certain influences (primarily cold or yin-influences) ascend in the body, contrary to their proper course. The reason for the application of *chüeh* in the context here is not clear.

46. The concept of *ku* appears to have been developed in a magical and demonological context (see section 2.4). Here, the term is applied to an illness caused by wind, the symptoms of which resemble those associated with the demonological concept, that is, swollen abdomen and internal pain.

47. *Huang-ti nei-ching su-wen,* 1971, chap. 6, pp. 4*b*–5*b*.

48. The first, major section of the excerpt quoted here appears only in the *Su-wen;* a treatise corresponding to the final section beginning with the words "The color of the liver is green" appears in *T'ai-su,* chap. 2.

49. *Huang-ti nei-ching su-wen,* 1971, chap. 7, pp. 3*b*–5*b*.

50. Ibid., pp. 7*b*–8*a*.

51. This excerpt appears only in the *Su-wen.*

52. *Huang-ti nei-ching su-wen,* 1971, chap. 7, pp. 12*a*–12*b*.

53. This treatise appears only in the *Su-wen. Yao*-illnesses have been interpreted as referring to malaria; cf. Miyashita 1979.

54. *Huang-ti nei-ching su-wen,* 1971, chap. 10, pp. 1*a*–2*b*.

55. *Chu-ping yüan hou lun,* 1964, chap. 1, pp. 1–2.

56. Ibid., chap. 2, p. 13.

57. Ibid., chap. 2, p. 18.

58. Ibid., chap. 13, pp. 1–2.

59. Ibid., chap. 22, p. 8.

60. Ibid., chap. 23, p. 1.

61. Ibid., chap. 23, p. 4.

62. Ibid., chap. 24, p. 5.

63. Ibid., chap. 29, p. 1.

64. Ibid., chap. 30, pp. 3–4.

65. Compare above pp. 39, 44.

66. *Ch'ien-chin i-fang,* 1965, p. 347.

67. Fan Wang lived around A.D. 400.

68. The abbreviation *Ch'ien-chin* refers to either the *Ch'ien-chin yao-fang* or the *Ch'ien-chin i-fang,* two prescription works compiled by Sun Ssu-miao (581–682?).

69. The *Chou-hou pei-chi fang* is a prescription work compiled by Ko Hung (281–341); *Wai-t'ai pi-yao,* 1964, pp. 97–98.

70. Ibid., pp. 105–106.

71. Ibid., p. 369.

72. Possibly an abbreviated title of the no longer existing *Chi-yen fang,* a prescription work by Yao Seng-t'an (fl. 535–580).

73. *Wai-t'ai pi-yao,* 1964, p. 1119.

74. These are: do not kill, do not steal, do not commit adultery, do not lie, do not drink alcohol.

75. These are: murder, theft, adultery, lying, duplicity, coarse language, obscene language, lust, anger, perverse views.

76. *Taishō Tripitaka,* 1914–1932, p. 793; cf. Sen 1945, pp. 76–84.

77. This and subsequent translations of "drug-" names reflect Chinese interpretations; they do not necessarily correspond to the original Indian meaning. Cf. Sen 1945, p. 85.

78. *Cure* is termed here with a character literally meaning "to expel," thus referring to the concept of exorcism.

79. The text says "1000"; this is probably an error.

80. *Taishō Tripitaka,* 1914–1932, p. 1059; cf. Sen 1945, pp. 85–95.

81. A point below the nose and above the lips.

82. *Ju-men shih-ch'in,* 1972, chap. 6, p. 16.

83. Ibid., chap. 6, p. 38.

84. Ibid., p. 45.

85. Ibid., pp. 46–47.

86. This sentence corresponds to an identical phrase in T'ao Hung-ching's *Pen-ts'ao ching chi-chu;* it may be, as Watanabe Kōzō has pointed out, an allusion to a statement in chap. 13 of Ko Hung's *Pao-p'u tzu, Nei-p'ien.* According to Ko Hung, willows are quite sturdy but once they are really hurt, even the best care cannot keep them from dying. Man, in contrast, is weak and vulnerable by nature; hence, he should care for his health all the more, beginning from his very youth. Cf. Watanabe Kōzō 1953, p. 2, and *Medicine in China: A History of Pharmaceutics,* p. 37.

87. On Li Tzu-yü see p. 41 above.

88. The *kao-huang*-case is recorded in the *Tso-chuan,* bk. 8, tenth year. In Marquis Ch'eng of Chin two demons had taken up a position below the throat (*kao*) and above the heart (*huang*), inaccessible to any therapy.

89. "Three Authors' *Materia Medica*" (?); an otherwise unidentifiable work. *Ku-chin i-t'ung ta-ch'üan,* 1570, chap. 3*b,* pp. 14*a*–14*b.*

90. The term *sui* used in the heading of this paragraph is identical to the pictogram "[to] curse" mentioned above on p. 21. The original emphasis on the cause appears, over time, to have yielded to an emphasis on the effect,

that is, the "injury." The continuing necessity to define the term, however, indicates that it remained associated with the concept of ancestor-caused illness, even if some authors, as the one cited here, endeavored to overcome these notions.

91. For Nagarjuna see above p. 146.

92. *Ku-chin i-t'ung ta-ch'üan,* 1570, chap. 49, p. 12*b*.

93. Ibid., p. 13*a*.

94. Compare above pp. 21 and 288.

95. *Tan* generally designates Taoist medicinal preparations in the form of a large pill that contains mineral ingredients.

96. A work by Lo T'ien-i (thirteenth century).

97. *Ku-chin i-t'ung ta-ch'üan,* 1570, chap. 49, pp. 15*b*–16*a*.

98. Ibid., p. 17*a*.

99. Compare above pp. 21, 288, and 326.

100. Another possible rendering of this passage would be "the old and the new evil influences turn against each other."

101. Compare above p. 288.

102. Cf. Steininger 1953, pp. 83–85.

103. This treatise is no longer extant.

104. *Chang-shih lei-ching,* 1975, pp. 246–248.

105. If, for instance, the liver (wood) suffers from a depletion of influences and the kidney (water), that is, the mother-depot, is replenished in order to transmit influences to its child-depot, it is a treatment "once removed." If, in such a case, the lung (metal), that is, the grandmother-depot, is replenished, it is a treatment "twice removed." If the spleen (soil), that is, the great-grandmother-depot, is replenished, it is a treatment "three times removed." The theoretical basis for this is the "Order of Mutual Generation" of the Five Phases.

106. *Shih-shih mi-lu,* 1974, p. 1.

107. The *ssu-mo* potion consists of four (*ssu*) drugs that are grated (*mo*) in water or wine and then boiled. The *ssu-ch'i* potion consists of four drugs that are boiled together with seven (*ch'i*) slices of ginger and two dates.

108. *Shih-shih mi-lu,* 1974, pp. 4–5.

109. See above pp. 000–000.

110. *Hsü Ling-t'ai i-shu ch'üan-chi,* 1969, chap. 1, pp. 71–72.

111. See appendix note 90.

112. *Hsü Ling-t'ai i-shu ch'üan-chi,* 1969, chap. 3, pp. 46–47.

113. Ibid., chap. 4, p. 204.

114. A derogatory designation for Confucius that utilizes Confucian values concerning the first- and second-born sons.

115. Cited according to the *Lun-yü* ("The Annals of Confucius"), bk. 7, chap. 8.

116. See p. 20 above.

117. Cited from the *Tso-chuan,* bk. 10, first year.

118. See p. 17 above.

119. Cited according to the *Han Fei-tzu,* chap. 19, sec. 49.

120. *Tso-chuan,* bk. 10, first year.

121. Cited according to the *Lieh-tzu,* bk. 6, sec. 6.

122. *Lun-yü,* bk. 3, chap. 13. The original quotation as used here is doubly misleading. First, the statement cited has no connection whatsoever to an illness of Confucius. Confucius replies with these words to the request of a man to interpret an old saying, metaphorically in the sense of "he who turns against the Supreme Power is beyond all help." Chu Hsi, the preeminent philosopher of Neo-Confucianism during the Sung period ascribed to the term *t'ien* ("heaven") in this statement of Confucius the meaning of *li* ("principle," "natural law"). Cf. Legge 1960, 1:159. Second, the authors of this article neglect to point out that Confucius, when he had once indeed fallen ill, and a disciple wished to pray for him, had responded: "Does such a thing exist?" To this the disciple replied: "Yes, such a thing exists. In the Eulogies it is written: Prayers were performed for the spirits above [in heaven] and below [on the earth]." To this Confucius responded: "[Then] have been praying for a long time!" (*Lun-yü,* bk. 7, chap. 24; Legge 1960, 1:206). The subtle rejection by Confucius of prayers thus followed from the conviction that the conduct of his life would have long since found favor with some spirits if, in fact, they existed.

123. A member of one of the three noble families that shared power in Confucius' native province of Lu.

124. *Lun-yü,* bk. 10, chap. 2. The quotation is used here in a false context, since Chi K'ang had sent the medications to Confucius as a present, without the latter being ill.

125. Cited according to the *Hsün-tzu,* chap. 11, sec. 17. See also pp. 62–65 above.

126. *Han Fei-tzu,* chap. 5, sec. 15.

127. Ibid., chap. 19, sec. 50.

128. Cited according to the *Shih-chi,* chap. 105, biography of Pien Ch'io.

129. See p. 287 above.

130. Prominent Confucian author of the early Han period (second century B.C.).

131. Cited according to the *Pen-ts'ao kang mu,* chap. 9, *shui-yin* ("quicksilver") monograph, section *fa-ming* ("commentaries"). The original quotation has been removed from its context and combined here with an inaccurate characterization of Li Shih-chen (1518–1593). The exact wording of the passage is as follows: "Quicksilver is pure yin-essence; its nature is immobility. When it is heated above fire, it ascends to heaven and is transformed into something spiritual. If the opportunity arises for quicksilver to vaporize together with the influences of man [in the body], it travels into the bones and penetrates the muscles. It interrupts the yang[-conduits] and consumes the

brain. [Quicksilver] is a poisonous substance without equal and yet Ta-ming [i.e., Jih Hua-tzu, medical author of the T'ang period) claims that it 'contains no poison.' In the *Pen-ching* [i.e., *Shen-nung pen-ts'ao ching*, the late Han classic of drug therapy] it is said that by 'taking it for a long period one can become a mountain hermit with the faculties of a spirit.' Chen Ch'üan [541?–643; an author of medical works] called it 'the real mother of the pill for transcending [to an immortal],' and Pao-p'u-tzu [i.e., Ko Hung, 281–341; Taoist, alchemist, and medical author] regarded it as a drug of longevity. I do not know how many people who value their lives have taken this substance since the time of the Six Dynasties (420–588) and developed terrible illnesses and ultimately died. The sorcerers are unworthy of any consideration, yet how was it possible for such false statements to find their way into medical literature? Quicksilver is not edible, but its effectiveness in treating illnesses is obvious. With black lead it forms a granular material that suppresses mucus, and with sulphur it forms a granular material that is of assistance in cases of grave illnesses. [Quicksilver] is like a soldier who adjusts easily; with its aid one is able to reach points of junction and attain the centers of power. Additional information can be found under 'white-lead frost' and 'cinnabar'" (*Pen-ts'ao kang mu*, 1933, chap. 3, p. 58).

The criticism expressed here is directed solely to quicksilver. Li Shih-chen did not reject the idea of longevity itself, but called for the greatest caution, since the necessary substances were so toxic. Thus, in his discussion of cinnabar he also cited the reports of some earlier authors of fatalities following the taking of such preparations; at the same time, however, he included opposing views, and himself reached the following conclusion: "The depots and palaces [in the body] of men are apparently of a widely diverse nature. Thus one must be knowledgeable when differentiating the symptoms of yin and yang, and no action should be taken on the basis of pre-conceived judgments. Only he who has penetrated into the deepest and most subtle secrets can understand such a course [i.e., the preparation and taking of immortality drugs]" (*Pen-ts'ao kang mu*, 1933, chap. 3, p. 54).

Following this warning against all forms of dilettantism Li Shih-chen recommended prescriptions based on cinnabar, which promised eventually first the liberation from all illnesses, followed by the blackening of graying hair, and then finally transcendence into a man with the faculties of spirits. Even Li Shih-chen's criticism of the sorcerers (*fang-shih*) must be viewed as relative. It is directed solely against those in groups competing with physicians like Li Shih-chen, but not against their ideas. Demonology and magic are amply represented in Li Shih-chen's work.

132. Shen Kua lived from 1030–1093. At one time a high Confucian official, he was exiled following a military defeat at the hands of foreign invaders. He wrote numerous works on various problems of nature and technology, including a book of prescriptions compiled together with the poet Su

Tung-p'o, an outspoken opponent of the reform plans of Wang An-shih, entitled *Su Shen liang-fang* ("Good Prescriptions by Su Tung-p'o and Shen Kua"). The work is marked by obvious Neo-Confucian elements.

133. Cited according to the *Su Shen nei-han liang-fang,* chap. 1, sec. "Lun t'ang san wan" ("On Boiled Potions, Powders, and Pills").

134. Ibid., chap. 1, sec. "Lun ts'ai-yao" ("On the Gathering of Drugs").

135. On Wu Yu-k'o (born Wu Yu-hsing) see section 8.2.2.2 above. The quotation is taken from the preface to *Wen-i lun* ("On Warmth Epidemics"). The conclusion "old prescriptions are unsuitable for today's illnesses" was first drawn by Chang Yüan-su (ca. 1180), the founder of Sung-Chin-Yüan medicine. Chang Yüan-su had received a Confucian education and attained the rank of *chin-shih.* But when he once used a prohibited character that constituted part of the name of a dead emperor, he was stripped of the *chin-shih* rank. Following this, he devoted himself solely to medicine. For further details see *Medicine in China: A History of Pharmaceutics,* pp. 101–104.

136. Shanghai Academy of Chinese Medicine Museum of Medical History 1974, pp. 84–92.

137. That is, solid, fluid, and gaseous waste products.

138. "Social-imperialistic country" is a common designation in the People's Republic of China for the Soviet Union.

139. One of the three laws of dialectics formulated by Engels is the unity of opposites.

140. *Tsen-yang chan-sheng man-hsing chi-ping,* 1978, pp. 1–7.

141. Ibid., pp. 110–111.

Bibliography

CHINESE PRIMARY SOURCES

Dates refer to editions used. The numbers in brackets following individual bibliographical entries refer to the list of Chinese characters on pp. 405–408.

Chang-shih lei-ching
1975   By Chang Chieh-pin. Taipei. [1]

Cheng-t'ung tao-tsang
1977   I-wen yin-shu-kuan, ed. Taipei. [2]

Ch'ien-chin i-fang
1965   By Sun Ssu-miao, Taipei. [3]

Chin-kuei yao-lüeh
1966   By Chang Chi. Taipei. [4]

Chu-ping yüan hou lun
1964   By Ch'ao Yüan-fang. Taipei. [5]

(Ch'in-ting) ch'üan T'ang-shih
1887   Shanghai [6]

Ch'uan-ya nei wai pien
1957   By Chao Hsüeh-min. Hong Kong. [7]

Ch'uan-ya nei-pien hsüan-chu
1980   By Chao Hsüeh-min; selection and commentary by anonymous committee. Peking. [8]

Ch'uan-ya wai-pien hsüan-chu
1977   By Chao Hsüeh-min; selection and commentary by anonymous committee. Peking. [9]

Ch'ung-chi hsin-hsiu pen-ts'ao
1964   Okanishi Tameto, ed. Taipei. [10]

Fu-chou ch'üan-shu
1977   Lin Hsien-chih, ed. Taipei. [11]

Han Fei-tzu
1966   By Han Fei; ed. Ssu-pu pei-yao. Taipei. [12]

Hsi-i lüeh-lun
1857   By Ho-hsin (B. Hobson) and Kuan Mao-ts'ai. Canton. [13]

Hsü Ling-t'ai i-shu ch'üan-chi
1969   By Hsü Ta-ch'un. Taipei. [14]

Hsün-tzu chi-chieh
1971   Yang Chia-lo, ed. Taipei. [15]

Huai-nan-tzu chu
1968   Yang Chia-lo, ed. Taipei. [16]

Huang-ti nei-ching su-wen
1971   By Wang Ping et al. Taipei. [17]

Huang-ti nei-ching t'ai-su
1981   By Yang Shang-shan. Peking. [18]

I-hsüeh hui-hai
1826   By Sun Te-jun. N.p. [19]

I-hsüeh ju-men
1973   By Li T'ing. Taipei. [20]

I-ku
1891   By Cheng Wen-cho. N.p. [21]

I-lin kai-ts'o
1849   By Wang Ch'ing-jen. N.p. [22]

I-lin kai-ts'o p'ing-chu
1976   By Wang Ch'ing-jen; annotated edition by anonymous
              committee. Peking. [23]

I-pu ch'üan-shu
1958   By Ch'en Meng-lei, ed. Ku-chin t'u-shu chi-ch'eng. Taipei.
              [24]

Ishimpō (I-hsin-fang)
1955   By Tamba Yasuyori. Peking. [25]

Ju-men shih-ch'in
1972   By Chang Ts'ung-cheng. Taipei. [26]

Ku-chin i-t'ung ta-ch'üan
1570   By Hsü Ch'un-fu. N.p. [27]

Kuan-tzu chiao-cheng
1954   By Tai Wang, ed.; ed. Chu-tzu chi-ch'eng. Peking. [28]

Lao-tzu Hsiang-erh chu chiao-chien
1956   Jao Tsung-i, ed. Hong Kong. [29]

Li-yang chi-yao
n.d.   By Hsüeh Chi. Shanghai. [30]

Ling-shu ching
1966   N.a., ed. Ssu-pu pei-yao. Taipei. [31]

Ling-yen fu-chu ch'üan-shu
1924   N.a. Shanghai. [32]

Lü-shih ch'un-ch'iu chi-shih
1969   Yang Chia-lo, ed. Taipei. [33]

Lun-heng
1974   By Wang Ch'ung. Shanghai. [34]

Mi-ts'ang i-shu chu-yu shih-san k'o
1895   By Lo Ch'i-ch'eng. Shanghai. [35]

Nan Ch'i-shu
n.d.   By Hsiao Tzu-hsien, ed. Chung-hua shu-chü, N.p. [36]

Nan-ching shu-cheng
1961   By Taki Mototane. Kao-hsiung. [37]

Pao-p'u-tzu
1969   By Ko Hung. Taipei. [38]

Pei-chi ch'ien-chin yao-fang
1965   By Sun Ssu-miao. Taipei. [39]

Pei-k'ao shih-wu pen-ts'ao kang mu
n.d.   By Yao K'e-ch'eng. N.p. [40]

Pen-ts'ao kang mu
1933   By Li Shih-chen. Shanghai. [41]

P'i-wei lun
1975   by Li Kao, ed. *I-t'ung cheng-mai ch'üan-shu* by Wang K'en-
              t'ang. Vol. 10. Taipei. [42]

P'i-wei lun chu-shih
1976   By Li Kao; annotated edition by anonymous committee.
              Peking. [43]

San-yin chi-i ping-cheng fang lun
1973   By Ch'en Yen. Taipei. [44]

Shan-hai ching chien-shu
1974   Shih I-hsing, ed. Taipei. [45]

Shang-han lun chin-shih
1931   By Chang Chi; annotated ed. by Lu Yüan-lei. Shanghai.
              [46]

Sheng-chi tsung-lu
1978   Ts'ao Hsiao-chung et al., eds. Taipei. [47]

Shih-chi
1969   By Ssu-ma Ch'ien; ed. Chung-hua shu-chü. Hong Kong.
              [48]

Shih-shih mi-lu
1974   By Ch'en Shih-to. Taipei. [49]

Shou-shih pao-yüan

1974   By Kung T'ing-hsien. Taipei. [50]

Su Shen nei-han liang-fang

n.d.   By Shen Kua and Su Tung-p'o; ed. Ssu-k'u ch'üan-shu. N.p. [51]

T'ai-p'ing yü-lan

1968   By Li Fang et al., eds. Taipei. [52]

Taishō Tripitaka

1914–32   Takakusu Junjiro and Watanabe Kaigyoku, eds. Tokyo. [53]

T'ang-yeh pen-ts'ao

1956   By Wang Hao-ku. Peking. [54]

Tsen-yang chan-sheng man-hsing chi-ping

1978   By Tuan Chen-li. N.p. (Cheng-chou?) [55]

Wai-t'ai pi-yao

1964   By Wang Tao. Taipei. [56]

Wen-i lun p'ing-chu

1977   By Wu Yu-hsing; annotated edition by anonymous committee. Peking. [57]

Wu-shih-erh ping fang

1979   Annotated edition by anonymous committee. Peking. [58]

Yen-k'o ta-ch'üan

n.d.   By Fu Jen-yü. Ming Shan-ch'eng-t'ang edition. N.p. [59]

Yung-yao hsin-te shih-chiang

1978   By Chiao Shu-te. Peking. [60]

CHINESE AND JAPANESE SECONDARY SOURCES

Akahori Akira

1979   *"Yin-yang shih-i mo-chiu ching* to *Su-wen." Nihon Ishigaku Zasshi* 25:277–287. [61]

1981   *"Yin-yang shih-i mo-chiu ching* no kenkyu." *Tōhō gakuhō* 53:299–339. [62]

Chang Tzu-kao

1962   "Chao Hsüeh-min *Pen-ts'ao kang mu shih i* chu-shu nien-tai chien-lun wo-kuo shou-tz'u yung ch'iang-shui k'o t'ung pan shih." *K'o-hsüeh shih chi-k'an* 4:106–109. [63]

Chao Kuei-hsin

1982   "TCM Modernization and My Understanding." *Medicine and Philosophy (I-hsüeh yü che-hsüeh)* 3:25–26. [64]

Ch'en Pang-hsien
    1920   *Chung-kuo i-hsüeh shih.* Shanghai. [65]
    1969   *Chung-kuo i-hsüeh shih.* Taipei.

Chou I-mou
    1980   "Ch'ien-t'an Huang-Lao che-hsüeh yü ku-tai i-hsüeh." *Ma-wang-tui i-shu yen-chiu chuan-k'an* 1:1–7. [66]

Committee of the Department of Hygiene of the Department of Logistics of the Army Unit Canton
    1972   *Hsin-pien chung-i-hsüeh kai-yao.* Peking. [67]

Hsieh Kuan
    1935   *Chung-kuo i-hsüeh yüan-liu lun.* Shanghai. [68]

Hu Hou-hsüan
    1944   "Yin-jen chi-ping k'ao." *Chia-ku-hsüeh Shang-shih lun-ts'ung.* Ch'eng-tu. [69]

Jen K'ang-t'ung
    1974   "Chen-tz'u ma-tsui chung ti pien-cheng fa." *Tzu-jan pien-cheng-fa* 1:62–79. [70]

Kanō Yoshimitsu
    1980   "Isho ni mieru kiron." In *Ki no shisō,* edited by Onozawa Seiichi et al., pp. 280–313. [71]

Ku Te-tao
    1979   *Chung-kuo i-hsüeh shih-lüeh.* T'ai-yüan. [72]

Kuo Ping-ch'üan and I Fa-yin
    1980   "Shih-lun Ma-wang-tui Han-mu ch'u-t'u ti liang-chung po-shu 'Lao-tzu' tui tsu-kuo i-hsüeh ti ying-hsiang." *Ma-wang-tui i-shu yen-chiu chuan-k'an* 1:8–11. [73]

Li Chung-wen
    1980   "*Wu-shih-erh ping fang* chung kao-yao-lei yao-wu ti t'an-t'ao." *Ch'ang-sha Ma-wang-tui i-shu yen-chiu chuan-k'an* 1:43–48. [74]

Liu Tun-yüan
    1972   "Han-hua-hsiang-shih shang ti chen-chiu-t'u." *Wen-wu ts'an-k'ao tzu-liao* 6:47f. [75]

Ma Chi-hsing
    1979   "T'ai Hsi ts'un Shang-mu chung ch'u-t'u te i-liao ch'i-chü pien lien." *Wen-wu* 6:54–56. [76]

Miyashita Saburo
    1959   "Medical Treatment and the People's Conception on Diseases in Ancient China." *Tōhō Gakuhō* 30:227–252. [77]

Okanishi Tameto
    1969   *Sung-i-ch'ien i-chi k'ao*. Taipei. [78]
Peking Academy of Chinese Medicine
    1968*a*   *Chung-kuo i-hsüeh-shih chiang-i*. Hong Kong. [79]
    1968*b*   *Chung-i ko-chia hsüeh-shuo chiang-i*. Hong Kong. [80]
Shang Chih-chün
    1980   "*Wu-shih-erh ping fang* chung yao-wu chih-pei kung-i k'ao-
                   ch'a." *Ch'ang-sha Ma-wang-tui i-shu yen-chiu chuan-k'an*
                   1:38–42. [81]
Shanghai Academy of Chinese Medicine Museum of Medical History
    1974   "Wo-kuo i-hsüeh-shang fan-t'ien-ming yü tsun-t'ien-ming
                   ti tou-cheng." *Tzu-jan pien-cheng-fa* 3:84–92. [82]
Shang-kuan Liang-fu
    1974   *Chung-kuo i-yao fa-chan-shih*. Hong Kong. [83]
Taki Mototane
    1956   *Chung-kuo i-chi k'ao*. Peking. [84]
Ting Shan
    1928   "Shih chi." *Chung-yang yen-chiu-yüan li-shih yü-yen yen-
                   chiu-so chi-k'an* 1:243–245. [85]
Watanabe Kōzō
    1953   "Honzō Shūchū joroku no yakuchū." *Kanpō* 2, no.
                   6:1–5. [86]
    1956   "General Remark on the Dissection and Anatomical Fig-
                   ures in China." *Nihon Ishigaku Zasshi* 7:88–182. [87]
Yamada Keiji
    1980   "Kyū-ku hachi-fu setsu to shōshiha no tachiba" *Tōhō ga-
                   kuhō* 52: 199–242. [469]
Yang Shou-i
    1982   "TCM Modernization Cannot Take the Principles of West-
                   ern Medicine as Its Evaluative Criterion." *Medicine and
                   Philosophy* (*I-hsüeh yü che-hsüeh*) 3:27. [88]
Yen I-p'ing
    1951   "Chung-kuo i-hsüeh chih ch'i-yüan chi k'ao-lüeh." *Ta-lu
                   tsa-chih* 2(8):20–22; (9):14–17. [89]

WESTERN SECONDARY SOURCES

Ackerknecht, Erwin H.
    1942   "Primitive Medicine and Culture Pattern." *Bulletin of the
                   History of Medicine* 12:545–574.
Ahern E. M.
    1973   *The Cult of the Dead in a Chinese Village*. Stanford.

Ardener, Edwin
1970   "Witchcraft, Economics and the Continuity of Belief." In *Witchcraft, Confessions and Accusations,* edited by Mary Douglas, pp. 141–160. London.

Balme, Harold
1921   *China and Modern Medicine.* London.

Bauer, Wolfgang
1976   *China and the Search for Happiness. Recurring Themes in Four Thousand Years of Chinese Cultural History.* New York.

Brown E. Richard
1976   "Public Health in Imperialism: Early Rockefeller Programs at Home and Abroad." *American Journal of Public Health* 66:897–903.

Bullock, Mary Brown
1980   *An American Transplant: The Rockefeller Foundation and Peking Union Medical College.* Berkeley.

Chan Wing-Tsit
1970   "The Ch'eng-Chu School of Early Ming." In *Self and Society in Ming Thought,* edited by William Theodore de Bary, pp. 29–52. New York.

Chang Tsung-Tung
1970   *Der Kult der Shang-Dynastie im Spiegel der Orakelinschriften.* Wiesbaden.

Ch'en, Kenneth
1964   *Buddhism in China.* Princeton.

"A Chinese View of the Plague."
1896   Medical Report on the Epidemics of Bubonic Plague 1894. Papers laid before the Legislative Council, 1895. Hong Kong Government Printers, pp. 55–58.

Chow Tse-tsung
1978   "The Childbirth Myth and Ancient Chinese Medicine: A Study of Aspects of the *Wu* Tradition." In *Ancient China: Studies in Early Civilization,* edited by David T. Roy and Tsuen-hsuin Tsien. Hong Kong.

Croizier, Ralph
1968   *Traditional Medicine in Modern China.* Cambridge, Mass.

De Bary, Wm. Theodore
1970*a*   "Introduction." In *Self and Society in Ming Thought,* edited by William Theodore de Bary pp. 1–28. New York.
1970*b*   "Individualism and Humanitarianism in Late Ming Thought." In *Self and Society in Ming Thought,* pp. 145–248.

De Groot, J. J. M.
    1892–1910   *The Religious System of China.* Vols. I–IV. Leiden.

Doré, Henry
    1966   *Researches into Chinese Superstitions.* Taipei.

Dubs, Homer H.
    1955   *The History of the Former Han Dynasty.* Baltimore.

Dudgeon, John
    1895   "Kung Fu or Medical Gymnastics." *Journal of the Peking Oriental Society* 3:341–565.

Eberhard, Wolfram
    1933   "Beiträge zur kosmologischen Spekulation Chinas in der Han-Zeit." *Baessler Archiv* 16:1–100.
    1942   *Die Lokalkulturen des Südens und Ostens.* Peking.

Edelstein, Ludwig
    1967   *Ancient Medicine.* Baltimore.

Eichhorn, Werner
    1954   "Descriptions of the Rebellion of Sun En and Earlier Taoist Rebellions." *Mitteilungen des Instituts für Orientforschungen der Deutschen Akademie der Wissenschaften* 2:325–352.
    1955   "Bemerkungen zum Aufstand des Chang Chio und zum Staate des Chang Lu." Ibid., 3:291–327.
    1973   *Die Religionen Chinas.* Stuttgart.
    1976   *Die alte chinesische Religion und das Staatskultwesen.* Leiden.

Epler, D. C.
    1980   "Bloodletting in Early Chinese Medicine and Its Relation to the Origin of Acupuncture." *Bulletin of the History of Medicine* 54:337–367.

Feng, H. Y., and J. K. Shryock
    1935   "The Black Magic in China Known as Ku." *Journal of the American Oriental Society* 55:1–30.

Filliozat, Jean
    1979   *Nagarjuna: Yogaśataka. Texte medical.* Pondicherry.

Foster, George M.
    1965   "Peasant Society and the Image of Limited Good." *American Anthropologist* 67:293–315.

Franke, Herbert, and Rolf Trauzettel
    1968   *Das Chinesische Kaiserreich.* Frankfurt am Main.

Franke, Otto
    1930–1952   *Geschichte des Chinesischen Reiches.* Vols. I–IV. Berlin.

Franz, Adolph
    1909   *Die kirchlichen Benediktionen im Mittelalter.* Freiburg.

Frazer, James G.
    1926   *The Golden Bough.* London.

Granet, Marcel
    1963   *Das chinesische Denken.* Munich.
    1976   *Die chinesische Zivilisation.* Munich.

Gulick, Edward V.
    1973   *Peter Parker and the Opening of China.* Cambridge, Mass.

Harnack, Adolf
    1892   "Medicinisches aus der Älteren Kirchengeschichte." In *Texte und Untersuchungen zur Geschichte der Altchristlichen Literatur,* edited by Oscar v. Gebhardt and A. Harnack, 8:37–147.

Hartner, Willy
    1941, 1942   "Heilkunde im Alten China." *Sinica* 16:217–265; 17:27–89.

Hintzsche, Erich
    1960   "Analyse des Berner Codex 350, ein bibliographischer Beitrag zur chinesischen Medizin und zu deren Kenntnis bei Fabricius Hildanus und Haller." *Gesnerus* 17:99–116.

Hōbōgirin
    1929   Sylvain Lévi, J. Takakusu, and Paul Demiéville, eds. Tokyo.

Hou, Ching-lang
    1979   "The Chinese Belief in Baleful Stars." In *Facets of Taoism,* edited by Holmes Welch and Anna Seidel, pp. 193–228. New Haven and London.

Hsu, Francis L. K.
    1973   *Religion, Science and Human Crisis.* Westport, Conn.

Hume, Edward H.
    1922   "Medical Education in China: A Survey and Forecast." In *Dedication Ceremonies and Medical Conference, Peking Union Medical College 1921.* Peking.

Hummel, Arthur W.
    1970   *Eminent Chinese of the Ch'ing Period.* Taipei.

Ishihara Akira and Howard S. Levy
    1968   *The Tao of Sex. Translation of the Twenty-eighth Section of Essence of Medical Prescriptions (Ishimpo).* Yokohama.

Jen Yu-wen
    1970   "Ch'en Hsien-chang's Philosophy of the Natural." In *Self and Society in Ming Thought,* edited by William Theodore de Bary, pp. 53–92. New York.

Jordan, D. K.
1972   *Gods, Ghosts, and Ancestors. Folk Religion in a Taiwanese Village.* Berkeley, Los Angeles, London.

Kaltenmarck, Max
1979   "The Ideology of the T'ai-p'ing ching." In *Facets of Taoism,* edited by Holmes Welch and Anna Seidel, pp. 19–52. New Haven and London.

Karlgren, Bernhard
1970   *Analytic Dictionary of Chinese and Sino-Japanese.* Taipei.

Keightley, David
1975   "Legitimation in Shang China." *Contribution to the Conference on Legitimation of Chinese Imperial Regimes, June 15–24, 1975, Monterey, Cal.*
1978   *Sources of Shang History: The Oracle-Bone Inscriptions of Bronze Age China.* Berkeley, Los Angeles, London.

Keupers, John
1977   "A Description of the *Fa-ch'ang* Ritual as Practiced by the *Lü Shan* Taoists of Northern Taiwan." In *Buddhist and Taoist Studies* I (Asian Studies at Hawaii 18), edited by Michael Saso and David W. Chappell, 79–94.

Kleinman, Arthur et al., eds.
1978   *Culture and Healing in Asian Societies.* Boston.

Kranz, Walther
1958   *Die griechische Philosophie.* Bremen.

Kwok, Daniel W. Y.
1965   *Scientism in Chinese Thought.* New Haven.

Lampton, David
1974   *Health, Conflict and the Chinese Political System.* Papers in Chinese Studies no. 18. Ann Arbor.

Legge, James
1960   *The Chinese Classics.* Hong Kong.
n.d.   *Tao Te Ching and the Writings of Chuang Tzu.* Taipei.

Levenson, Joseph R., and F. Schurmann
1969   *China: An Interpretative History.* Berkeley.

Levy, Howard
1956   "Yellow Turban Religion and Rebellion at the End of the Han." *Journal of the American Oriental Society* 76:214–227.

Li Lun
1975   "Acupuncture Develops in the Struggle between the Confucian Thinking and the Legalist Thinking." *Scientia Sinica* 18:581–590.

Liu Ts'un-yan
  1970   "Taoist Self-Cultivation in Ming Thought." In *Self and Society in Ming Thought*, edited by William Theodore de Bary, pp. 291–326. New York.

Lu Gwei-djen and Joseph Needham
  1980   *Celestial Lancets: A History and Rationale of Acupuncture and Moxa*. Cambridge.

Mao Tse-tung
  1967   *Selected Works*. Peking.

Michaud, Paul
  1958   "The Yellow Turbans." *Monumenta Serica* 17:47–127.

Miyashita Saburo
  1979   "Malaria (*yao*) in Chinese Medicine during the Chin and Yüan Periods." *Acta Asiatica* 36:90–112.

Needham, Joseph
  1961, 1956,   *Science and Civilization in China*. Vols. I, II, and V/2. Cambridge.
  1970, 1974   *Clerks and Craftsmen in China and the West*. Cambridge.

Opitz, Peter J.
  1972   *Chinas große Wandlung*. Munich.

Pascoe, Richard
  1980   "Chinese Reviving Old Superstitions. Newspapers Publishing Detailed Accounts." *Japan Times*, April 9, p. 9.

Porkert, Manfred
  1965   "Die energetische Terminologie in den chinesischen Medizinklassikern." *Sinologica* 8:184–210.
  1974   *The Theoretical Foundations of Chinese Medicine*. Cambridge, Mass.

Prunner, Gernot
  1973   *Papiergötter aus China. Wegweiser zur Völkerkunde*. Heft 14. Hamburg.

Read, Bernard E.
  1931   "Treatment of Worm Diseases with Chinese Drugs." *National Medical Journal of China* 17:644–654.

Sakai Tadao
  1970   "Confucianism and Popular Educational Works." In *Self and Society in Ming Thought*, edited by William Theodore de Bary, pp. 331–366. New York.

Schipperges, Heinrich
  1977   "Einheitsbestrebungen und Normbegriff auf der Naturforscherversammlung im 19. Jahrhundert." *Sudhoffs Archiv* 61:313–330.

Schmidt-Glintzer, Helwig, trans.
1975   *Mo Ti: Gegen den Krieg.* Düsseldorf.

Schoeck, Helmut
1974   *Der Neid und die Gesellschaft.* Freiburg.

Schram, Stuart R.
1969   *The Political Thought of Mao Tse-Tung.* Harmondsworth, England.

Seidel, Anna
1978   "Der Kaiser und sein Ratgeber. Lao Tzu und der Taoismus der Han Zeit." *Saeculum* 29:18–50.

Sen Satiranjan
1945   "Two Medical Texts in Chinese Translations." *Visva-Bharati Annals* I:70–95.

Sigerist, Henry E.
1963   *Anfänge der Medizin.* Zurich.

Sivin, Nathan
1968   *Chinese Alchemy. Preliminary Studies.* Cambridge, Mass.

Spence, Jonathan D.
1969   "Peter Parker, Bodies or Souls?" In *To Change China. Western Advisers in China 1620–1960*, pp. 34–56. Boston.

Stein, Rolf A.
1963   "Remarques sur les movements du Taoisme politico-religieux au IIe siècle ap. JC." *T'oung Pao* 50:1–78.
1979   "Religious Taoism and Popular Religion from the Second to Seventh Centuries." In *Facets of Taoism,* edited by Holmes Welch and Anna Seidel, pp. 53–81. New Haven and London.

Steininger, Hans
1953   *Hauch- und Körperseele und der Dämon bei Kuan Yin-tzu.* Leipzig.

Stinchcombe, Arthur L.
1965   "Social Structure and Organizations." In *Handbook of Organizations,* edited by J. J. March. Chicago.

Tang Chun-I
1970   "The Development of the Concept of Moral Mind from Wang Yang-ming to Wang Chi." In *Self and Society in Ming Thought,* edited by William Theodore de Bary, pp. 93–120. New York.

Thomson, J. C.
1887   "Historical Landmarks of Macao." *The Chinese Recorder* 18:392–393.

Topley, Marjorie
    1970   "Chinese Traditional Ideas and the Treatment of Disease: Two Examples from Hongkong." *Man* 5:421–437.

Tu Wei-ming
    1979   "The 'Thought of Huang-Lao': A Reflection on the Lao Tzu and Huang Ti Texts in the Silk Manuscripts of Ma-wang-tui." *The Journal of Asian Studies* 39:95–110.

Unschuld, Paul U.
    1975   "Zur Bedeutung des Terminus *tu* in der traditionellen medizinisch-pharmazeutischen Literatur Chinas." *Sudhoffs Archiv* 59:165–183.
    1978*a*   *Medical Ethics in Imperial China.* Berkeley, Los Angeles, London.
    1978*b*   "Die konzeptuelle Überformung der individuellen und kollektiven Erfahrung von Kranksein." In *Krankheit, Heilkunst, Heilung,* edited by H. Schipperges, E. Seidler, and P. U. Unschuld, pp. 491–516. Freiburg.
    1978*c*   "Das *Ch'uan-ya* und die Praxis chinesischer Landärzte im 18. Jahrhundert." *Sudhoffs Archiv* 62:378–402.
    1982*a*   "Ma-wang-tui *Materia Medica.* A Comparative Analysis of Early Chinese Pharmaceutical Knowledge." *Zinbun: Memoirs of the Research Institute for Humanistic Studies, Kyoto University* 18:11–63.
    1982*b*   "Der Wind als Ursache des Krankseins. Einige Gedanken zu Yamada Keijis Analyse der *Shao-shih* Texte des *Huang-ti nei-ching.*" *T'oung-Pao* 68:91–131.
    1983*a*   "Die Bedeutung der Ma-wang-tui Funde für die chinesische Medizin- und Pharmaziegeschichte." *Festschrift für Rudolf Schmitz,* pp. 389–417. Graz.
    1983*b*   "Frühe christliche Missionshospitäler in China im 19. Jahrhundert." In *Krankenhausmedizin im 19. Jahrhundert,* edited by H. Schadewaldt and J. H. Wolf, pp. 98–111. Munich.

Unschuld, Ulrike
    1972   *Das T'ang-yeh pen-ts'ao und die Übertragung der klassischen chinesischen Medizintheorie auf die Praxis der Drogenkunde.* Munich.
    1977   "Traditional Chinese Pharmacology: An Analysis of Its Development in the Thirteenth Century." *Isis* 68:224–248.

Wasson, R. Gordon
    1968   *Soma: Divine Mushroom of Immortality.* New York.

Watson, Burton, trans.
    1963   *Hsün-Tzu. Basic Writings.* New York.

Welch, Holmes
    1972   *Taoism: The Parting of the Way.* Boston.

White, Andrew D.
    1897   *A History of the Warfare of Science with Theology.* New York.

Wilhelm, Hellmut
    1948   "Eine Chou Inschrift über Atemtechnik." *Monumenta Serica* 13:385f.

Wilhelm, Richard
    1924   *I Ging. Das Buch der Wandlungen.* Jena.
    1930   Li Gi. Das Buch der Sitte des Älteren und Jüngeren Dai. Jena.
    1940   *Dschuang Dsi. Das wahre Buch vom Südlichen Blütenland.* Jena.
    1941   *Lao Tse Tao Te King. Das Buch des Alten vom Sinn und Leben.* Jena.

Wright, A. F.
    1948   "Fo-Thu-Teng: A Biography." *Harvard Journal of Asian Studies* 11:321f.

Yamada Keiji
    1979   "The Formation of the *Huang-Ti Nei-Ching.*" *Acta Asiatica* 36:67–89.

Young, Theron Kue-Hing
    1973   "A Conflict of Professions: The Medical Missionary in China, 1835–1890." *Bulletin of the History of Medicine* 47:250–272.

List of Chinese Characters

This list refers to Bibliography (p. 391) and General Index (p. 415).

[1] 張氏類經　張介賓　　[2] 正統道藏　藝文印書館　[3] 千金翼方　孫思邈　[4] 金匱要略張機　[5] 諸病源候論　巢元方　[6] 欽定全唐詩　[7] 串雅內外編　趙學敏　[8] 串雅內編選注　[9] 串雅外編選注　[10] 重輯新修本草岡西為人　[11] 符咒全書　林先知　[12] 韓非子韓非　[13] 西醫略論　合信　管茂材　[14] 徐靈胎醫書全集　徐大椿　[15] 荀子集解　楊家駱　[16] 淮南子注　楊家駱　[17] 黃帝內經素問　王冰　[18] 黃帝內經太素　楊上善　[19] 醫學匯海　孫德潤　[20] 醫學入門李梴　[21] 醫故　鄭文焯　[22] 醫林改錯王清任　[23] 医林改錯评注　王清任　[24] 醫部全書　陳夢雷　古今圖書集成　[25] 醫心方　丹波康賴　[26] 儒門事親　張從正[27] 古今醫統大全　徐春甫　[28] 管子校正

戴望　諸子集成　[29] 老子想爾注校牋

饒宗頤　[30] 瘍瘍機要　薛己　[31] 靈樞經

四部備要　[32] 靈驗符咒全書　[33] 呂氏春

秋集釋　楊家駱　[34] 論衡　王充　[35] 秘

藏醫書祝由十三科　雄奇成　[36] 南齊書

蕭子顯　中華書局　[37] 難經疏證　丹波元

胤　[38] 抱朴子　葛洪　[39] 備急千金要方

孫思邈　[40] 備考食物本草綱目　姚可成

[41] 本草綱目　李時珍　[42] 脾胃論　李杲

醫統正脈全書　王肯堂　[43] 脾胃论注释

李杲　[44] 三因極一病證方論　陳言　[45]

山海經箋疏　郝懿行　[46] 傷寒論今釋

張機　陸淵雷　[47] 聖濟總錄　曹孝忠

[48] 史記　司馬遷　[49] 石室秘錄　陳士鐸

[50] 壽世保元　龔廷賢　[51] 蘇沈內翰良方

沈括　蘇東坡　四庫全書　[52] 太平御覽

李昉　[53] 大正新修大藏經　高楠順次郎

渡邊海旭　[54] 湯液本草　王好古　[55] 怎

样战胜慢性疾病　段振离　[56] 外臺秘要

王燾　[57] 温疫论评注　吴有性　[58] 五十

二病方　[59] 眼科大全　傅仁宇　明善咸堂

[60] 用药心得十讲　焦树德　[61] 赤堀昭

陰陽十一脈灸經と素問　日本医史学雜誌

[62] 陰陽十一脈灸經の研究　東方學報

[63] 張子高　趙學敏〝本草綱目拾遺〞著述年代兼論我國首次用強水刻銅版事　科學史集刊　[64] 赵桂馨　中医现代化之我见　医学与哲学　[65] 陳邦賢　中國醫學史

[66] 周一谋　浅谈黄老哲学与古代医学　马王堆医书研究专刊　[67] 广州部队后勤部卫生部组织　[68] 謝觀　中國醫學源流論

[69] 朗厚宣　殷人疾病考　甲骨學商史論叢

[70] 任康同　针刺麻醉中的辩证法　自然辩证法　[71] 納喜光　医書に見える気論

小野沢精　気の思想　[72] 賈得道　中国医学史略　[73] 郭兵权　易法银　试论马王堆汉墓出土的两种帛书《老子》对祖国医学的影响　马王堆医书研究专刊

[74] 李钟文　五十二病方中膏脂类药物的探讨　马王堆医书研究专刊　[75] 劉敦愿漢畫象石上的針灸圖　文物参考資料

[76] 马继兴　台西村商墓中出土的医疗器具砭镰　文物　[77] 宮下三郎　東方學報

[78] 岡西為人　宋以前醫籍考　[79] 北京中醫學院　中國醫學史講義　[80] 中醫各家學說講義　[81] 尚志钧　五十二病方中药物制备工艺考察　长沙　马王堆医书研究专刊　[82] 上海中医学院医史博物馆

我国医学上反天命与尊天命的斗争　自然、
辩证法　[83] 上官良甫　中國醫藥發展史
[84] 丹波元胤　中國醫籍考　[85] 丁山　釋
狀　中央研究院歷史語言研究所集刊　[86]
渡邊幸山　本草集注序錄の訳注　漢方
[87] 渡邊幸三　現存する中國近世までの五
藏六府圖の概説　日本醫史學雜誌　[88]
杨守义　中医现代化不能以西医的是非为标
准　医学与哲学　[89] 嚴一萍　中國醫學
之起源及考畧　大陸雜誌　[90] 張機
（字仲景）　[91] 張介賓　[92] 張角　[93]
張脩　[94] 張一楷　[95] 張魯　[96] 張道陵
[97] 張載　[98] 張從正　[99] 張子高　[100] 腸
胃　[101] 張元素　[102] 趙獻可　[103] 趙學敏
[104] 巢元方　[105] 折衷派　[106] 臣　[107] 珍
珠囊　[108] 珍珠囊補遺藥性賦　[109] 甄權
[110] 陳獻章　[111] 貞人　[112] 陳士鐸
[113] 陳獨秀　[114] 陳言　[115] 正　[116] 乘
[117] 正氣　[118] 程顥　[119] 正一　[120] 正
醫法　[121] 正名　[122] 鄭文焯　[123] 成
無已　[124] 程頤　[125] 佈；疾　[126] 氣
[127] 氣　[128] 氣　[129] 祭酒　[130] 七慶三
觀經　[131] 氣口　[132] 岐伯　[133] 焦樹德
[134] 千金翼方　[135] 姦令　[136] 芝　[137] 赤

脚医生杂志　　[138] 治躄大祭酒　　[139] 禁經

[140] 金匱玉函要略　　[141] 禁術　　　[142] 禁藥

[143] 經　　　[144] 精　　　[145] 精氣　　[146] 經脈

[147] 靜室　　　[148] 經水　　[149] 求　　[150] 九宮八

風　　　[151] 肘後方　　　[152] 肘後百一方　　　[153]

周敦頤　　　[154] 咒　　[155] 主　　[156] 朱震亨

[157] 主氣　　[158] 諸風狀論　　[159] 諸風數類

[160] 諸風雜論　　[161] 朱熹　　[162] 諸病源候論

[163] 注忤　　[164] 祝由　　[165] 串雅　　[166] 莊周

[167] 莊子　　[168] 君　　[169] 羣众　　[170] 君火

[171] 群药　　[172] 中　　[173] 中醫　　[174] 衝脈

[175] 中惡　　[176] 發泄　　[177] 發熱　　[178] 方士

[179] 方有執　　[180] 風穴　　[181] 風痺　　　[182]

風水　　[183] 佛圖澄　　　[184] 府；腑　　[185] 輔

[186] 傅仁宇　　[187] 傅奕　　　[188] 豰改　　[189] 韓

非　　[190] 漢學　　[191] 寒涼派　　[192] 韓愈

[193] 河圖紀命符　　[194] 西醫略論　　[195] 西域

名醫所集藥方　　[196] 相火　　[197] 小心

[198] 蕭子顯　　[199] 邪　　[200] 瀉　　[201] 邪氣

[202] 邪鬼　　[203] 邪魔鬼祟　　[204] 邪祟

[205] 仙；僊　　[206] 新修本草　　[207] 心包絡

[208] 虛　　[209] 洫　　[210] 徐景輝　　[211] 徐春

甫　　[212] 徐福　　[213] 徐大椿　　[214] 穴

[215] 薛己　　[216] 荀子　　[217] 胡適　　[218] 華

佗 [219] 淮南子 [220] 黃帝 [221] 黃帝內經 [222] 黃帝內經靈樞 [223] 黃帝內經素問 [224] 黃帝內經太素 [225] 黃帝素問宣明論方 [226] 惠民藥局 [227] 魂 [228] 毉 [229] 義 [230] 易經 [231] 醫學正傳 [232] 醫學入門 [233] 醫故 [234] 醫林改錯 [235] 義舍 [236] 醫心方 [237] 仁 [238] 人迎 [239] 儒門事親 [240] 溉 [241] 康有為 [242] 告 [243] 剋 [244] 客氣 [245] 葛洪 [246] 格物致知 [247] 鉤割除之 [248] 寇宗奭 [249] 蠱 [250] 古今醫統大全 [251] 古今錄驗方 [252] 顧炎武 [253] 灌 [254] 貫衆 [255] 管茂材 [256] 管子 [257] 觀音 [258] 關尹子 [259] 鬼 [260] 鬼擊 [261] 鬼氣 [262] 鬼擊徹痛 [263] 鬼箭 [264] 鬼臼 [265] 鬼客忤擊 [266] 鬼卒 [267] 歸有光 [268] 公 [269] 攻下派 [270] 龔廷賢 [271] 國粹 [272] 老舍 [273] 老子 [274] 老子想爾注 [275] 類經 [276] 理 [277] 李翺 [278] 禮記 [279] 厲氣 [280] 李中梓 [281] 李杲 [282] 李時珍 [283] 李斯 [284] 李梴 [285] 梁啟超 [286] 良知 [287] 靈蘭秘典論 [288] 劉安 [289] 劉邦 [290] 六韜 [291] 劉敦愿 [292] 劉完素 [293] 劉溫舒 [294] 劉禹錫 [295] 絡 [296]

絡渠 [297] 盧復 [298] 魯迅 [299] 呂氏春秋

[300] 呂望 [301] 龍木論 [302] 龍樹眼論

[303] 秘藏醫書祝由十三科 [304] 命門 [305] 明

堂 [306] 繆希雍 [307] 脈法 [308] 墨翟

[309] 難經 [310] 逆醫法 [311] 倪維德 [312]

農家 [313] 惡 [314] 八陣 [315] 八正 [316] 八

正風候 [317] 巴金 [318] 配合 [319] 配伍 [320]

本草綱目 [321] 本草綱目拾遺 [322] 本草 [323]

瘅 [324] 辟邪 [325] 脾胃論 [326] 辨證 [327]

辯証法 [328] 辯証論治 [329] 扁鵲 [330] 魄

[331] 撥 [332] 婆羅門藥方 [333] 補 [334] 不及

[335] 補脾胃派 [336] 不死之草 [337] 補土派

[338] 三虛三實 [339] 三因極一病證方論 [340] 山

海經 [341] 傷寒 [342] 傷寒論 [343] 傷寒論

條辯 [344] 上古天真論 [345] 上帝 [346] 射魃

[347] 神箭 [348] 神農 [349] 神農經 [350] 神農

黃帝食禁 [351] 神農本草經 [352] 神農本草經

集注 [353] 聖濟總錄 [354] 使 [355] 使 [356]

實 [357] 史記 [358] 時氣病 [359] 詩經 [360]

師君 [361] 始皇帝 [362] 石室秘錄 [363] 壽世保

元 [364] 壽夭剛柔 [365] 書經 [366] 淳于意

[367] 說文 [368] 搜神後記 [369] 司馬遷 [370]

祟 [371] 燧 [372] 孫星 [373] 孫一奎 [374] 孫

思邈 [375] 孫德潤 [376] 戴震 [377] 太一

[378] 太過　　[379] 太平經　　[380] 太平道　　[381] 戴思恭　　[382] 丹波康賴　　[383] 丹經要訣　　[384] 譚壯　　[385] 膻中　　[386] 湯液本草　　[387] 道　　[388] 陶弘景　　[389] 道德經　　[390] 道藏　　[391] 導引　　[392] 德　　[393] 帝　　[394] 地仙　　[395] 調食　　[396] 天　　[397] 天忌　　[398] 地支　　[399] 天仙　　[400] 天干　　[401] 丁文江　　[402] 藏 臟　　[403] 怎樣戰勝慢性疾病　　[404] 佐　　[405] 左傳　　[406] 驪行　　[407] 卒中惡忤　　[408] 足臂十一脈灸經　　[409] 寸口　　[410] 毒　　[411] 瀆　　[412] 段振離　　[413] 通　　[414] 動氣　　[415] 刺禁論　　[416] 自然辯証法　　[417] 自得　　[418] 外臺秘要　　[419] 萬病回春　　[420] 王安石　　[421] 王清任　　[422] 王充　　[423] 王好古　　[424] 王冰　　[425] 王叔和　　[426] 王燾　　[427] 王陽明　　[428] 味　　[429] 衛　　[430] 衛氣　　[431] 衛矛　　[432] 胃厭　　[433] 溫疫論　　[434] 溫補　　[435] 巫　　[436] 武　　[437] 五常　　[438] 五行　　[439] 無病　　[440] 五十二病方　　[441] 五德　　[442] 五斗米道　　[443] 無為　　[444] 吳有性　　[445] 五運六氣　　446 楊朱　　447 楊上善　　448 楊超　　[449] 養陰　　[450] 藥　　[451] 瘧　　[452] 嚴一萍　　[453] 眼科大全　　[454] 眼論　　[455] 炎帝　　[456] 顏元　　[457] 印　　[458] 陰陽十一脈灸經　　[459] 營　　[460] 營氣　　[461] 禦　　[462] 禹　　[463] 于吉　　[464] 虞

博　　[465]元氣　　[466]用藥法象　　[467]用药
心得十讲　　　[468]素問玄機原病式
[469]山田慶兒　　九宮八風説と少師派の
立場　　東方學報

General Index

The numbers in brackets following individual entries refer to the list of Chinese characters on pp. 408–413.

Ackerknecht, Erwin, 3, 4
acupuncture, 45, 92–99, 130, 167,
  168, 173, 175, 212, 216, 252,
  255, 261, 262
acupuncture anesthesia, 255, 262
alchemistic, alchemy, 43, 112
American Board of Commissioners
  for Foreign Missions, 239
amulets, 39, 143, 222, 224, 225,
  232
analytical world view, 6
anatomical, 78, 82, 213
ancestor(s), 7, 18, 19, 21, 22, 24,
  26–28, 30, 32, 35, 36, 55, 68,
  232
ancestor medicine, ancestral healing,
  22, 27, 36, 122, 222
anesthesiology, 151
anthroposophy, 235
Avalokitesvara, 136
ayurveda, 141

bathing, 93
Bauer, Wolfgang, 138, 230
Bible, 232
black magic, 25
bleeding, 96
blood, 75–79, 82, 83, 96, 198, 205,
  236
bloodletting. See bleeding
bodhisattva, 136
breath magic, breathing techniques,
  38, 44, 106, 110, 143, 212
Buddha, 134–136, 138–140, 147,
  159

Buddhism, Buddhist, 40, 43, 45,
  122, 132–160, 162–165, 173,
  191, 193, 196, 224, 225, 227,
  251, 252
Buddhist medicine, 4, 260

cataract surgery, 145–147, 152
cause-and-effect relations, 5, 7, 54
Chang Chi (tzu: Chung-ching) [90],
  168, 169, 173–175, 206, 209,
  210
Chang Chieh-pin [91], 199, 200,
  220–222
Chang Chüeh [92], 119–122, 124
Chang Hsiu [93], 127–129
Chang I-ch'a [94], 224
Chang Lu [95], 122, 124, 127–130,
  132, 133
Chang Tao-ling [96], 39, 40, 44,
  127–129
Chang Tsai [97], 165
Chang Ts'ung-cheng [98], 174–175,
  177, 205, 216
Chang Tzu-kao [99], 211
"Ch'ang-wei" [100], 78
Chang Yüan-su [101], 173, 177,
  181, 183, 184, 187, 202, 210
Chao Hsien-k'o [102], 200–202
Chao Hsüeh-min [103], 211, 216
Ch'ao Yüan-fang [104], 176
che-chung p'ai [105], "school of
  compromise," 203
chemotherapy, 238
ch'en [106], "minister"-drugs, 115,
  259

Chen-chu nang [107], 177, 183, 184
Chen-chu nang pu-i yao-hsing fu
[108], 177
Chen Ch'üan [109], 41
Ch'en Hsien-chang [110], 196
chen-jen [111], "the true man," 105,
107
Ch'en Shih-to [112], 206–208, 222
Ch'en Tu-hsiu [113], 247
Ch'en Yen [114], 175–177, 205
cheng [115], "proper," "to correct,"
67, 83
ch'eng [116], "to seize," 67
cheng-ch'i [117], "correct
influences," 254
Ch'eng Hao [118], 165, 190
cheng-i [119], school of Taoism,
163
cheng-i-fa [120], "direct healing,"
206–207
cheng-ming [121], "rectification of
names," 62
Cheng Wen-cho [122], 224
Ch'eng Wu-i [123], 181
Ch'eng Yi [124], 165, 190
chi [125], "illness," 20
ch'i [126], "finest matter
influences," "vapors," 67, 68, 71,
72, 74–77, 82, 83, 85, 88, 92,
93, 96, 97, 124, 126, 165
ch'i [127], "climatic influences,"
170, 171
ch'i [128], "thermo-influences,"
180–182
chi-chiu [129], "libationers," 127,
129
"Ch'i-ch'u san-kuan ching" [130],
142
ch'i-k'ou [131], "influence-
opening," 86
Ch'i Po [132], 73, 100, 206
Chiao Shu-te [133], 257–259
Ch'ien-chin i-fang [134], 42, 43, 45,
96
chien-ling [135], "soldiers against
immorality," 129
chih [136], herb of immortality,
112, 115
Ch'ih-chiao i-sheng tsa-chih [137],
257
chih-t'ou ta chi-chiu [138], "district
governor, grand libationer," 129

Chin-ching [139], 43
Chin-kuei (yü-han) yao-lüeh [140],
168, 175
Ch'in Shih Huang-ti. *See* Shih
Huang-ti
chin-shu [141], "the art of
interdictions," 224
chin-yao [142], "repelling drugs,"
212
Chin-Yüan medicine, 114, 168
China Medical Missionary
Association, 241
ching [143], "conduits,"
"transportation channels," 75,
81–83
ching [144], "essence," "finest
matter," 82, 110, 124, 126, 142,
178
ching-ch'i [145], "finest matter
influences," 110
ching-mo [146], "conduit-vessels,"
75, 77
ching-shih [147], "chambers of
silence," 129
"Ching-shui" [148], 78, 82
ch'iu [149], "conjuration," 21
"Chiu-kung pa-feng" [150], 68
Chou-hou fang [151], 149
Chou-hou pai-i fang [152], 149
Chou Tun-i [153], 165
Christian, Christianity, 139, 149,
152, 157, 232, 233, 238, 240,
243
Christian dogma, 10
Christian missionaries, 230
Christian science, 235
chu [154], "priests," "supplicants,"
35
chu [155], "leader"-drugs, 259
Chu Chen-heng [156], 187, 195,
198, 199, 210
chu-ch'i [157], "primary
influences," 171
"Chu-feng chuang-lun" [158], 71
"Chu-feng shu-lei" [159], 71
"Chu-feng tsa-lun" [160], 71
Chu Hsi [161], 164–166, 190, 196
Chu-ping yüan hou lun [162], 176
chu-wu [163], "possessed by the
hostile," 36
chu-yu [164], "exorcism of the
cause," 21, 217, 220, 224

Ch'uan-ya [165], 211, 212
Chuang-Chou [166], 103, 105–109, 111
Chuang-tzu [167]. *See* Chuang Chou
chün [168], "ruler"-drugs, 115, 259
ch'ün-chung [169], "folk masses," 258
chün-huo [170], "ruler-fire," 171
ch'ün-yao [171], "drug masses," 258
chung [172], "to be hit," 67
chung-i [173], "Chinese medicine," 250
ch'ung-mo [174], "through-way vessel," 81
chung-o [175], "struck by evil," 36
cinnabar, 40, 42, 111, 223
circulation of *ch'i* and blood, 75, 77, 82, 85, 92, 97, 98
Communist Party, 245, 251
Confucian, Confucianism, 10, 34, 36, 43, 50, 51, 56, 60–68, 99, 101, 103, 107, 108, 113, 114, 116, 122, 133, 152–180, 190–193, 197, 203, 208, 210, 218, 225, 227, 243, 245, 249, 250, 254, 259
Confucius, 45, 61, 62, 65, 101, 102, 138, 149, 210, 244
contact magic, 7, 52
correspondences, paradigm of, 52
cosmobiological, cosmobiology, 160, 168, 170
Cultural Revolution, 259
cupping, 93
curse, 19. See also *sui*

Darwin, Charles, 234
deductive reasoning, 91
demon(s), 7, 19, 35–37, 40–45, 65, 68, 69, 71, 73, 96, 116, 122–124, 128, 129, 143, 144, 166, 216–223, 233
demonic medicine, 4, 8, 19, 25, 36, 40, 43, 45–47, 51, 67, 68, 120, 128, 166, 216, 217, 251, 252, 260
demonological, demonology, 38, 39, 52, 69, 71, 73, 74, 93, 94, 97, 116, 134, 138, 143, 160, 163, 173, 195, 204, 212, 215, 218,

220, 224, 232
dharanis, 143
dialectical materialism, 245, 248, 249, 253, 254
diet, 231, 232
dietetics of systematic correspondence, 180
disease, definition of, 19
dissection, 78, 83
divination, diviners, 26, 27, 68, 148, 156
Doré, Henry, 224
dosa theory, 141–143
drug(s), 4, 22, 33, 40, 42, 47, 53, 93, 99, 101–116, 130, 138, 168, 169, 173, 175, 176, 179–188, 198, 205, 207, 208, 210, 211, 216–218, 220, 221, 224, 232, 250, 252, 257–259, 261, 262. *See also* materia medica.

Edelstein, Ludwig, 2, 3
Eichhorn, Werner, 35, 128
energetics, energy, 2, 72, 111
envy, 23, 48, 50
epidemic(s), 21, 39, 44, 118, 119, 205, 212, 223, 226
Epler, D. C., 75, 96
evil eye, 48
exorcism, exorcistic techniques, exorcists, 34, 39, 40, 42, 43, 45, 160, 163, 167, 212, 220, 224, 225

fa-hsieh [176], "dissipating," 182–183
fa-je [177], "heating," 182, 183
fang-shih [178], "prescription scholars," 113
Fang Yu-chih [179], 209
Feng, H. Y., 48
feng-hsüeh [180], "wind caves," 71
feng-pi [181], 71
feng-shui [182], "wind and water," 27
feudal, feudalism, 29, 30, 32–34, 36, 79, 100, 103, 104, 247
Five Phases of Change theory, 6, 7, 34, 51, 52, 54, 57–61, 65–67, 70, 71, 83, 84, 86, 88, 98, 115, 126, 130, 134, 150, 160, 170–172, 178–181, 186, 206, 207,

Five Phases of Change (*continued*) 211, 217, 221–223, 228, 245, 250, 253, 257, 260
Fo-t'u-teng [183], 148
Foster, George, 22
Four Elements, doctrine of, 134, 141, 143, 145, 150, 151
Franke, Herbert, 62, 133, 161
Frazer, James G., 52
Freud, Sigmund, 215
fu [184], the body's "palaces," 77, 78, 81, 83
fu [185], "helper"-drugs, 259
fumigation, 93
Fu Jen-yü [186], 147
Fu Yi [187], 159

gandhara myth, 97
"Gang of Four," 260–261
germ theory, 234
god(s), 7, 55, 65, 109, 112, 124, 143, 144, 232
Granet, Marcel, 24, 56
gymnastics, 93, 110

hai-ssu [188], "amulets," 39
Han Fei [189], 37, 63
Han-hsüeh [190], "(return to) the teachings of the Han," 209
han-liang p'ai [191], "school of cooling," 173
Han Yü [192], 159
Harper, Donald, 38
heliotherapy, 9
Hippocrates, 231
Ho-t'u chi-ming fu [193], 124
Hobson, Benjamin, 236
holistic perspective, thought, 6, 234
homeopathic magic, 7, 52–54, 56, 60, 67
Hong Kong, 27, 260
hospitals, 149, 240, 242
Hsi-i lüeh-lun [194], 236
Hsi-yü ming-i so-chi yao-fang [195], 149
hsiang-huo [196], "minister-fire," 171
hsiao-hsin [197], "the minor-heart," 200
Hsiao Tzu-hsien [198], 137
hsieh [199], "evil," "harmful," "heterodox," 67, 83, 113, 174, 218
hsieh [200], "purgative," 182–183

hsieh-ch'i [201], "evil influences," 68
hsieh-kuei [202], "evil demons," 68
hsieh mo kuei sui [203], "curse of malevolent demons and pathogenic agents," 222
hsieh-sui [204], "curse of evil," 222
hsien [205], "immortal," 109
Hsin-hsiu pen-ts'ao [206], 160
hsin pao-lo [207], "the heart-enclosing network," 208
hsü [208], "depletion," 83
hsü [209], "gutter," 82
Hsü Chin-hui [210], 224
Hsü Ch'un-fu [211], 216, 220
Hsü Fu [212], 112
Hsü Ta-ch'un [213], 85, 209, 210, 216, 222
hsüeh [214], "caves," "holes," 71
Hsüeh Chi [215], 198–200, 202
Hsün-tzu [216], 63–65
Hu Shih [217], 230
Hua T'o [218], 151, 251
Huai-nan tzu [219], 71, 110, 113
Huang-Lao political philosophy, 108
Huang-ti [220], 72, 103, 107, 113, 225
Huang-ti nei-ching [221], 56, 58, 63, 74–76, 78, 81–85, 93, 94, 96–98, 100, 107, 108, 114, 115, 166–169, 173, 175, 177–179, 188, 195, 197, 199, 200, 204, 209, 218, 221, 259
Huang-ti nei-ching ling-shu [222], 71, 77, 78, 207
Huang-ti nei-ching su-wen [223], 107, 160, 170, 173, 180, 181, 183, 185, 200, 201, 208
Huang-ti nei-ching t'ai-su [224], 68–71, 179, 180
Huang-ti su-wen hsüan-ming lun fang [225], 173
hui-min yao-chü [226], "charitable apothecaries," 149
humoral pathology, 232
hun [227], ethereal soul, 36, 83

i [228], "healer," 37
i [229], "righteousness," 103
I-ching [230], 124
I-hsüeh cheng-ch'uan [231], 219
I-hsüeh ju-men [232], 217
I-ku [233], 224

I-lin kai-ts'o [234], 213
i-she [235], "free hostels," 129
illness, definition of, 19
immortality, 109–112, 115, 121
incantations, 143, 173, 222
inductive reasoning, 6
influences of finest/subtle matter, 7,
    51, 67, 178. See also *ch'i; ching-
    ch'i*
Ishimpō [236], 146
Islam, 157

Jaspers, Karl, 215
jen [237], "benevolence," 103, 165
jen-ying [238], location for pulse-
    diagnosis, 86, 88
Jenner, Edward, 233
Jesuits, 235
Jesus Nazareth, 139
Jivaka, 151
Ju-men shih-ch'in [239], 174, 175,
    216

kai [240], "to irrigate," 82
Kaltenmarck, Max, 130
K'ang Yu-wei [241], 246
kao [242] "conjuration," 21
karma, 134–136, 144, 150, 156
k'e [243], "to subdue," 67
k'e-ch'i [244], "guest influences,"
    171, 174
Keightly, David, 26
Ko Hung [245], 124, 127, 133, 149
ko-wu chih-chih [246], "to achieve
    an understanding of things by
    investigating them," 166, 195,
    196
kou-ko ch'u-chih [247], "to remove
    through cutting with a sickle,"
    145
K'ou Tsung-shih [248], 181
ku [249], spirit, 25, 46–50
Ku-chin i-t-ung ta-ch'üan [250], 220
Ku-chin lu-yen fang [251], 41
Ku Yen-wu [252], 193, 208
kuan [253], "to pour," 82
kuan-chung [254], Rhizome
    Cyrtonii, 228
Kuan Mao-ts'ai [255], 236
Kuan-tzu [256], 82, 110
Kuan-yin [257], 136, 148, 150
Kuan yin tzu [258], 221
kuei [259], "demons," 35
kuei-chi [260], "assaulted by

demons," 36
kuei-ch'i [261], "demonic
    influences," 217
kuei-chi ch'en-t'ung [262], "piercing
    pain caused by the attack of a
    demon," 217
kuei-chien [263], "demon arrow,"
    42, 218
kuei-chiu [264], "demon-vessel"
    plant, 223
kuei-k'o wu-chi [265], "possessed
    by the hostile influence of
    demonic guests," 36
kuei-tsu [266], "warriors against
    demons," 129
Kuei Yu-kuang [267], 191
Kuhn, Thomas, 57
kung [268], "civic spirit," 128
kung-hsia p'ai [269], "school of
    attack and purgation," 175, 205
Kung T'ing-hsien [270], 204, 205,
    216, 218, 223
kuo-ts'ui [271], "spirit of the
    nation," 251
Kuomintang, 245, 251

Lao She [272], 247
Lao-tzu [273], 40, 43, 102, 104,
    107, 120, 127, 136, 138, 155,
    157
Lao-tzu Hsiang-erh chu [274], 122
Legalists, school of, 32, 61, 63, 100,
    108, 254
Lei-ching [275], 220
li [276], "principle," 196
Li Ao [277], 159, 164
Li-chi [278], 37, 56, 82
li-ch'i [279], "evil influence," 205
Li Chung-tse [280], 202, 203, 210
Li Kao [281], 177–179, 181, 198,
    199, 202, 205
Li Shih-chen [282], 53, 216, 237
Li Ssu [283], 63
Li T'ing [284], 216, 217
Liang Ch'i-ch'ao [285], 246
liang-chih [286], "knowledge
    existing a priori in man," 196
"Ling-lan mi-tien (lun)" [287], 107,
    200
Liu An [288], 113, 114. See also
    Huai-nan tzu
Liu Pang [289], 33
Liu-t'ao [290], 52
Liu Tun-yüan [291], 97

Liu Wan-su [292], 172–175
Liu Wen-shu [293], 171, 172
Liu Yü-hsi [294], 146
Livingston, J., 235, 236
lo [295], "network"-conduits, 81
lo-chü [296], "gutters," 82
longevity, 109, 111–114, 121, 125, 148
Lu Fu [297], 209
Lu Hsün [298], 242
Lu Gwei-djen, 2
Lü-shih ch'un-ch'iu [299], 82
Lü Wang [300], 52, 53
Lung-mu lun [301], 147
Lung-shu yen-lun [302], 146

Ma-wang-tui graves/scripts, 38, 74, 75, 77, 81, 85, 93, 94, 96, 97, 99, 108, 112, 152
macrobiotics, 108, 110, 111, 133
madness, 222
magical concepts/powers/skills, 32, 35, 38–40, 44, 51, 56, 62, 66, 74, 93, 121, 129, 148, 224, 235, 245
magic correspondence, 5–7, 52
magician, 127
Manicheism, 157
Mao Tse-tung, 230, 245, 248, 249, 251, 252, 256, 257, 259
Marxism, Marxists, 10, 230, 231, 245, 247, 248, 251, 252, 254, 256–258, 260, 261
massage, 93
materia medica, 1, 53, 99, 112, 116, 237, 252
matter, 109, 111
Maxwell, J. L., 240
medical missionaries, 235, 238–241, 246
Mencius, 64, 244
Mi-ts'ang i-shu shih-san k'o [303], 224
Michaud, Paul, 118
ming-men [304], "gate of life," 200–202
ming-t'ang [305], "hall of light," 126
Miu Hsi-yung [306], 209
Mo-fa [307], 74
Mo Ti [308], 122–124
Moists, 61, 122, 124
moisture, 6, 7

Morrison, Robert, 235, 236
moxabustion, moxa-cauterization, 93, 94, 96, 97, 130, 174, 212

Nagarjuna, 146
Nan-ching [309], 78, 84–86, 89–91, 98, 167, 169, 197, 200, 201
Needham, Joseph, 2, 9, 112
Nei-ching. See Huang-ti nei-ching
Neo-Confucianism, 154–188, 190–194, 208–210
"New (Democratic) Medicine," 247, 254–257, 260, 261
Nestorian Christianity, 157
ni i-fa [310], "reversing treatment," 207
Ni Wei-te [311], 203
nirvana, 135, 136, 139
nung-chia [312], agrarian school, 113

o [313], "malevolent," 67
ophthalmology, 144–147, 152
oracle, 18, 20–22, 25–27, 33, 34, 47, 68, 69
oracular therapy, 4, 150, 251

pa-chen [314], "the eight strategic formations," 199
pa-cheng [315], "the eight seasonal turning points," 69
"Pa-cheng feng-hou" [316], 69
Pa Chin [317], 247
Parker, Peter, 152, 238, 239
p'ei-ho [318], "to combine," 258
p'ei-wu [319], "to combine," 258
Pen-ts'ao ching. See Shen-nung pen-ts'ao ching
Pen-ts'ao ching chi-chu. See Shen-nung pen-ts'ao ching chi-chu
Pen-ts'ao kang mu [320], 237
Pen-ts'ao kang mu shih-i [321], 211
pen-ts'ao [322], pharmaceutical literature, 93, 168, 180, 250
pharmaceutical, 181, 184, 250, 259, 260
pharmaceutical literature, 114. See also pen-ts'ao
pharmacological, pharmacologists, pharmacology, 179, 181, 182, 186–188, 211, 238, 252, 257, 259, 262
pharmacology of systematic

correspondence, 99, 169, 177, 179, 180, 195

pi [323], rheumatic illness, 71

pi-hsieh [324], "banishers of evil," 39

P'i wei lun [325], 178

pien-cheng [326], "diagnosis," 258

pien-cheng fa [327], "dialectic," 258

pien-cheng lun-chih [328], "differential diagnostic therapy," 258

Pien Ch'io [329], 45, 97, 201, 204

p'o [330], corporeal soul, 36, 83

po [331], "to poke," 147

Po-lo-men yao-fang [332], 149

Porkert, Manfred, 2

possession, 41

"psychiatry," 215

"psychoanalysis," 215

psychologists, 175

pu [333], "to replenish," 179

pu-chi [334], "insufficient," "partly developed," 171

pu p'i wei p'ai [335], "school of replenishing spleen and stomach," 179

pu-ssu chih ts'ao [336], "herb of immortality," 112

pu-t'u p'ai [337], "school of replenishing the soil (phase)," 179

public health measures, 96

pulse diagnosis, 76

religious healing, religious medicine, 4, 8, 117–131

Rockefeller Foundation, 242, 248

"San-hsü san-shih" [338], 69, 70

San-yin chi i-ping cheng fang lun [339], 175

science, scientific, 230, 231, 233, 242–246, 249, 251, 252

Scientism, 243, 244

sexual practices/techniques, 93, 111, 125

shamans, 25, 35, 37, 54, 56, 65, 109, 113, 216, 219, 224

Shan-hai ching [340], 53

shang-han [341], "cold-induced maladies," 205

Shang-han lun [342], 168, 173, 174, 177, 209

Shang-han lun t'iao-pien [343], 209

"Shang-ku t'ien-chen lun" [344], 107

Shang-ti [345]. See Ti

she-ch'i [346], "projectiles against demons resembling a child," 39

shen-chien [347], "divine arrow," 42

Shen-nung [348], 113, 114, 209, 225, 237

Shen-nung ching [349], 114

Shen-nung Huang-ti shih-chin [350], 113

Shen-nung pen-ts'ao (ching) [351], 114, 115, 166, 167, 209

Shen-nung pen-ts'ao ching chi-chu [352], 53, 167

Sheng-chi tsung-lu [353], 147

shih [354], "aide"-drugs, 115

shih [355], "emissary"-drugs, 259

shih [356], "repletion," 83

Shih-chi [357], 60, 68, 75, 92–94

shih-ch'i ping [358], "illness caused by seasonal influence," 171

Shih-ching [359], 55

shih-chün [360], "master of masters," 129

Shih Huang-ti [361], 32, 33, 63, 80, 112, 115

Shih-shih mi-lu [362], 206, 222

Shou-shih pao-yüan [363], 218

"Shou yu kang jou" [364], 71

Shryock, J. K., 48

Shu-ching [365], 59

Shun-yü I [366], 75, 92, 93

Shuo-wen [367], 39, 72

soma, "toadstool," 112

Sou-shen hou-chi [368], 41

spirits, spiritual agents, 6, 7, 25, 28, 35, 36, 38–40, 42, 44, 46, 47, 65, 68, 71, 96, 122–124, 127–129, 166, 216, 222–224

Ssu-ma Ch'ien [369], 75, 92

Su-wen. See *Huang-ti nei-ching su-wen*

Su-wen hsüan-chi yüan-ping-shih [468], 172

sui [370], "curse," 21

sui [371], "underground passage," 82

Sun Hsing-yen [372], 209

Sun I-k'uei [373], 202

Sun Ssu-miao [374], 42–45, 150, 151, 160, 225

Sun Te-jun [375], 216, 222
surgery, surgical, 144–146, 151, 152, 251, 262
systematic correspondence, medicine of, 4, 43, 51, 61, 63, 66–100, 107, 114–116, 134, 137, 138, 144, 145, 167, 210, 212, 215, 216, 218, 223, 250
systematic correspondence, framework of, paradigm of, 5–7, 52, 54–61, 115, 160, 167–169, 173, 175, 179, 195, 197, 208, 220, 224, 243, 245, 253, 254, 259, 261

Tai Chen [376], 208
T'ai-i [377], 68, 69
t'ai-kuo [378], "too much," "excessively developed," 171
T'ai-p'ing ching [379], 120, 122, 124, 127, 130
t'ai-p'ing (tao) [380], "the way of great peace," 118, 120
Tai Ssu-kung [381], 198
T'ai-su. See Huang-ti nei-ching t'ai-su
Taiwan, 27, 260
talismans, 39, 40, 43, 147, 224
Tamba Yasuyori [382], 146
Tan-ching yao-chüeh [383], 42
T'an Chuang [384], 247, 251
tan-chung [385], 208
T'ang-yeh pen-ts'ao [386], 181, 184, 187
tao [387], "the law/way of nature," 101, 102, 105, 124–126, 130, 159, 197
T'ao Hung-ching [388], 53, 114, 149, 167
Tao-te ching [389], 102, 122, 124, 129
Tao-tsang [390], 130
tao-yin [391], gymnastic techniques 110
Taoism, Taoist(s), 10, 34, 39, 40, 43, 45, 61, 63, 74, 101–116, 122, 124, 133, 134, 136, 137, 145, 149, 150, 155, 157, 163–167, 191, 193, 210, 216, 221, 224, 259
te [392], "potential," "power of virtue," 56, 62, 102, 130

Ti [393], 18, 25, 35
ti-hsien [394], "terrestrial immortals," 109
"T'iao-shih" [395], 179
T'ien [396], "heaven," celestial deity, 35
"T'ien-chi" [397], 71
ti-chih [398], "terrestrial branches," 171
t'ien-hsien [399], "celestial immortals," 109
t'ien-kan [400], "celestial stems," 170
Ting Wen-chiang [401], 244
Trauzettel, Rolf, 62, 133, 161
tsang [402], the body's "depots," 77, 78, 81, 83
Tsen-yang chan-sheng man-hsing chi-ping [403], 260
tso [404], "assistant"-drugs, 115, 259
Tso-chuan [405], 41, 48, 59
Tsou Yen [406], 58–60, 65
tsu-chung o-wu [407], "sudden attack by evil agents," 217
Tsu-pi shih-i mo-chiu ching [408], 74
ts'un-k'ou [409], "inch-opening," 88, 91
tu [410], "poison," 142
tu [411], "ditch," 82
Tu Wei-ming, 108
Tuan Chen-li [412], 260
t'ung [413], "penetrating," 182–183
tung-ch'i [414], "driving influence," 202
"Tz'u-chin lun" [415], 200
Tzu-jan pien-cheng-fa [416], 248, 254
tzu-te [417] "personal experience," 196

Virchow, Rudolf, 243, 246

Wai-t'ai pi-yao [418], 145, 160, 204
Wan-ping hui-ch'un [419], 223
Wang An-shih [420], 162
Wang Ch'ing-jen [421], 79, 212, 213, 215
Wang Ch'ung [422], 60, 61, 82
Wang Hao-ku [423], 181, 184, 187

Wang Ping [424], 160, 170, 180
Wang Shu-ho [425], 168, 209
Wang Tao [426], 145, 150, 160, 204
Wang Yang-ming [427], 191, 193, 196, 244
Wasson, K. Gordon, 112
wei [428], "flavor," 181, 182
wei [429], "guards," 67
wei-ch'i [430], "protective influences," 77
wei-mao [431], "protective spear," 42
wei-yen [432], "the stomach flap," 207
Wen-i lun [433], 205
wen-pu [434], "to fill with warmth," 198, 205
wind, 6, 7, 25, 67–73, 84, 87, 151, 169, 173, 174, 176, 204, 205, 222, 231
wind-spirits, 25
wu [435], "shamans," "magicians." *See* shamans
Wu [436], Han-Emperor, 33, 63, 68, 112
wu-ch'ang [437], "the five normal (elements of all existence)," 176
wu-hsing [438], "Five Phases of Change." *See* Five Phases
wu-ping [439], "nirvana," 139
Wu-shih-erh ping fang [440], 38, 39, 41, 99, 112
wu-te [441], 60
wu-tou mi tao [442], "the five pecks of rice movement," 127
wu-wei [443], "no active intervention," 101
Wu Yu-hsing [444], 205, 206
wu-yün liu-ch'i [445], "five circulatory (phases) and six

(seasonal) influences," 160, 168, 170–172

Yang Chu [446], 109
Yang Shang-shan [447], 70
Yang Ch'ao [448], 247
yang yin [449], "to nourish the yin," 198
yao [450], "drug," 179
yao [451], "intermittent fevers," 44, 45
Yellow Turban Revolt, 117, 118, 120, 127, 132
Yen I-p'ing [452], 22
Yen-k'o ta-ch'üan [453], 147
Yen-lun [454], 146
Yen-ti [455], 113
Yen Yüan [456], 193, 208
Yersin, A., 226
yin [457], "seals," 39
Yin-yang shih-i mo-chiu ching [458], 74
yinyang dualism, theory, 6, 7, 34, 51, 52, 54–58, 65, 67, 70, 71, 83, 84, 98, 110, 115, 130, 160, 170–172, 180, 181, 183, 186, 188, 199, 208, 211, 217, 223, 228, 245, 250, 253, 257, 260
ying [459], "army camps," 67
ying-ch'i [460], "constructive influences," 77
yü [461], "conjuration," 21
Yü [462], the steps of, 39, 44
Yü Chi [463], 120
Yü Po [464], 216, 219
yüan-ch'i [465], "primordial influences," "original influences," 77, 202
Yung-yao fa-hsiang [466], 177
Yung-yao hsin-te shih-chiang [467], 257

Designer: Robert S. Tinnon
Compositor: Publisher's Typography
Text: 10/13 Sabon
Display: Sabon